FOOD AND NUTRITION IN PRACTICE

ISOBEL COLE-HAMILTON · ANN LIVERMORE
JACQUIE WATSON

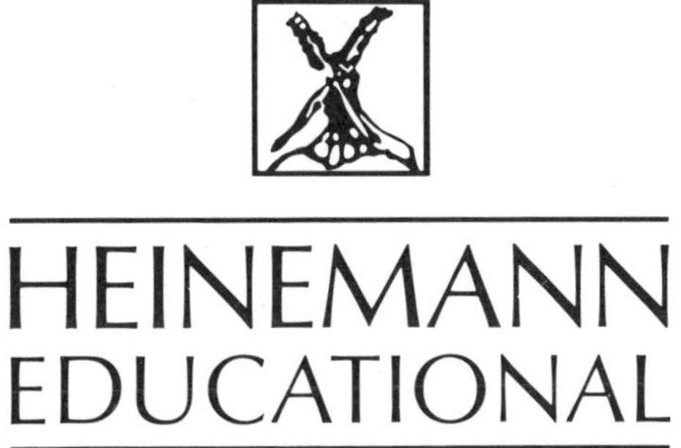

Heinemann Educational Ltd
a division of Heinemann Educational Books Ltd
Halley Court, Jordan Hill, Oxford OX2 8EJ

OXFORD LONDON EDINBURGH MADRID
ATHENS BOLOGNA PARIS MELBOURNE
SYDNEY AUCKLAND SINGAPORE TOKYO
IBADAN NAIROBI HARARE GABORONE
PORTSMOUTH NH (USA)

First published 1987
95 15 14 13 12 11 10 9

British Library Cataloguing in Publication Data

Cole-Hamilton, Isobel
Food and nutrition in practice.
1. Nutrition
I. Title II. Livermore, Ann III. Watson, Jacquie
613.2 TX354

ISBN 0 435 42040 2

Designed, typeset and illustrated by Gecko Limited, Bicester, Oxon

Printed in Great Britain by Thomson Litho Ltd, East Kilbride, Scotland

Cover illustration by Pat Thorne

Thanks are due to the following for permission to reproduce photographs:

Judith Aldridge p. 64; Peter Allen/*Farmers Weekly* p. 52; Allied Mills Ltd p. 79 (fig. 2); Barnaby's Picture Library p. 136 (fig. 1); Andrew Besley/Barnaby's p. 138 (fig. 2); Bird's Eye Walls Ltd p. 105 (fig. 1, bottom); Anthony Blake Photo Library p. 81; Claire Booker/Age Concern p. 8 (fig. 2); Tony Boxall/Barnaby's p. 7 (bottom right); J. Allan Cash p. 148; The Commissioner for New Zealand/ Barnaby's p. 120 (fig. 2); Elliott, Service & Co. p. 105 (fig. 1, centre); *Farmer's Weekly* pp. 65, 69 (fig. 3b), 93, 138 (fig. 1); The Federation of Bakers p. 22 (fig. 2); Melanie Friend/Format, pp. 6 (bottom), 24 (fig. 1); Elida Gibbs p. 45; Sheila Gray/Format pp. 11 (fig. 3a), 63 (fig. 3), 130 (fig. 1a); Sally and Richard Greenhill pp. 6 (top right), 7 (bottom left), 9, 14 (fig. 2), 22 (fig. 1), 24 (fig. 2), 34 (fig. 2), 39 (fig. 3), 50, 51, 54, 55, 58 (fig. 1), 86 (figs 4 and 5), 102, 112, 114 (fig. 1a), 130 (fig. 1b); Jeremy Hartley/Oxfam pp. 34 (fig. 1), 74; The Health Education Council p. 61; IAZ International p. 11 (fig. 3b); John Watney Photo Library p. 43; Camilla Jessel p. 60; Sri Kanth/Oxfam p. 128 (fig. 1); David Kirby/ Barnaby's p. 14 (fig. 1); Douglas Low/*Farmers Weekly* p. 114 (fig. 1b); Jenny Matthews/Format p. 89; Metropolitan Police Public Information Department p. 47; Michael Ann Mullen/Format p. 122; Maggie Murray/Format pp. 8 (fig. 1), 108 (fig. 1), 129 (fig. 3); Joanne O'Brien/Format pp. 56, 108 (fig. 2); Oxfam pp. 127 (fig. 2), 129 (fig. 5); Raissa Page/Format pp. 7 (top), 62; Brenda Prince/ Format pp. 7 (centre), 63 (fig. 2); James Read p. 131; Rex Features p. 117; Chris Ridgers pp. 23, 28, 30 (fig. 1), 32, 33, 36, 39 (fig. 2), 40 (figs 1 and 2), 42, 49, 75, 77, 79 (fig. 3), 80, 82, 83, 96, 97, 105 (fig. 1, top), 106 (fig. 3), 109, 110 (figs 1 and 2), 115, 116, 119, 120 (fig. 1), 121, 133, 136, (fig. 2), 137, 139 (figs 3 and 4), 140, 144, 145; Suzanne Roden/Format p. 30 (fig. 2); The RSPCA p. 31; B. Russell/ Oxfam p. 126; St Bartholomew's Hospital pp. 19, 103; David Alexander Simson/ Barnaby's p. 6 (top left); Ann Dalrymple Smith/Oxfam p. 73; Liz Somerville p. 25; Sporting Pics p. 58 (fig. 2); The Sugar Bureau p. 69 (fig. 3a); M. Thompson/Oxfam p. 127 (fig. 3); Charles Topham/*Farmers Weekly* p. 85; Peter Wiles/Oxfam p. 128 (fig. 2); Val Wilmer/Format p. 57.

The authors also wish to thank Annie Tomlin for typing the manuscript.

Contents

Introduction 6

Section 1. Food and health 8
1.1 Why what we eat matters 8
1.2 Food and health in the UK 10
1.3 Guidelines for a healthy balanced diet 12
1.4 Types of food in a healthy balanced diet 14
1.5 Nutrients provided by a healthy balanced diet 16
1.6 Human digestion 18

Section 2. Choosing a healthy balanced diet 20
2.1 Classifying foods for choosing a healthy balanced diet 20
2.2 Cereal foods and starchy vegetables (food group 1) 22
A Identifying cereal foods and starchy vegetables 22
B The place of cereal foods and starchy vegetables in the diet 24
2.3 Fruit and vegetables (food group 2) 26
A Identifying fruit and vegetables 26
B The place of fruit and vegetables in the diet 28
2.4 Meat and alternatives (food group 3) 30
A Identifying meat and alternatives 30
B The place of meat and alternatives in the diet 32
2.5 Milk and milk products (food group 4) 34
2.6 Sugar, sugary foods and drinks (food group 5) 36
A Identifying sugar, sugary foods and drinks 36
B The place of sugar, sugary foods and drinks in the diet 38
2.7 Fats and oils (food group 6) 40
A Identifying fats and oils 40
B The place of fats and oils in the diet 40
2.8 Salt in the diet 42
2.9 Water and fluids in the diet 44
2.10 Alcohol in the diet 46
2.11 Food additives in the diet 48

Section 3. Eating patterns and special needs 50
3.1 Eating patterns in the UK 50
3.2 Availability of food 52
3.3 Individual choice 54
3.4 The special needs of infants and toddlers 56
3.5 The special needs of teenagers 58
3.6 The special needs of women who are pregnant or breastfeeding 60
3.7 The special needs of the elderly 62
3.8 The special needs of vegetarians and vegans 64

Section 4. The nutrients in our food 66
4.1 Dietary energy 66
4.2 Carbohydrates 68
4.3 Fats 70

4.4 Protein 72
4.5 Protein-calorie deficiency 74
4.6 Vitamins and minerals 75
4.7 The nutritional role of cereal foods and starchy vegetables 76
A Dietary energy, starch and protein 76
B Dietary fibre 78
C Iron, zinc and calcium 80
D Vitamins 82
E Effects of cooking and processing 84
F Digestion 88
4.8 The nutritional role of fruit and vegetables 89
A Dietary energy, dietary fibre and carbohydrate 89
B Vitamin C 90
C Vitamins A and K 92
D B vitamins and minerals 94
E Effects of processing, storage and cooking 96
F Digestion 98
4.9 The nutritional role of meat and its alternatives 99
A Dietary energy, protein, dietary fibre and fat 99
B B group vitamins 100
C Fat soluble vitamins 102
D Minerals 104
E Effects of cooking and processing 105
F Digestion 107
4.10 The nutritional role of milk and milk products 108
A Infant feeding 108
B Dietary energy, protein, carbohydrates and fat 110
C Minerals 112
D Vitamins 113
E Effects of cooking and processing 114
F Digestion 115
4.11 The nutritional role of sugar, sugary foods and drinks 116
A Dietary energy and health 116
B Effects of cooking and processing 118
4.12 The nutritional role of fats and oils 120
A Dietary energy and fat soluble vitamins 120
B Effects of cooking and processing 122
C Digestion 123
4.13 Nutrient and energy density 124

Section 5. Feed the world 126
5.1 Hunger and food aid 126
5.2 Long term aid 128

Section 6. Kitchen skills and hygiene 130
6.1 Food hygiene 130
6.2 Hygienic practices 132
6.3 Food storage 134
6.4 Food spoilage 136
6.5 Food preservation 138
6.6 Cooking (heat movement) 142
6.7 Cooking methods 144

6.8 Equipment and safety 146
6.9 Aesthetics and food 148

Section 7. Food tables 150
Some typical nutritional values per 100 g of food 150
Recommended daily intakes of energy and nutrients for the UK 155
Summary of the importance and dietary sources of different nutrients 156

Index 168

Introduction

How many times a day do you think about what you will eat or drink? Next time you do, stop and think for a minute or two. What are you choosing? Why are you choosing it? How is it affecting your body?

Food, like air and water, is basic to human life. Without it we would soon die. But does it really matter how, what, when and why we eat? Yes it does. This book will answer many of your questions.

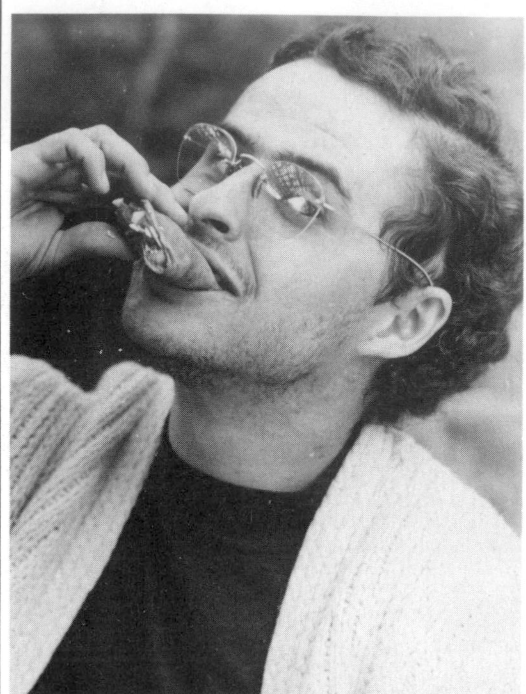

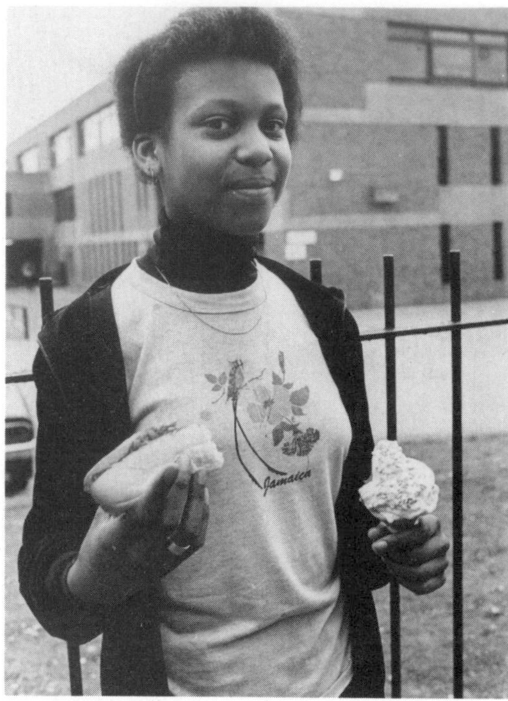

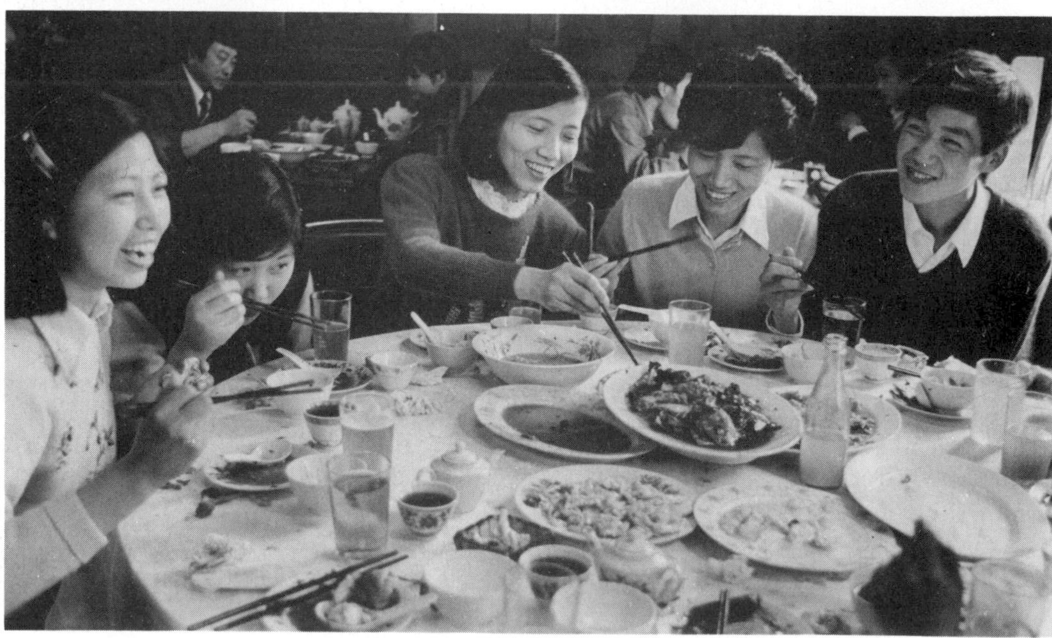

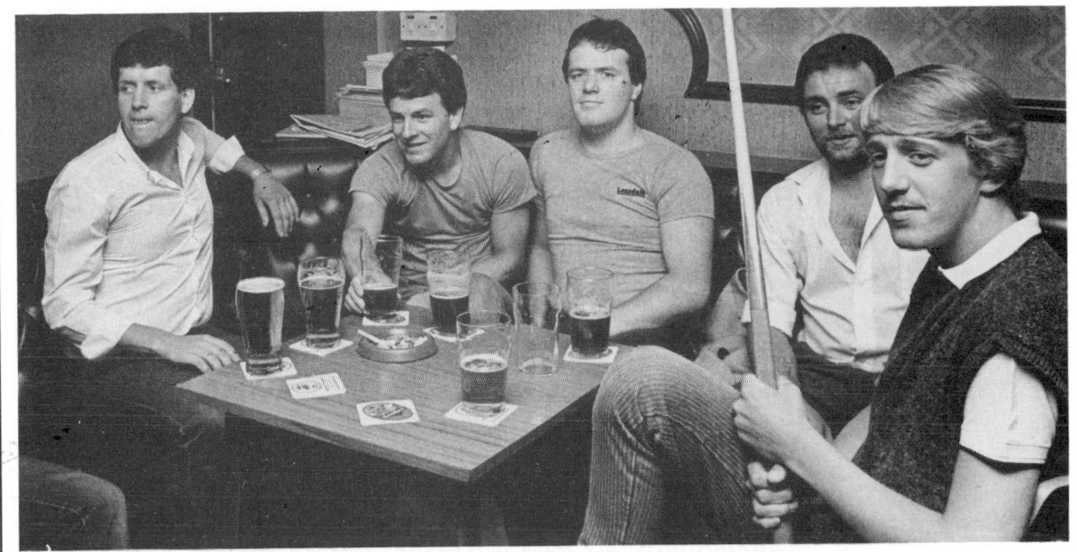

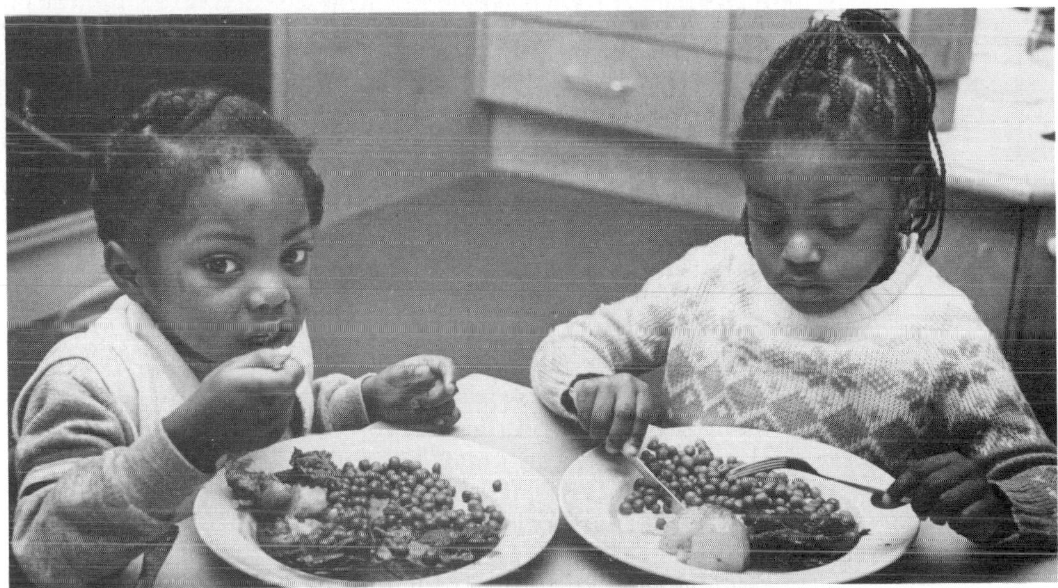

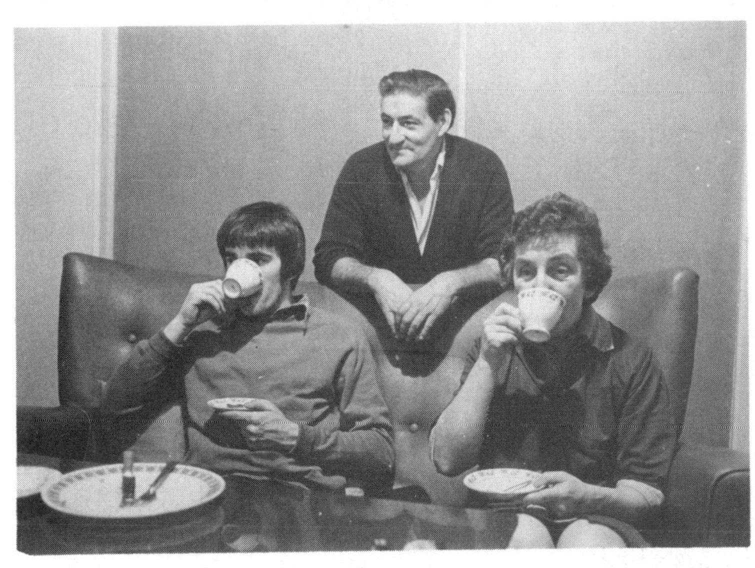

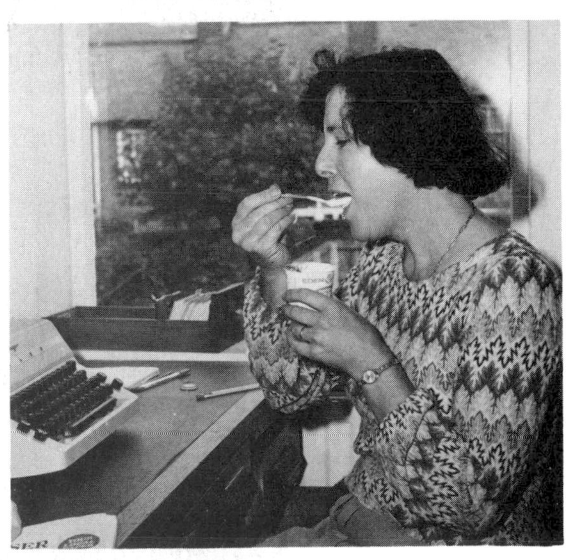

SECTION 1 Food and health

1.1 Why what we eat matters

Wouldn't it be nice and simple if we could just eat whatever we wanted, whenever we fancy it, and stay fit and healthy? Unfortunately it's not quite that easy. These days it helps to understand something about food and drink. The food and drink we consume is called our **diet**. From our diet we must get all the **nutrients** we need to stay healthy. Nutrients are the parts of food and drink which build, repair and protect our bodies and keep us fit, active and healthy. The study of people's diets and how they affect health is called **nutrition**.

Nobody is completely sure what is the best diet for any one person. It depends on many factors. What we do know is that throughout the world there are many people who simply do not have enough to eat. At the same time, there are many other people who have too much. There are still others who have enough food, but it is of poor quality nutritionally. The health of all these groups of people is damaged by their diets. They are all said to be suffering from **malnutrition**, i.e. bad nutrition.

Undernutrition

Undernutrition is most common in poor countries where the poorest people do not have enough food. In many of these countries people grow their own food (Fig. 1), but the climate is unpredictable and crops are often destroyed. Inadequate roads to rural areas, low incomes and other social and political factors often mean that, even if food is available in the country, it does not reach the people who need it most. The result is that people, especially children, become weak and thin. They pick up infections easily and show all the signs of not having enough nutrients. This topic is discussed more fully in Section 5, 'Feed the World'.

Some people in richer countries like the UK also suffer from undernutrition (Fig. 2). They tend to be children and elderly people, from households where there are often social problems associated with having a low income. Food costs money and so do most other things we need. Sometimes there is just not enough to go round and diets may suffer.

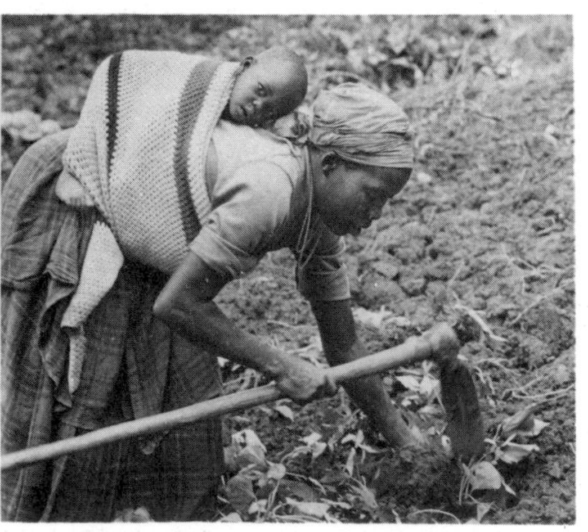

Fig. 1 Tilling the soil in Rwanda, Africa

Overnutrition

In many countries where people are suffering from undernutrition, there are also people who are **overnourished**. They have more food than they need and become overweight and unhealthy. In the UK, nearly four out of every ten men and over three out of every ten women are overweight (Fig. 3). This type of overnutrition is therefore common. It is a result of eating too much of the wrong sorts of foods. People who are overweight are more likely to become ill as they get older than those who are not.

Poor quality diets

In most rich countries many people become ill or die prematurely from a variety of diseases. Many of the diseases seem to be associated with the type of diet eaten. These diets tend to have the wrong combinations of food, providing an imbalance of nutrients. This is why it is important to understand something about nutrition when we are deciding what to eat or drink.

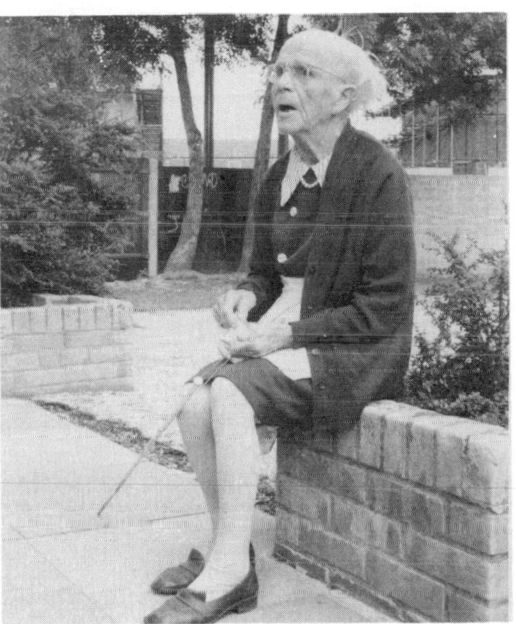

Fig. 2 Undernourishment in the UK

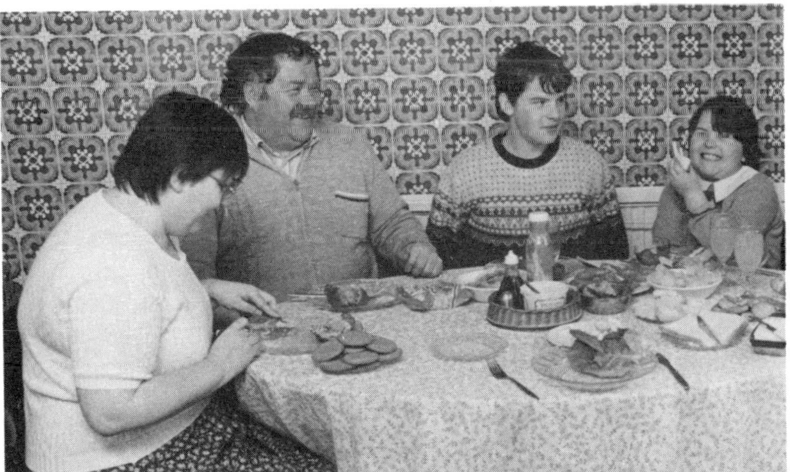

Fig. 3 Overnutrition in the UK

Nutritional recommendations for the public

Since the mid-1970s there has been increased interest in the links between diet and health in the UK. The Government and the Health Education Council have published books and reports which advise us to think carefully about the way we eat. They have given guidelines about what is currently thought to be the best type of diet for our health. This book explains the current guidelines and how they can be put into practice.

A changing world

All the time nutritionists and doctors are studying the links between diet and health. As they learn more, their ideas change slightly. What is understood now is different from what was thought ten years ago. In ten years' time, new information may have changed some of the ideas about what is now accepted. We must be prepared either to accept or to question these changes in current knowledge. Perhaps the most important part of learning about nutrition is learning to evaluate the information we are given. We can then make up our minds about how and what we will eat.

Summary

- Food is related to health.
- In the UK there is both overnutrition and undernutrition.
- In the UK there are nutritional recommendations for the public.
- It is important to understand and evaluate the information we receive about food and health.

Questions

1. Write a few sentences to explain how you would persuade someone that it is important to learn about food and health.
2. Many people confuse the word 'diet' with trying to lose weight. What is its correct meaning?
3. Explain the difference between malnutrition (i.e. bad nutrition) in poor countries and rich countries.

1.2 | Food and health in the UK

YEAR	1970	1972	1974	1976	1978	1980	1982	1984
White bread	914	811	801	751	710	623	615	568
Brown bread	69	68	59	84	79	94	94	186
Wholemeal bread	14	13	16	18	29	57	59	
Other breads	84	83	74	89	92	99	112	112
Total bread	1080	975	950	942	911	872	880	867
Potatoes	1529	—	—	1002	1149	1276	1236	1129

Fig. 1 Consumption of bread and potatoes in the UK

These figures are taken from 'Household Food Consumption and Expenditure' MAFF for appropriate years. They represent grams per person per week.

Eating patterns in the UK

In the UK, there have been major and rapid changes in diet over the last 40 years or so. We now eat much less bread, potatoes and other fresh foods and much more meat, meat products and processed foods than our grandparents and their parents did (Fig. 1). **Processed foods** (Fig. 2) are those which have been changed in some way from their natural state. There are wide variations in the extent of processing. Some foods, such as wholemeal bread and frozen vegetables, have been processed in simple ways. They contain most of the nutrients found in the original product. Other foods, such as dessert mixes and canned foods, have been highly processed. Their nutrient composition is usually much poorer than for fresh foods. Most processed foods contain chemical **additives** which are used to enhance the keeping qualities and give extra colour and flavour. The effects of these additives are discussed later in this book. Generally, the diets of most people in the UK now contain too much fat, sugar and salt and not enough foods providing bulk. Recently, the way in which we eat has also changed. Nowadays, it is possible to buy 'fast food' and 'take-aways' in almost every town, and many people literally eat in the street, while doing other things.

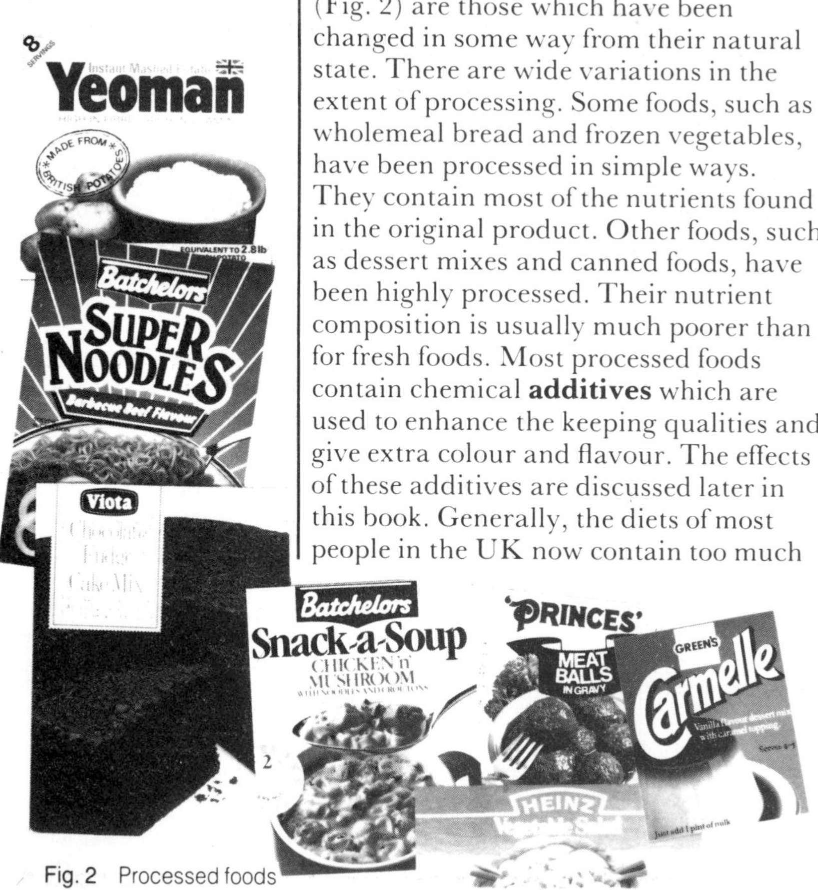

Fig. 2 Processed foods

Health patterns in the UK

At the beginning of this century the main health problems in the UK were connected with infectious diseases. People died from illnesses which now no longer exist in the UK. The main causes were poor sanitation and poor nutrition.

Nowadays the health problems due to diet are different. People die prematurely from **heart disease** and **cancer**. They can become disabled because of **high blood pressure** and **strokes**, and many people suffer because their **digestive systems** are unhealthy. Many people are also **overweight** or suffer from **tooth decay**.

Life-styles in the UK

Food and health patterns are not all that have changed in recent years. Labour-saving devices in the home and mechanization of industry mean fewer people have to do very hard physical work (Fig. 3). Most households also have televisions. In general, therefore, people take much less exercise than they did in the past. This has an effect on health patterns, along with the dietary changes.

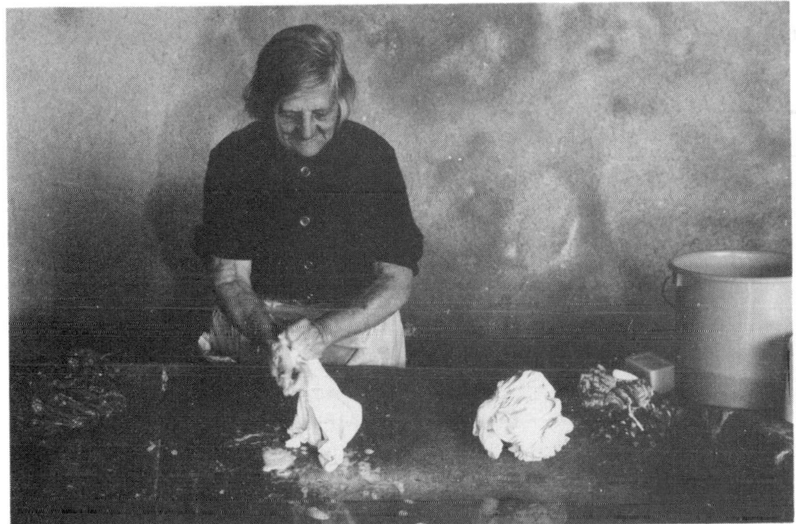

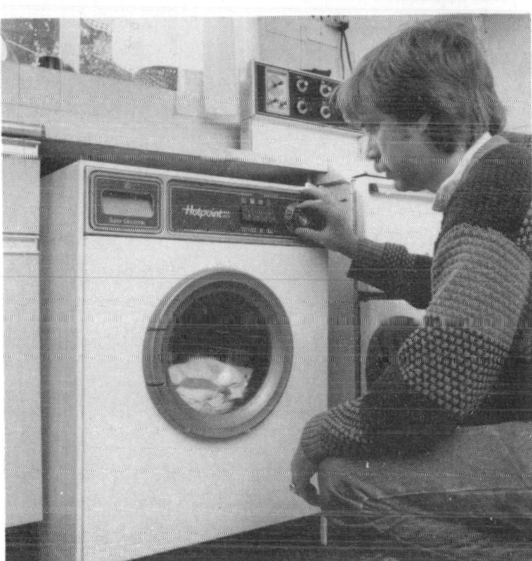

Fig. 3 (a) Using a washboard
(b) using a washing machine

We're not all the same

People's health, food and life-style are different depending on their circumstances. Many people in the UK still live in poverty. They have to buy cheaper food and may not have fridges or decent kitchens and cooking facilities. Because there is not enough housing, some people have to live in bed and breakfast accommodation and have nowhere to cook. They have to eat all their meals in cafés and restaurants. This can be very expensive and affect their nutritional state and health. Some elderly people are lonely, isolated and immobile and have difficulty in shopping. They may also lose their interest in food. This can result in undernutrition.

It is important to remember that no two people are the same. Everyone has different needs, different priorities and lives in different circumstances. Diets differ in a similar way.

Summary

- Food patterns have changed a lot in the last 40 years.
- Health patterns have also changed.
- Life-styles have changed.
- People's health, food and life-style are different depending on their circumstances.

Questions

1. Explain what is meant by 'processed' foods. Give examples of five 'highly processed foods' and five foods which have been through simple processing.
2. Make a list of the commonest causes of health problems at the beginning of this century.
3. Draw a graph to show how total bread consumption changed between 1970 and 1984.
   How many grams of bread were eaten per person per week in (a) 1970 (b) 1974 (c) 1979 (d) 1984?

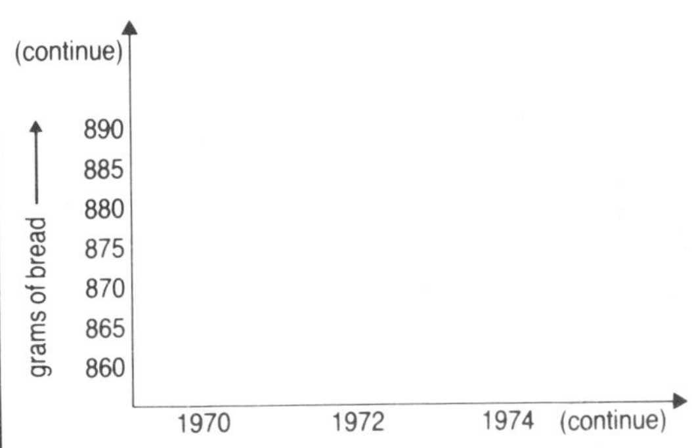

4. Give three examples of circumstances which can prevent people from cooking and eating the kind of food they would like.

1.3 Guidelines for a healthy balanced diet

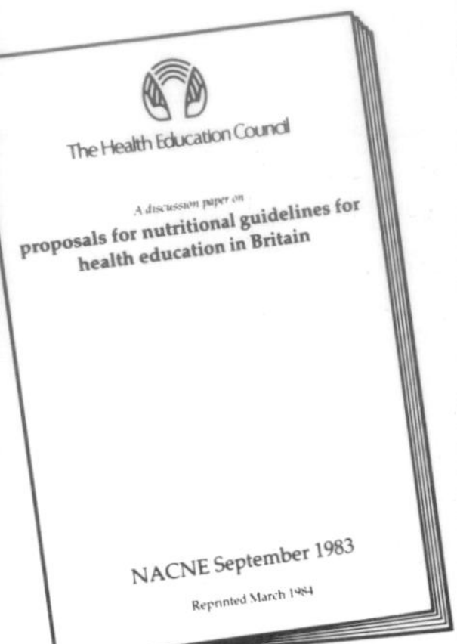

Fig. 1 The NACNE report

In the UK there are scientifically based guidelines about the amounts of each nutrient we need. These guidelines have three main uses. Firstly, they provide a yardstick against which diets can be measured. The food intake of different groups of the population can be compared with these recommendations. Secondly, the standards give a guide to caterers and dietitians who are planning to feed people in large numbers. Thirdly, they are necessary for any planning of agricultural policies and the organized food trade. In the UK, nutritional recommendations exist in two forms: **recommended daily amounts** of nutrients and **dietary goals**.

Recommended Daily Amounts of nutrients (RDAs)

RDAs were last published in 1979 by the Department of Health and Social Security. They are figures for the intake of food energy and certain nutrients necessary to avoid **deficiencies** and to ensure health for different **population groups**. In general, the figures provide a liberal margin of safety. They need regular checking and updating. For example, in the UK the recommendation for energy intake has been reduced in recent years, because people are now less active.

RDAs are given for specific groups of the population, but not for individuals. For example, most children and pregnant women need more calcium than most adults. The RDAs reflect these needs.

RDAs in the UK leave a safety margin for groups of people who may be at particular risk of vitamin or mineral deficiencies. RDAs in other countries are based on different criteria.

Dietary goals

Dietary goals have been produced more recently than RDAs. These are concerned with health problems related to **overconsumption** as well as **underconsumption**, and with ensuring a healthy balance of nutrients in the diet.

(i) Eating for Health Dietary goals in the UK were first given by the Government in 1978 in a DHSS publication called *Eating for Health*. The recommendations were that:

- As far as possible, babies should be breastfed so that they would have the 'best possible start in life', even if this was for only a few days.
- People should try to avoid becoming overweight.
- The population as a whole should try to
  - increase its intake of dietary fibre and starch
  - reduce its intake of fat, sugar, salt and alcohol.

Unlike RDAs, these general guidelines did not recommend specific amounts.

(ii) NACNE In 1983 the Health Education Council published a document called *Proposals for Nutritional Guidelines for Health Education in Britain*

	Current intakes	*Short term guidelines*	*Long term guidelines*
Total fat (% energy)	38	34	30
Saturated fat (% energy)	18	15	10
Sugar (kg per year)	38	34	20
Dietary fibre (g per day)	20	25	30
Salt (g per day)	12	11	9
Alcohol (% energy)	6	5	4
Energy – should be maintained at current levels and people should take more exercise			

Fig. 2 The NACNE guidelines

(Fig. 1). This was a discussion paper from a sub-group of the National Advisory Committee on Nutrition Education (NACNE). It suggested that to reduce the amount of ill health related to poor diet in the UK, the intake of some **dietary components** should change significantly. (They estimated it would take about 15 years for this to happen.) It also gave interim targets for the end of the 1980s (Fig. 2).

Fig. 3 COMA recommendations

Fats

2.1.1 The ratio of polyunsaturated to saturated fats should be approximately 0.45.
Saturated fats should provide 15% dietary energy.
Total fat should provide 35% dietary energy.

Sugar

2.1.4 The intake of simple sugars should not be increased further. (Restriction has been recommended on other health grounds, e.g. dental caries.)

Alcohol

2.1.5 Excessive intake of alcohol should be avoided.

Salt

2.1.6 The intake of salt should not be increased further and consideration should be given to ways of decreasing it.

Fibre

2.1.7 Reduced fat intake should be compensated for with increased fibre rich carbohydrates.

Energy

2.1.8 Obesity should be avoided.

Remember that the NACNE recommendations are for averages of the whole population and not for individuals or even groups of individuals. For example, they are not necessarily relevant to babies or young children, or to the elderly population. The NACNE recommendations are useful for planning food production, assessing dietary change and planning large scale meal provision.

(iii) COMA In 1984, the DHSS committee which had been set up to study **heart disease** published a report on diet and **cardiovascular** disease. This is known as the *COMA* report. It only considered components of the diet connected with diseases of the heart and blood system. Its primary recommendations were about fat and salt (Fig. 3).

Summary

- Nutritional recommendations for the public in the UK are in two forms: recommended daily amounts of food energy and nutrients (RDAs) and dietary goals.
- The RDAs are set at levels to prevent deficiency of particular nutrients.
- The RDAs are given for groups of people within the population and are not specific to individuals.
- Dietary goals are set at levels to prevent overconsumption and underconsumption of different dietary components.
- Dietary goals are aimed at the population as a whole and may not apply to specific groups of the population.

Questions

1. Look at the table of RDAs. What are the RDAs for Energy, Iron and Vitamin C for someone in your group?
2. Are these figures personal advice on the amount of particular nutrients to eat? Explain your answer.
3. Use a computer program like 'Nu-Pack' or a nutrition table to find out whether your class's diets yesterday gave you your RDAs of the three components named in Q1.
4. Why is it thought necessary for people in Britain to change their diets?
5. What are the main recommendations of (a) the NACNE report, (b) the COMA report?
6. Is your diet a healthy one? Explain your answer and say how it might be improved if you think it needs to be.

1.4 Types of food in a healthy balanced diet

A healthy balanced diet is one which provides the right combination of food and nutrients for optimum growth and health. The only food which supplies everything a person needs is human breast milk (Fig. 1). Even this is only enough for the first few months of life. To get a balanced diet it is therefore important to eat a mixture of foods. Foods rich in one nutrient 'balance' the lack of that nutrient in another.

In the UK there is an increasing **variety** of foods available. These range from fresh foods to highly processed foods. Twenty years ago, for example, food like instant meals in pots did not exist. Now there are a number of different types to choose from. However, when we look at these foods, how much variety are we really being offered?

Food manufacturers take a few basic foods. They refine them and add different chemical **additives**. Suddenly we have a 'new' type of food. This sort of increase in the variety of foods is not necessarily a good thing. It can make it more difficult for people trying to choose a healthy balanced diet. Food traditions are formed over centuries and, until recently, have changed very little and very slowly. Many of the foods available today are not part of dietary traditions from anywhere in the world, and they do not always fit in well with traditional eating patterns.

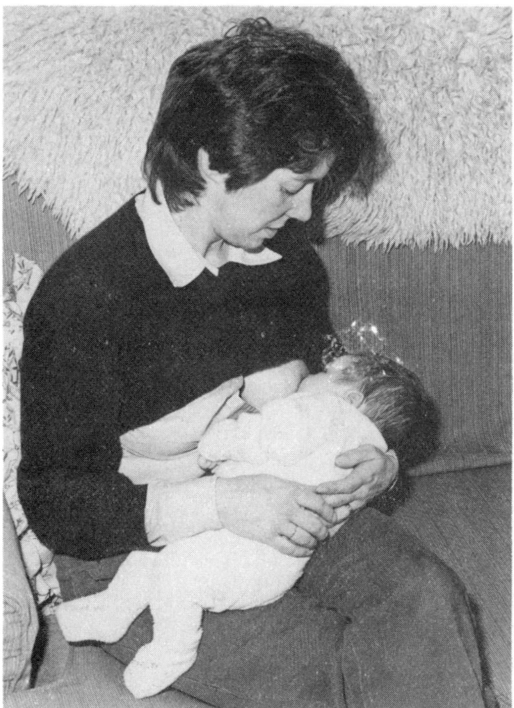

Fig. 1 Breastfeeding a child

Food processing

The vast majority of the food available to us is **processed** in some way. The degree of processing varies from the simple freezing of fresh food, to prevent it going bad, to complicated technical procedures which totally alter the structure and nutritional composition of the food. Some highly processed foods have extra nutrients added to replace those lost in processing. Many do not.

Cooked foods

As the variety of foods in shops increases so does the number of places where we can buy food ready to eat away from home. Eating out and the consumption of snacks has gone up rapidly in the last few years. When eating these foods we are relying on the food manufacturers and caterers to make healthy food available to us. Often this does not happen. Much of the food in snack bars and fast food restaurants is very fatty and salty (Fig. 2). They rarely provide really healthy food. Some places have salad bars, but the vegetables are often covered in oil or mayonnaise based dressing. Once again, increased variety does not in itself make it easier to choose a healthy balanced diet.

Ethnic and cultural changes

Over the last 30 years the variety of foods available in the UK has also grown as a result of the multicultural nature of our society, increased travel and advances in methods of transporting food. Indian, Chinese, Italian, Greek and Turkish restaurants are now common in many towns (Fig. 3). The use of spices and different flavourings has increased, and many more kinds of fruit, vegetables, bread, cereal and pulses are now available. In most parts of the country it is easy to buy vegetables such as peppers, aubergines, okras and courgettes, whereas 20 years ago it was very difficult.

Fig. 2 A fast food restaurant

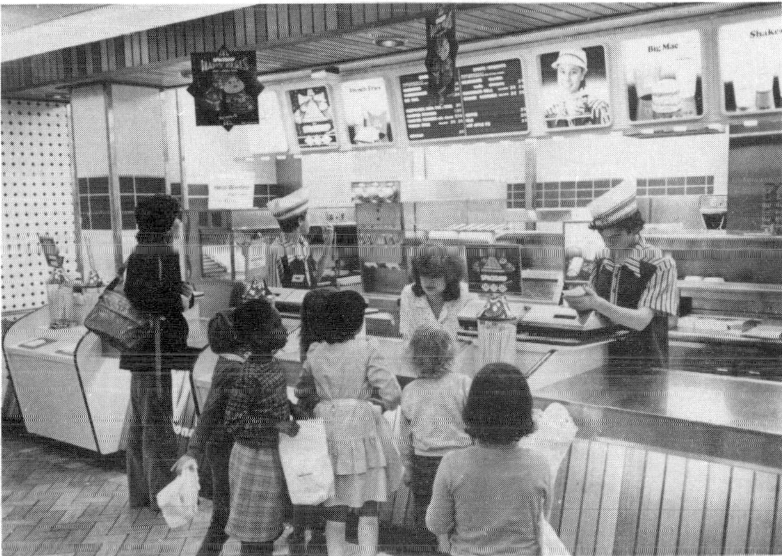

Choosing a healthy balanced diet from the variety available

Unfortunately, merely eating a wide variety of foods does not guarantee a balanced diet. Many of the foods we can easily buy are naturally high in fat and sugar which are the components of the diet we are trying to limit. Also, the highly processed foods which are readily available often contain very few of the more useful nutrients. Therefore, to make sure we are choosing a healthy balanced diet we need some guidelines about how to choose and combine different types of foods.

Summary

- In the UK, a very wide variety of foods is available.
- Most of the food we eat is processed in some way.
- A healthy balanced diet needs a variety of food.
- Variety has to be chosen within careful guidelines.

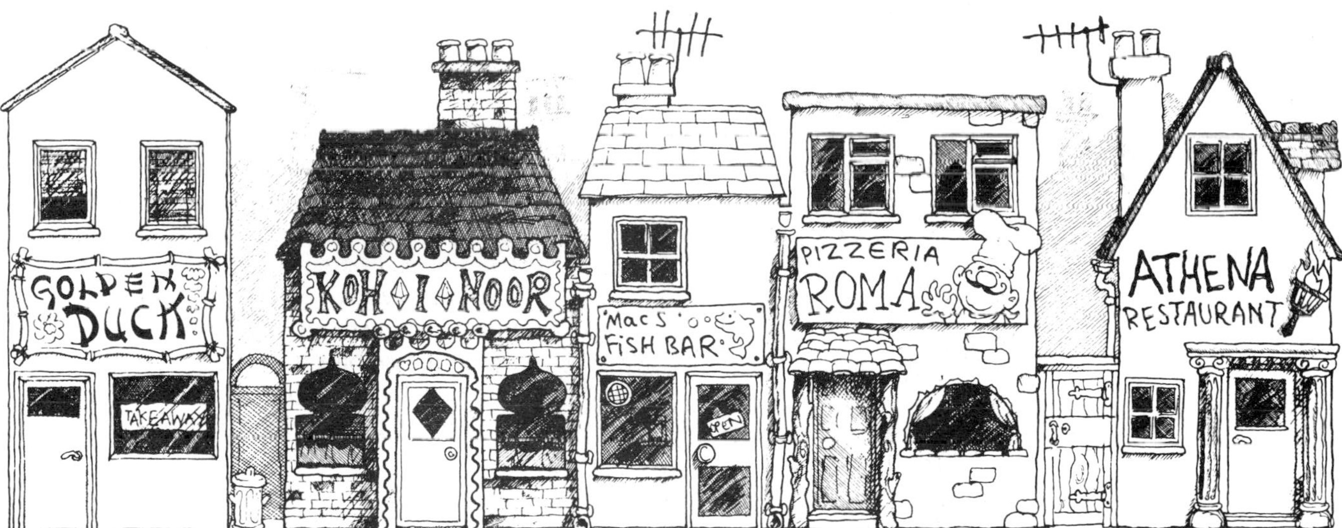

Fig. 3 Multicultural food

Questions

1. Why does eating a variety of foods not necessarily ensure a balanced diet?
2. Give four examples of foods you eat which were not available here 20 years ago.
3. Give three reasons why many of the foods you eat were not available 20 years ago.

1.5 Nutrients provided by a healthy balanced diet

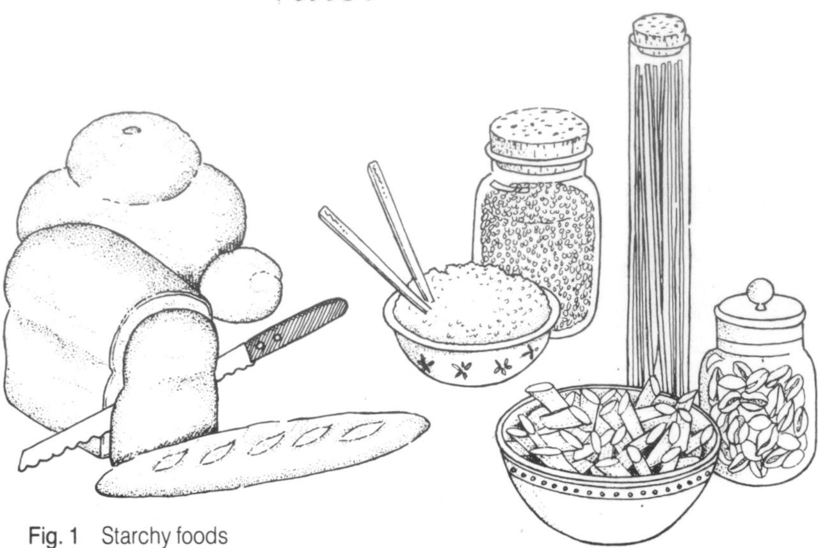

Fig. 1 Starchy foods

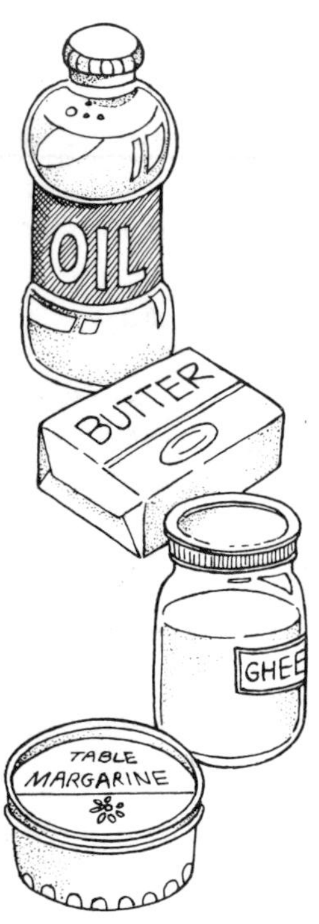

Fig. 2 Fatty foods

There are three reasons why we have to eat and drink. Like any other living creature, and any machine, our bodies need fuel to provide us with energy. This energy comes from our diet. At the same time, every cell in our body needs to be regularly repaired, and those which die need to be replaced. Also, people who are growing need the 'building blocks' for the new cells to grow and develop.

The nutrients in food and drink all have very individual, specific functions. Some provide energy, some are the building blocks for growth and repair, and some protect our cells. They also help each other out. For example, some of the 'protective' nutrients help the energy giving nutrients to produce their energy. The building blocks cannot build without the help of the protective nutrients, and so on.

The main nutrients in food are protein, fats, carbohydrates, vitamins and minerals. Protein, fats and carbohydrates can all provide **dietary energy**, but the most important sources are carbohydrates and fats.

Carbohydrates

There are three types of carbohydrates used by our bodies. They are used differently and have different effects. The most complicated chemically is **dietary fibre**. This is so complex that it cannot be fully digested in the gut and is passed out in the stool. It is important in keeping the gut healthy and our diets should contain plenty.

Starch is also a 'complex' carbohydrate, but is not too complicated to be digested and absorbed into our bodies. It is the most important energy source we have (Fig. 1). In its natural state, starch is found in foods together with the vitamins that are needed for energy production (see below). Sometimes starch is refined and the vitamins are removed. It is not necessarily so good for you if this has happened.

The third type of carbohydrate is **sugars**. One of these is the sugar we have all heard of and use regularly. This is purified or **refined** sugar. The sugar we eat comes mainly from sugar beet, but some is made from sugar cane.

It is well known that refined sugar is one of the causes of tooth decay, and we should try to eat less of it. There are, however, a number of other sugars which are found in unrefined foods. These include the sugar in milk, called lactose, and the main sugar in fruit, called fructose. These sugars are usually consumed with plenty of water (as in milk), or with water and dietary fibre (as in fruit), so they are not considered harmful to health. Milk and fruit also provide a whole range of other useful nutrients.

Fats

Fats are another useful source of energy (Fig. 2). Some types are essential for the working of the body; others are not. The most useful fats are **polyunsaturated** fats. In general, we eat more fat than we need to and most of us should eat much less of the non-essential types.

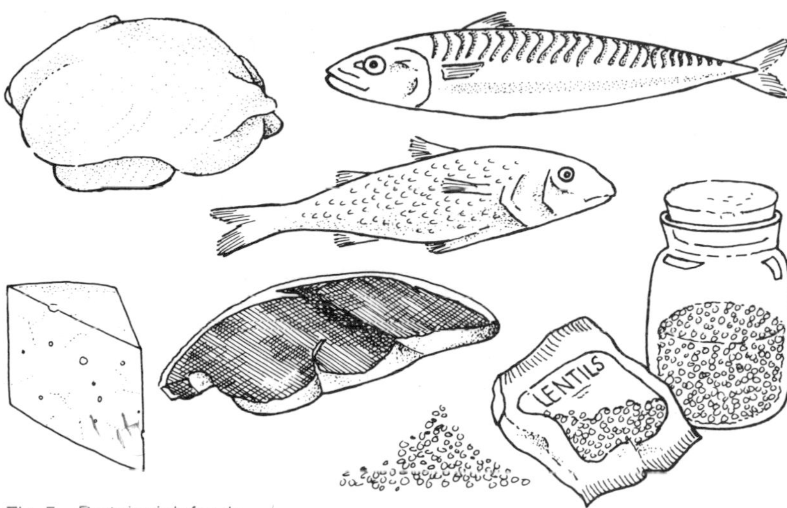

Fig. 3 Protein rich foods

Protein

Protein also provides energy, but its main function is in building and repairing the structure of all the cells in the body. However, if there is not enough fat and carbohydrate in the diet, protein will be used to provide energy instead. (This happens in starvation.) Protein is found in a wide variety of foods (Fig. 3) and it is very unusual for people in the UK not to get enough. Many people, however, eat much more than they need to.

Vitamins

We need many different vitamins to keep us healthy (Fig. 4). These are usually given letters of the alphabet as names, although they also have chemical names. Some vitamins are **water soluble** and are found in foods which contain water.

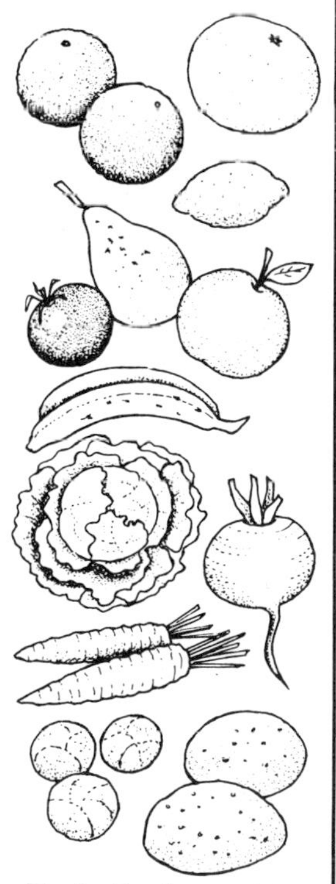

Fig. 4 Foods containing vitamins

Other vitamins are **fat soluble** and are only found in some fatty foods.

Water soluble vitamins are the vitamin B complex (a number of different vitamins with different uses but mostly connected with producing energy and keeping the nervous system healthy) and vitamin C, which helps general **resistance** of the cells to infections. The fat soluble vitamins are vitamins A, D, E and K. These too have important individual functions and are vital for keeping the body fit and healthy.

Minerals

A number of minerals are needed to protect and keep our bodies healthy. The ones we know most about are calcium, iron, phosphorus, potassium and sodium. All the time new research is discovering the importance of other minerals. These are sometimes called **trace elements**.

Summary

- A healthy balanced diet provides the right amount of dietary energy.
- Protein, fat and carbohydrate all provide dietary energy.
- Protein's main function is to build and repair the structure of cells.
- Vitamins are important in many functions including energy production and protecting the body.
- New research is discovering the importance of tiny amounts of different minerals in the diet.

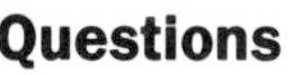

Questions

1. What are the three main reasons why we need food?
2. Copy and complete this table.

Nutrient	*Main function*
Carbohydrates 1. 2. 3. Sugars Fats 1. Saturated 2. Protein	

3. Which vitamins are water soluble, and which are found in fatty foods?

1.6 Human digestion

The food we eat is used as a source of energy, to grow and repair all the body's cells and tissues, and to protect us from disease. Before we can make use of it, food needs to go through physical and chemical changes. These changes we call **digestion** (Figs 1 and 2).

(a) It is broken into small pieces and mixed with fluids to turn it into a solution called **chyme**.

(b) It is acted on by various **enzymes**, which break the large and complex molecules into small simple ones which can pass through membranes into the blood. There they can be transported to the sites where they are used for the three functions outlined above.

An enzyme is a biological **catalyst**, i.e. a substance which brings about a change without itself changing. Enzymes are made up of proteins and are sensitive to heat and to the chemical conditions

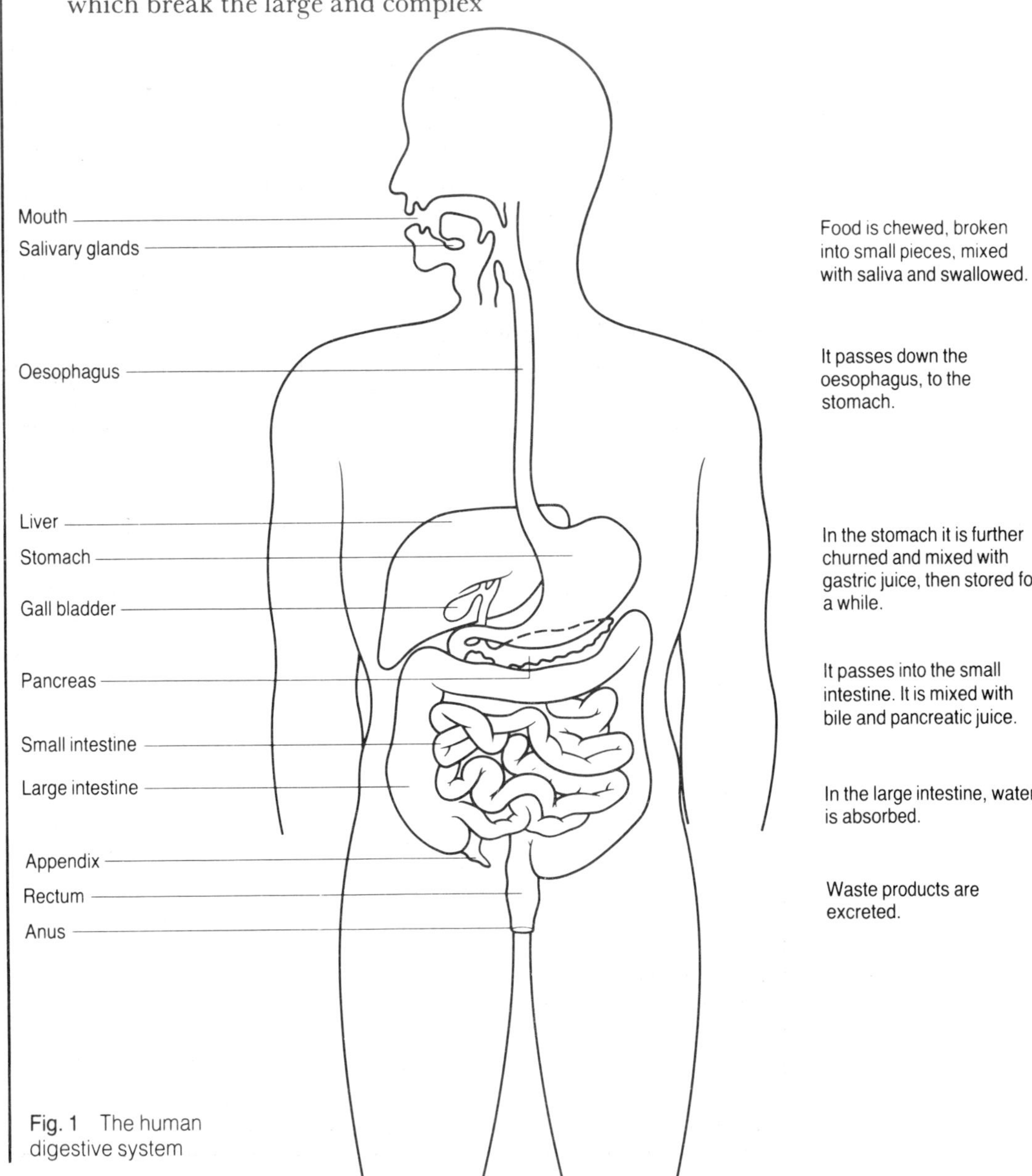

Fig. 1 The human digestive system

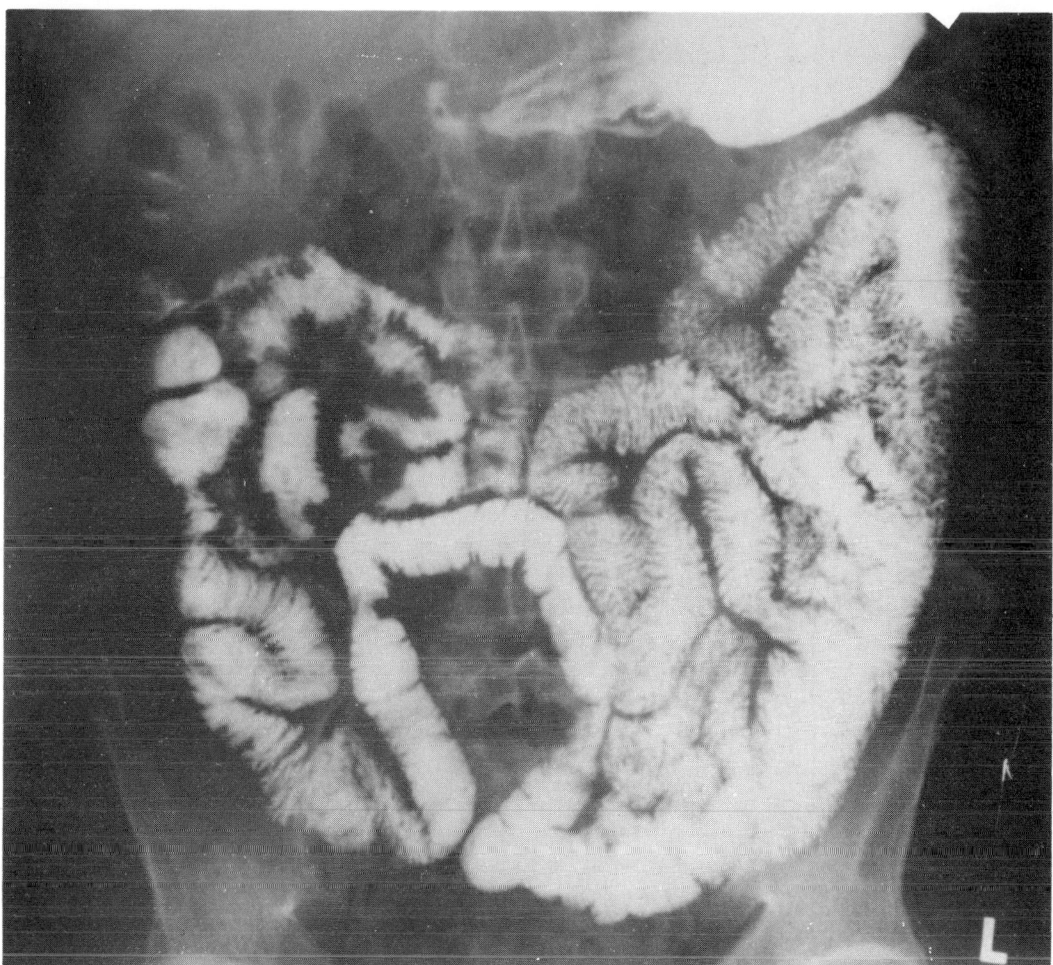

Fig. 2 X-ray photograph of the lower part of the human digestive system

surrounding them. Some enzymes act only in acidic surroundings, some only in alkaline, but they all require a warm temperature to operate, i.e. body temperature of 37°C.

The enzymes which are important in digestion are:
– lipase (fat splitting)
– amylase (carbohydrate splitting)
– proteases (protein splitting)
Only a few of the simplest molecules found in our foods are used without needing to be split. Glucose, a simple type of sugar, is absorbed directly into blood, and vitamins do not have to be digested before being useful. Minerals also are not subject to digestion. Some of the mineral salts we take in are in an insoluble form, and these are changed into a soluble form. Others are already soluble and go directly into the blood system.

Summary

- We need food to keep the body alive, active and in good health.
- Before it can be used food needs to be broken down into simple molecules.
- Enzymes bring about digestion.

Questions

1. Describe what happens to food during digestion.
2. What do enzymes do during digestion? Describe the conditions they need.
3. What are the three kinds of enzymes which digest food?
4. Which substances do not need to be digested?

SECTION 2 *Choosing a healthy balanced diet*

2.1 *Classifying foods for choosing a healthy balanced diet*

To help choose a healthy balanced diet it is possible to divide foods into six main **food groups** – two from plants, two from animal sources and two of refined foods.

First look carefully at the **plant foods**. Divide these up according to which part of the plant they come from. For examples, see Fig. 1. We can then divide these into two or more groups based on nutritional factors and their use in the diet – those which contain significant amounts of starch and those which do not (Fig. 2). This separates the cereals, tubers and a few fruits from the fruit and vegetables group. The tubers and starchy fruits, such as green bananas, we call 'starchy vegetables'. Nuts and pulses are considered separately.

Now look at the **animal foods** (Fig. 3). These can also be divided into two groups – the milk and milk products, and the foods from the animal itself or its eggs. These two groups of food have different nutritional uses and are used in different ways. Many people, however, do not eat meat or fish. For them, pulses and nuts from the plant foods become especially important for their protein. Pulses and nuts are therefore grouped with meat and fish. A few people do not drink any milk or eat milk products. For them plant milks like that from soya beans (which are a type of pulse) may be particularly useful. Soya milk is therefore put in this group.

The third group is the **highly refined foods** (Fig. 4). These also can be divided into two groups – foods and drinks containing relatively large amounts of sugar, and fats and oils. Fats and oils may be of animal origin, for example butter, cream, lard or suet, or of vegetable origin, for example cooking oil and many margarines.

We are now left with six basic food groups (Fig. 5).

A healthy balanced diet contains plenty of foods of plant origin, some from animals and only a small amount of highly refined foods. That is, it should contain plenty of cereal foods and starchy vegetables, plenty of fruit and vegetables, a variety of fish, meat and eggs, and some milk and milk products. Small amounts of polyunsaturated vegetable fats are important to ensure that there are sufficient essential fatty acids and fat soluble vitamins in the diet.

Fig. 1 Plant foods

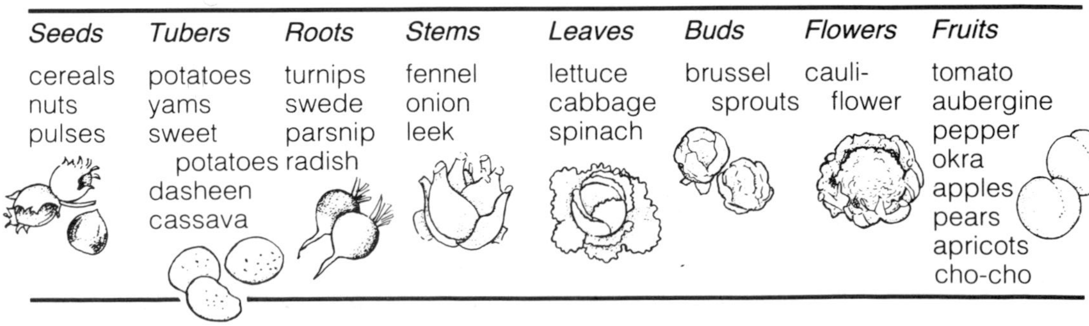

Seeds	*Tubers*	*Roots*	*Stems*	*Leaves*	*Buds*	*Flowers*	*Fruits*
cereals nuts pulses	potatoes yams sweet potatoes dasheen cassava	turnips swede parsnip radish	fennel onion leek	lettuce cabbage spinach	brussel sprouts	cauli-flower	tomato aubergine pepper okra apples pears apricots cho-cho

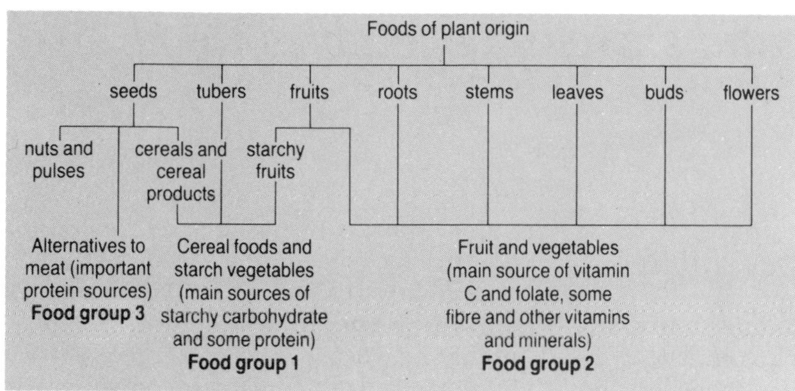

Fig. 2 Foods of plant origin

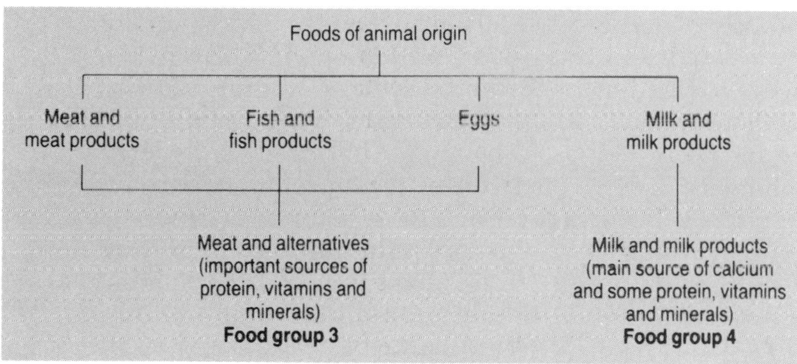

Fig. 3 Foods of animal origin

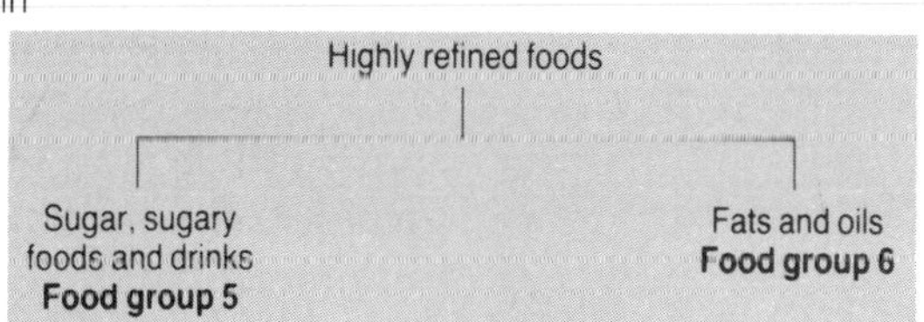

Fig. 4 Highly refined foods

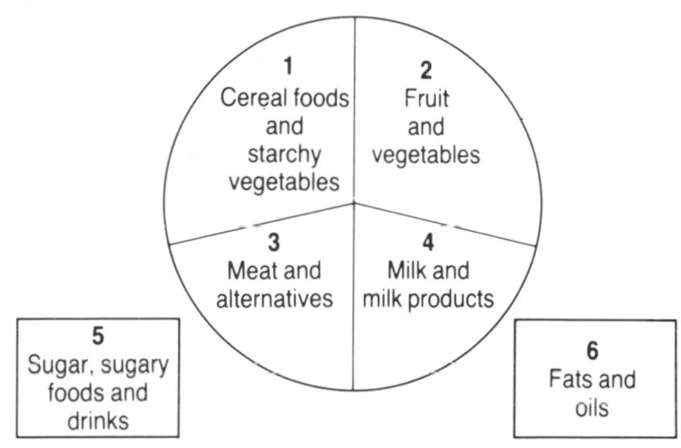

Fig. 5 The six basic food groups

Summary

- Foods can be broadly divided into those from plant and those from animal origin, and those which have been highly refined.
- We can divide food into six basic food groups.
- For most people to achieve a healthy balanced diet they need to eat plenty of food from plant origin, some from animal origin and only a small amount of highly refined foods.
- A few foods cross the food group boundaries because of their nutrient content and their use in the diet.
- Highly refined foods have only a small part to play in the diet.

Questions

1. This arrangement of boxes represents the way we divide foods into groups. Fill in each space with the appropriate word or words.

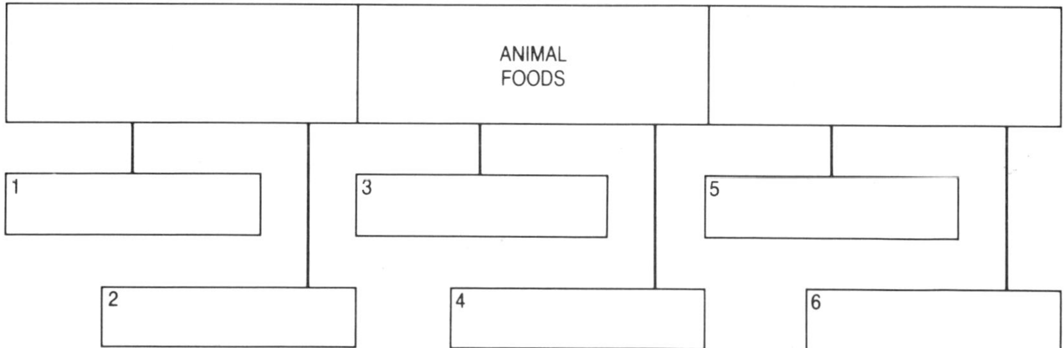

2. List all the foods you ate yesterday and put each food into its correct group.
3. Write a sentence to explain the importance in the diet of food groups 1–4.
4. What advice is given about groups 5 and 6?
5. List ten foods of animal origin, and ten of plant origin. List five which are a mixture of both.

2.2 Cereal foods and starchy vegetables (food group 1)

A Identifying cereal foods and starchy vegetables

The foods in this group come from plants and contain significant amounts of **starch**. Starch is used as a food store in growing plants.

Cereals and cereal foods Cereals are seeds and contain both starch and protein, as well as a variety of vitamins and minerals. Cereals include wheat, rice, oats, barley, maize and rye.

Wheat is the most commonly used cereal in the UK (Fig. 1). It is milled to produce **flour**, which is used in a wide variety of foods including bread, biscuits, cakes and pastry. Wheat can be **roller milled** or **stoneground**. During roller milling the wheat grain is broken down and separated out. The bran and wheat germ are removed (see page 79). If wholemeal flour is required these are then mixed in again. If brown flour is required some of the bran and wheat germ are added back, and if white flour is required the bran and wheat germ are used for other purposes. Stone milling crushes the wheat grains between two stones, producing wholemeal flour.
In the shops you see some flour and bread marked 100% wholemeal and some marked 100% stoneground.
The difference is in the milling process.

Fig. 1 Growing wheat

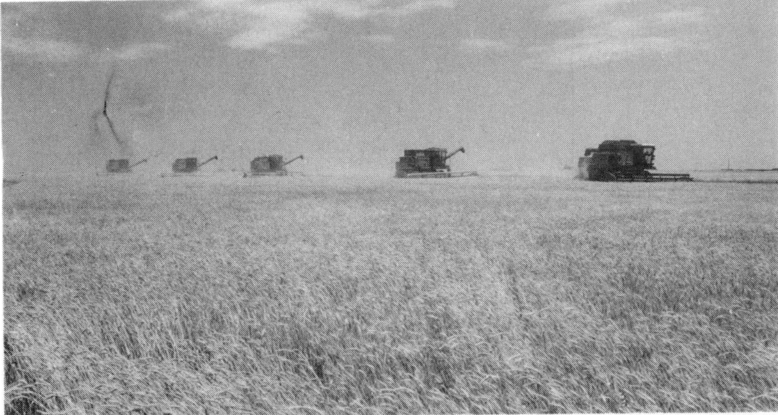

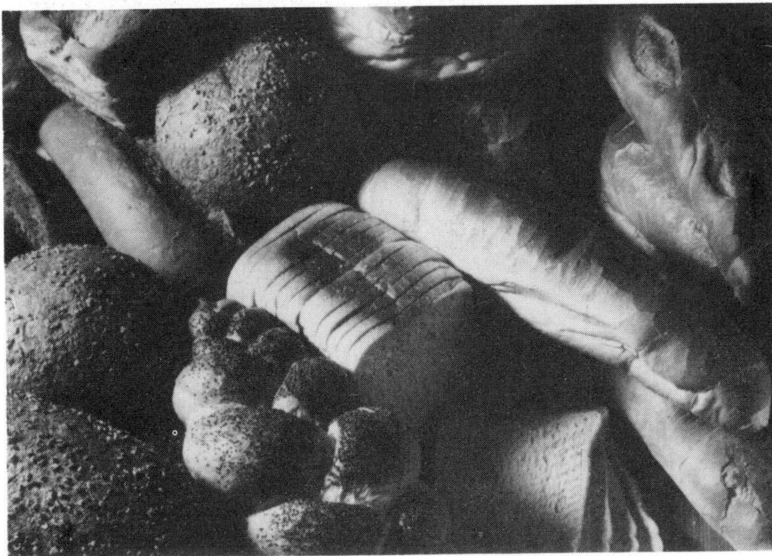

Fig. 2 Different breads

Flour differs depending on the quality of the wheat grain and its protein content. The protein in flour is called **gluten** (see page 86). Flour with a high protein content is called 'strong' flour and is good for making most bread. It keeps its shape well after rising. 'Weak' flour has a lower protein content and it is better for baking. It produces a lighter product. The wheat grown in the UK is generally fairly low in protein, therefore much of the flour used for breadmaking in the UK is imported from the USA and Canada. Flour also has important properties affecting its uses in cooking (see page 85).

Bread is the main product made from wheat. There are hundreds of different types available. These different breads include the more familiar white, brown and wholemeal bread, as well as risen breads like high bran, wheat germ and granary breads. Other breads include pitta bread, chapattis, puris and parathas, rye breads and sweetened breads (Fig. 2).

Pasta is made from the 'middings' (semolina) of strong wheat. The semolina is made into a paste with water and

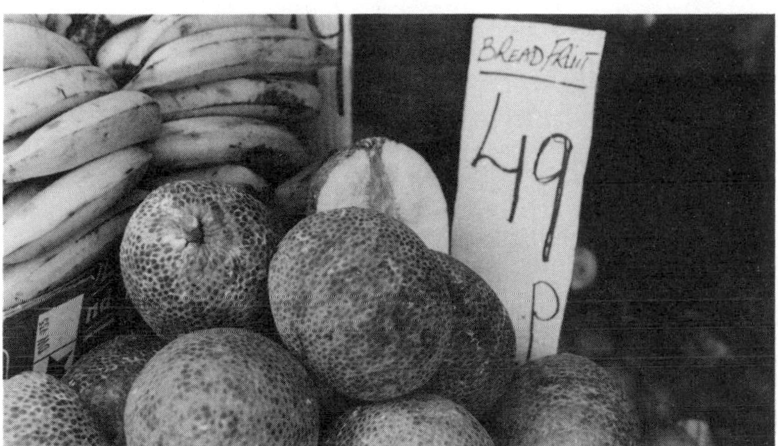

Fig. 3 Plantains and breadfruit

sometimes an egg. This paste is then extruded or moulded to make a variety of different shapes and sizes, e.g. spaghetti and macaroni. It can be made from white flour to produce ordinary white pasta, wholemeal flour to produce brown pasta, or coloured with tomato or spinach to make it pink or green.

Breakfast cereals are made from a variety of different cereals, for example 'Puffed Wheat' and 'Weetabix' from wheat, 'Cornflakes' from maize and 'Rice Krispies' from rice.

Rice is mainly used boiled whole. It can become the basis of a savoury meal, or as a sweet cooked with milk. It can also be ground and used to make porridges and doughs.

Oats are mainly eaten in the form of porridge. They are occasionally used in other cooking.

Maize is often ground and made into cornmeal and is widely used as a staple food in many parts of the world. It can also be made into cornflour, which is used as a thickening agent in cooking as it is almost 100% starch.

Rye can also be milled into a flour. It is used in rye bread and crispbreads.

Barley is used mainly in the form of pearl barley in soups and stews.

Starchy vegetables are those which contain significant amounts of starch. They are the swollen food storage organs of the plants. Many are tubers, for example potatoes, sweet potatoes and yam. **Potatoes** are mostly bought fresh and cooked in the home, although they are available in cans, frozen, dried or already cooked. There are ten species of **yam**, several of which are available in this country. The commonest one is the large tropical yam. Confusion arises when the name 'yam' is applied to any tropical root crop. Some starchy vegetables are swollen roots, e.g. cassava (which is called tapioca in Asia), taro (known as eddo or dasheen in the West Indies and coco yam in West Africa) and arrowroot, which is not commonly eaten as a vegetable but used as a valuable source of starch. Sago is produced from the starchy pith of sago palm trees in SE Asia. It is consumed locally as flour and exported as pearl sago. In this form it is eaten in milk puddings.

Starchy fruits Two of the foods in this group are actually fruit, i.e. green banana or plantain and breadfruit (Fig. 3). Bananas used for cooking have a higher starch and lower sugar content than those used for dessert. They are picked and used when their flesh is too hard to eat. Some would sweeten if left to ripen, but some would not. Cooking bananas are sometimes called plantains, but this is confusing since eating bananas are called plantains in some countries. Breadfruit is normally eaten roasted and forms the main part of the diet of the Pacific Islands.

Summary

- The foods in this group are the plant foods which contain significant amounts of starch.

Questions

1. What do all the foods in this group have in common?
2. Why must strong flour be used when making bread?
3. Name one use of the following grains: (a) oats, (b) barley, (c) rye, (d) maize.
4. Give five examples of starchy vegetables and say how they are used in the diet.

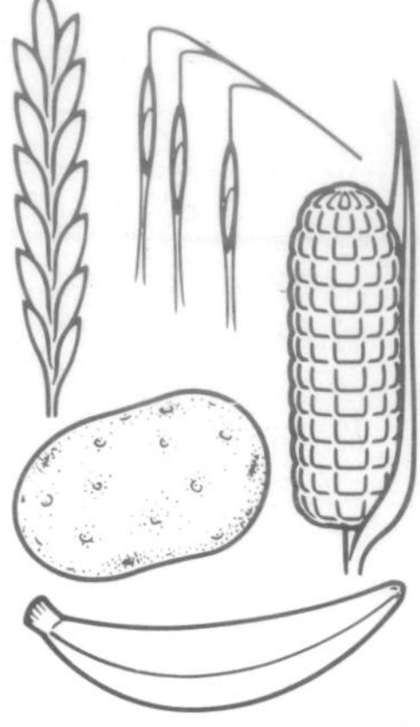

B *The place of cereal foods and starchy vegetables in the diet*

A balanced diet contains plenty of cereal foods and starchy vegetables. They are most important for the **dietary fibre** they give us. They are also our main source of **starch** (see page 76). Cereals are also an important source of **protein** especially for vegetarians and people who eat only a small amount of food of animal origin. Try to eat some kind of bread, potatoes, or other starchy vegetable, rice or other cereal, pasta, or breakfast cereals with a meal or snack at least three times a day. The best sources of dietary fibre are the whole grain cereal foods such as wholemeal bread, brown rice, wholewheat pasta and dishes made with wholemeal flour. These can include shortcrust pastry for flans and pies, scones and dumplings. Eating the skins of starchy vegetables, such as potatoes and sweet potatoes, also helps to increase dietary fibre. Try to eat these high fibre foods rather than their more refined equivalents – white flour, white rice, white bread and instant potato. If you do your own cooking you can combine whole grain cereals with refined cereal foods in a way that still provides enough dietary fibre. It also allows for a greater variety of textures and flavours.

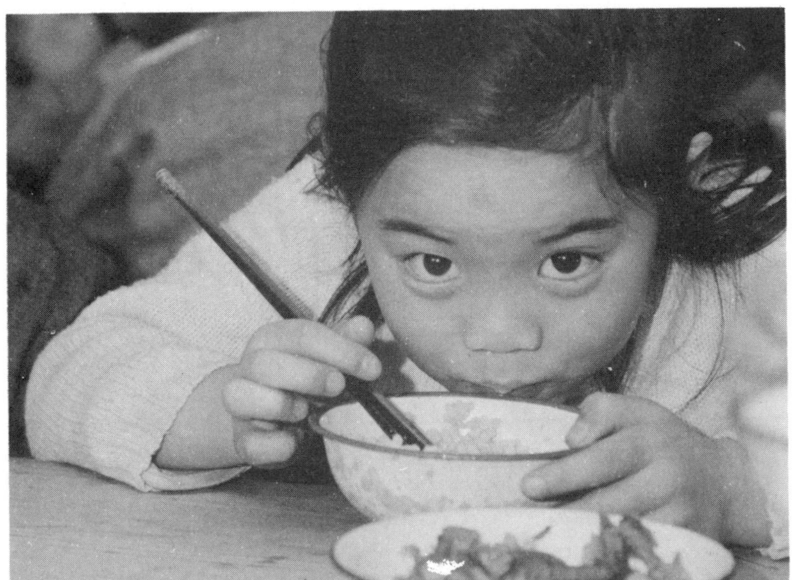

Fig. 1 Rice is a staple food for Chinese people

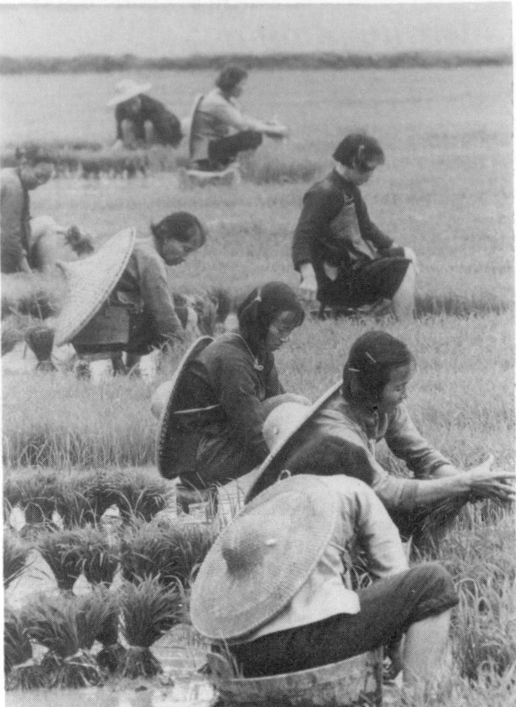

Fig. 2 Rice growing in China

Cereal foods and starchy vegetables are often known as **staple foods**. They are usually the cheapest and most readily available sources of dietary energy. They form the basis and main bulk of a balanced diet. Staple foods like potatoes, rice, pasta, maize or cassava are often boiled and served as the main part of the meal (Fig. 1). Taste and palatability are added by smaller amounts of fruit, vegetables, meat or pulses, often in a sauce.

In societies where transport systems are poor and cultural diversity is limited, there are usually only one or two staple foods. This depends on what cereal foods or starchy vegetables grow best in that particular climate and soil (Fig. 2).

In the UK where transport systems are well developed and the society is culturally very mixed, it is possible to find a wide variety of staple foods (Fig. 3). Those eaten mostly by the indigenous population are bread (based on wheat) and potatoes. Other traditional staple foods now often available in the UK include rice, pasta, cornmeal and starchy vegetables, such as yam, cassava and sweet potatoes.

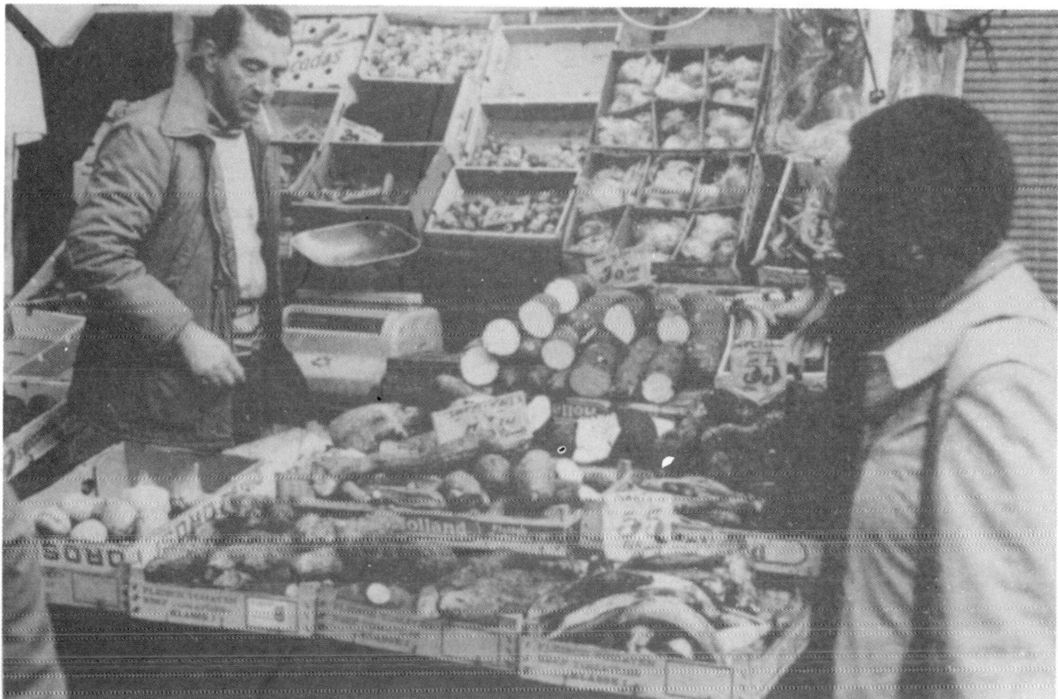

Fig. 3 Many staple foods are available in the UK

Refining of cereal foods

Cereal foods and starchy vegetables are very important sources of dietary fibre, However, cereal foods are often **processed** and **refined** and much of the dietary fibre is removed. For a balanced diet it is important to include some of the less refined cereal foods which are higher in dietary fibre.

Over the past 20 years there has been a rapid increase in processed cereal foods such as breakfast cereals, instant pasta and rice meals. The amount of cereal foods and starchy vegetables eaten often depends on the amount of money available for food within the household. Bread and potatoes are consumed in greater quantities in households with low incomes. However, in households with high incomes wholemeal bread is often chosen in preference to white bread. Wholemeal bread can be as much as ten pence a loaf more expensive than white bread.

Current guidelines suggest that most people should try to eat more cereal foods and starchy vegetables than they have in the past and that they try and eat particularly those high in dietary fibre.

Summary

- A healthy diet contains plenty of cereal foods and starchy vegetables, especially those high in dietary fibre.
- The most commonly eaten cereal foods and starchy vegetables in the UK are potatoes, bread, rice and pasta.
- People with low incomes eat more of these foods than those on higher incomes.
- Whole grain cereal foods are often more expensive than their white refined equivalents.

Questions

1. Explain how cereal foods and starchy vegetables make an important contribution to the diet.
2. How could you use foods from this group to increase the amount of dietary fibre in your diet?
3. What is meant by 'staple' foods? Describe any two staples and say how they are used in traditional diets.

2.3 Fruit and vegetables (food group 2)

A Identifying fruit and vegetables

All fruit and vegetables are parts of plants. They are very important for good health because of the **dietary fibre** and **vitamins** they contain. Different types of fruit and vegetables contain different nutrients in differing amounts. It is therefore very important to eat a variety. In the UK many people do not eat enough fruit and vegetables, even though there is a wide variety available. It is possible to get many fruit and vegetables at all times of the year. Most of the vegetables eaten in the UK are grown here. Less than 10% are imported. Only one third of fresh fruit eaten here is grown here.

A **fruit** is the ripened ovary of the flower which enclosed the seeds (Fig. 1). Therefore tomato, cucumber, chilli, marrow and drumstick are fruits (whereas rhubarb is not since it is a stem). The term fruit when used in cooking and eating is less precise than this biological definition and would not include foods like tomatoes, marrows or cucumbers. These are called vegetables or salad vegetables. Most fruits have a sweet flavour and are generally eaten on their own. They are relatively cheap, easily available snack foods.

A **vegetable** may be one of several parts of the plant or indeed a whole plant. Edible fungi are also used as vegetables. The vegetables we eat in the UK may either be leaves, stems, roots, buds, flowers or fruits.

Fruits

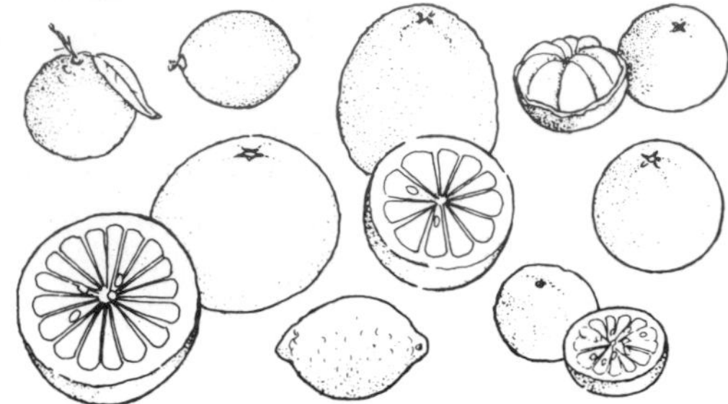

Fig. 2 Citrus fruits

Citrus fruits (clementines, grapefruits, lemons, limes, oranges, satsumas, tangerines, ugli fruit) do not grow in the UK and are imported from a number of different countries. Oranges, lemons and grapefruit are usually available all year round while satsumas, clementines and tangerines tend to be available only in the winter months (Fig. 2).

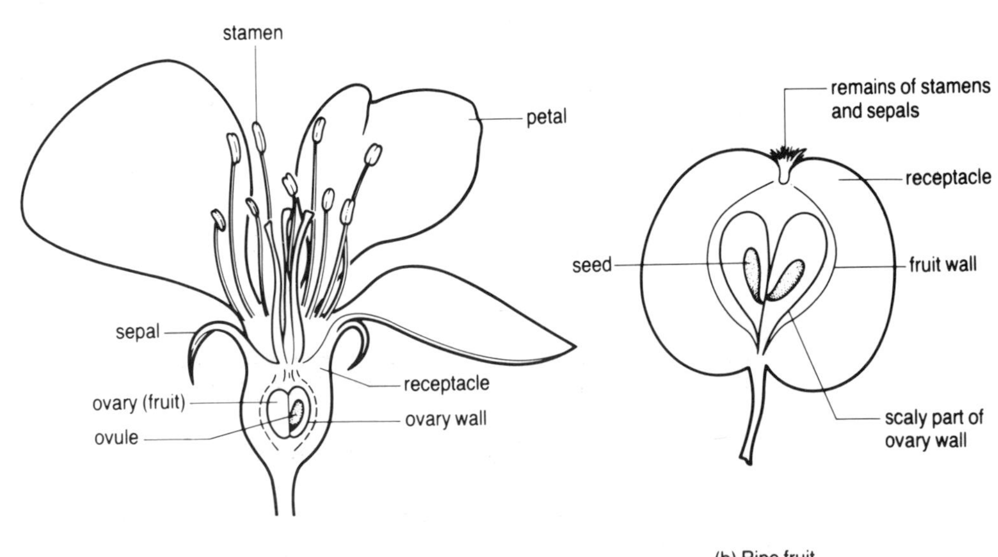

Fig. 1 The formation of an apple

Berries and **soft fruits** (blackberries, blackcurrants, gooseberries, grapes, loganberries, raspberries, redcurrants, strawberries) all grow in the UK, although grapes are harder to cultivate as they need extended periods of sunshine. Surprisingly though, they are the only fruits of this kind which are found fresh all year round in UK shops. They are imported from other countries. The other berries and soft fruits do not keep for long and have, traditionally, been preserved in the form of jam. They are seasonal and widely available only in the summer months.

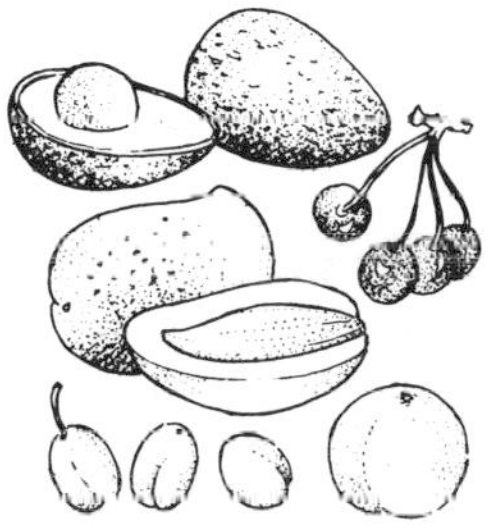

Fig. 3 Stone fruits

Stone fruits (ackees, apricots, avocado pears, cherries, damsons, dates, mangoes, nectarines, peaches, plums) are generally imported into the UK and, with the exception of ackees, mangoes and avocado pears, are not usually available all year round (Fig. 3).

Dried fruits – apples, apricots, currants, figs, peaches, pears, prunes (plums), raisins, sultanas (grapes) – are used in cooking or as snacks. Drying is a method of preserving them.

Other fruits vary in their origin and nature (apples, bananas, kiwi fruit, melon, pears, persimmon, pineapple, pomegranate, rhubarb).

Vegetables

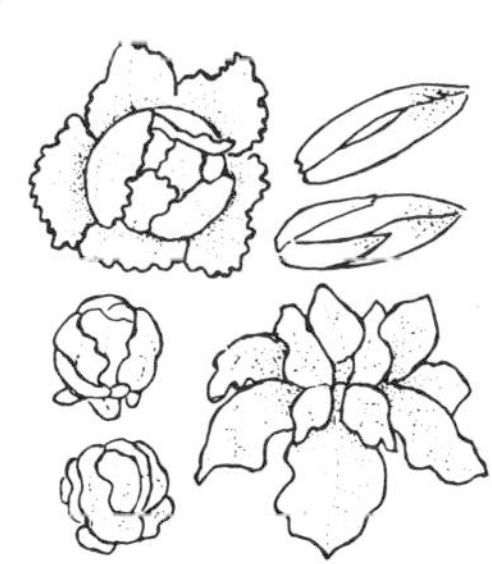

Fig. 4 Leafy vegetables

Leafy vegetables (cabbage, chicory, endive, kale, lettuce, spinach, watercress) grow above the ground and are the leaf structure of the plant (Fig. 4).

Stems (asparagus, celery, rhubarb, leeks) are generally eaten cooked. Celery can be eaten either raw or cooked.

Roots (beetroot, carrots, mooli, parsnips, radishes, salsify, swede, turnips) grow under the ground. They are not high in starch like tubers and are therefore included in this food group.

Flowers (broccoli, calabrese, cauliflowers) are generally eaten cooked, although cauliflower is sometimes eaten raw in salads and in dips (Fig. 5).

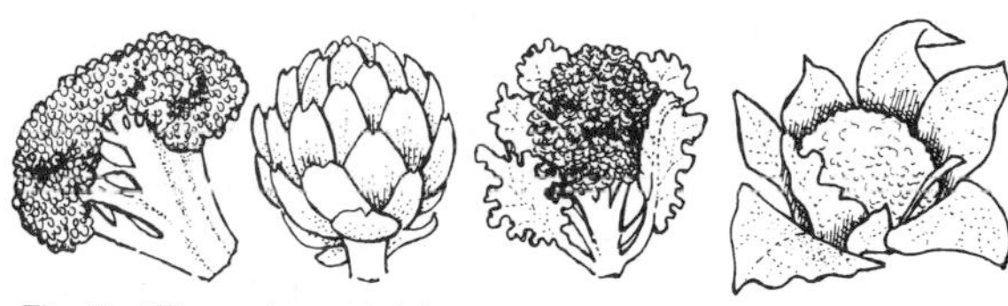

Fig. 5 'Flower' vegetables

Fruits (aubergines, courgettes, cucumbers, marrows, peppers, pumpkins, tomatoes, drumstick) are usually cooked before eating. Some grow in the UK but others are imported. Most of them are available all year round but prices vary according to the season and whether or not they are imported (Fig. 6).

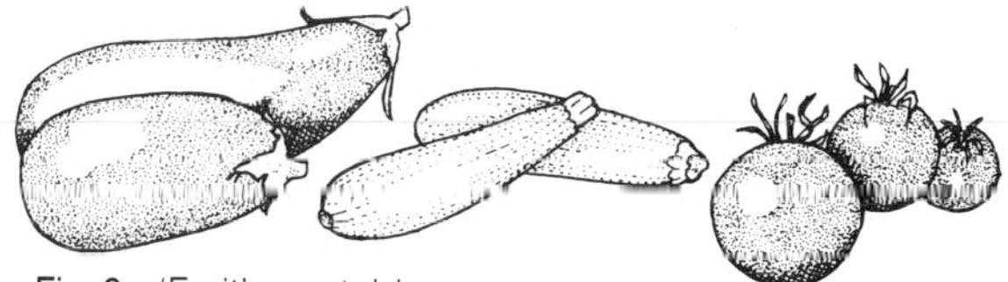

Fig. 6 'Fruit' vegetables

Bulbs (onions and shallots) grow at the surface of the ground and form the bulb of the plant, which is a 'condensed' stem with leaves. They are generally eaten cooked although they can be eaten raw. Both onions and shallots grow readily in the UK.

Summary

- The foods in this group are all from plants.
- They grow seasonally, but technological advances make these foods available all year round in most parts of the UK.

Questions

1. The term 'fruit' can mean different things to a biologist and a cook. Explain how each would use the word and give some examples.
2. In the UK many fruits have a short season. How are they made available all the year round?
3. Which fruits and vegetables could you use to make (a) a summer salad, (b) a winter salad?

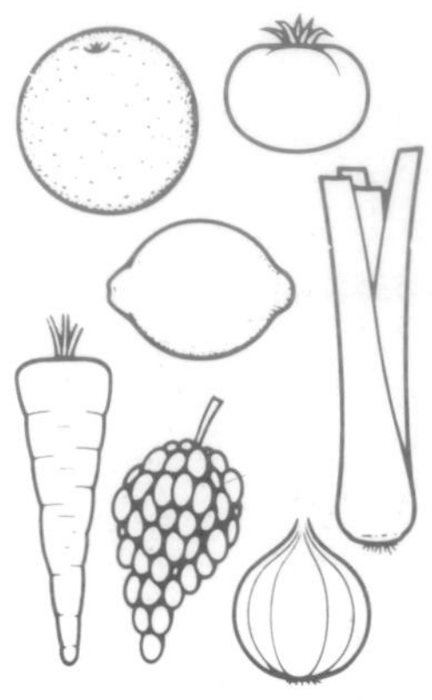

B The place of fruit and vegetables in the diet

It is important to eat at least three portions of vegetables or fruit a day. They provide many vitamins, especially **vitamin C**, and **minerals**, as well as important **dietary fibre**. Most people do not eat enough. Most fruit and some vegetables are eaten uncooked. Preparation and cooking destroys some of the vitamins so great care must be taken. Try to eat some sort of fresh fruit or salad vegetables at least once a day (Fig. 1).

There is no recommended daily intake for fruit and vegetables but the diet should provide at least 30 mg of vitamin C a day. For some people levels of 60 mg a day are advised. These include pregnant women and women who are breastfeeding. The quantity of fruit and vegetables required to supply these amounts of vitamin C depends on the combination eaten.

Fruit and vegetables can be very expensive and on the whole people with high incomes eat more of them than people with low incomes. People living in households with children seem to eat less fruit and vegetables than those who do not have children.

Fruit in particular can be a very convenient, readily available snack food. The price of fruit when compared with other snack foods such as chocolate and crisps is not so great.

Vitamin supplementation

If you are eating a balanced diet, including plenty of fruit and vegetables, there is no need for **vitamin supplements**. Vitamin C tablets may make someone suffering from a cold feel better. However, there is little evidence to show that large doses of vitamin C taken on a regular basis actually protect against colds and flu. When body tissues are saturated with vitamin C any extra is excreted in the urine.

There are some groups of people who may be at risk of having low levels of vitamin C in their blood. This might be because of low intake or because of increased requirement. Low intake is

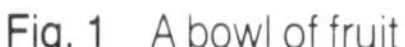

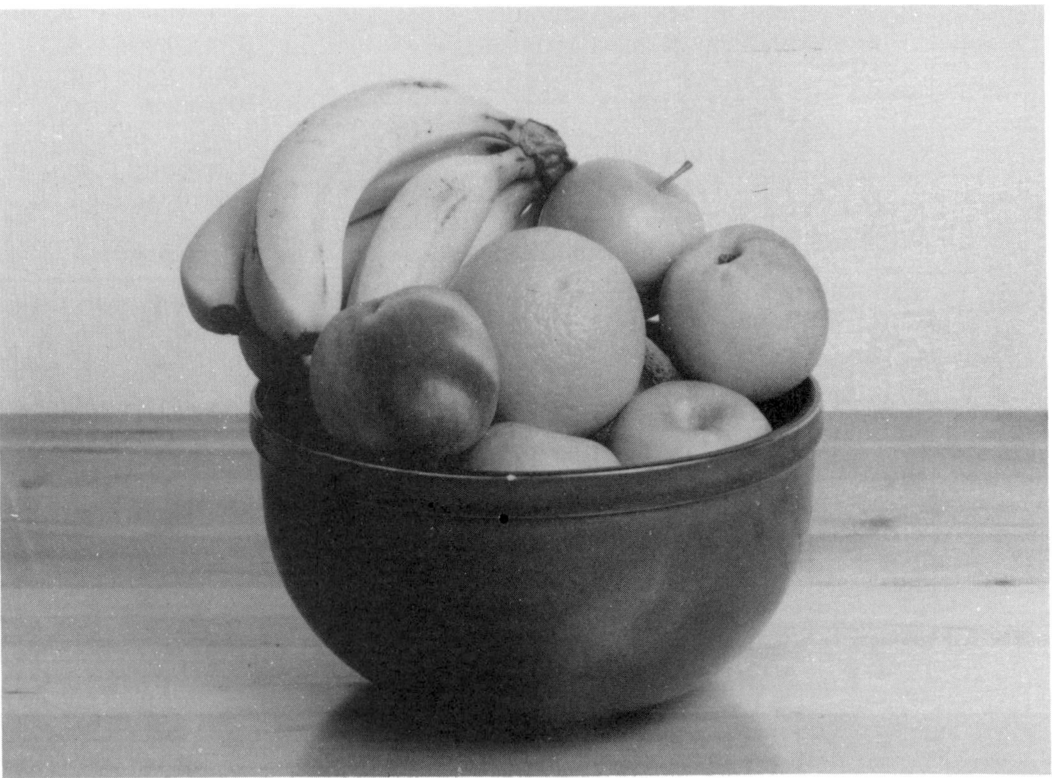

Fig. 1 A bowl of fruit

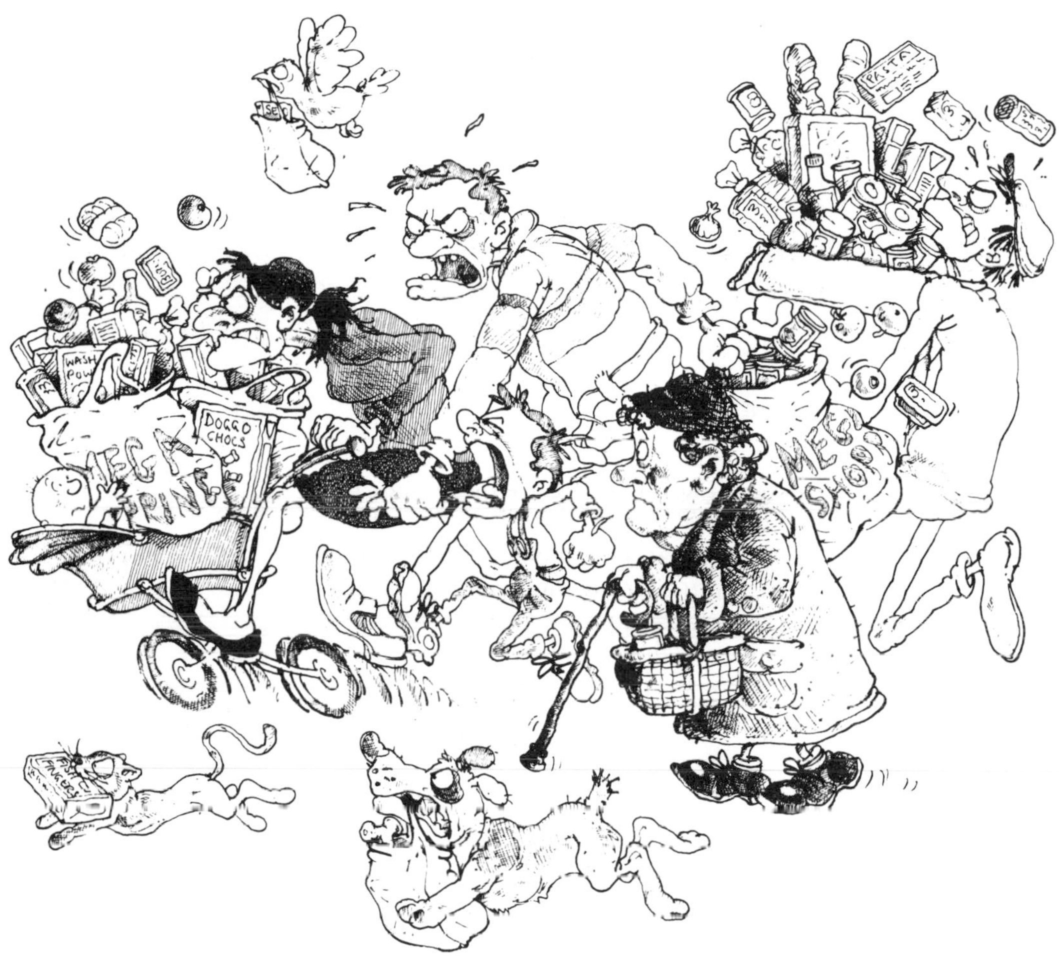

Fig. 2 Elderly people can have difficulty shopping

often found among elderly people who have difficulty buying and eating fruit and vegetables (Fig. 2). Increased requirements are found amongst smokers, alcoholics, drug addicts and women taking the contraceptive pill. Some of these people may need extra vitamin C. If so, it should be prescribed by the doctor.

Summary

- A healthy balanced diet contains plenty of fruit and vegetables.
- The amount and types of foods eaten in this group differ widely between individuals.
- Fruit and vegetables can be expensive compared to some other foods.
- People with low incomes tend to eat much less of these foods than people with high incomes.

Questions

1. Why is it important to eat plenty of fruit and vegetables?
2. What is the RDA for vitamin C for (a) teenagers, (b) pregnant women?
3. Which groups of the population might have a need for larger amounts of vitamin C?
4. Why do some people take 'megadoses' of vitamin C? What happens to excess vitamin C when our body tissues are saturated?

2.4 Meat and alternatives (food group 3)

A Identifying meat and alternatives

There is a wide variety of foods in this group. Some of them come from animals and some from plants. Some of them are eaten fresh with very little processing and some are eaten highly processed.

Meat

Meat is the flesh of animals which are eaten (Fig. 1). There are more than 100 different types of animal which are regularly eaten by human beings. In the UK there are only three mammals that are eaten commonly as food. These are cattle, which provide **beef**, pigs, from which we get **pork** and **bacon**, and sheep, from which we get **lamb** and **mutton**. Goat and rabbit meat is sometimes eaten, but it is less common.

Meat products

Much of the meat we eat is in the form of manufactured meat products. These include such foods as beefburgers, sausages, tinned meat, pies and meat pasties. These products are usually high in fat, but the fat is not visible. Meat products generally include parts of the animal which would not otherwise be used, e.g. gristle and excess fat. They also often contain polyphosphates which are used to bind water in the product. Colours, flavours and preservatives are added so that poor quality parts of the animal are made edible and saleable.

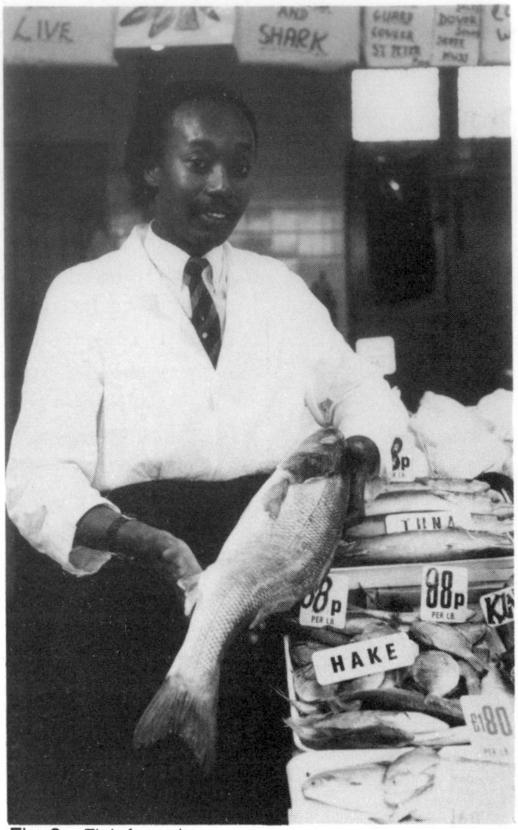

Fig. 1 Meat for sale at a butcher's

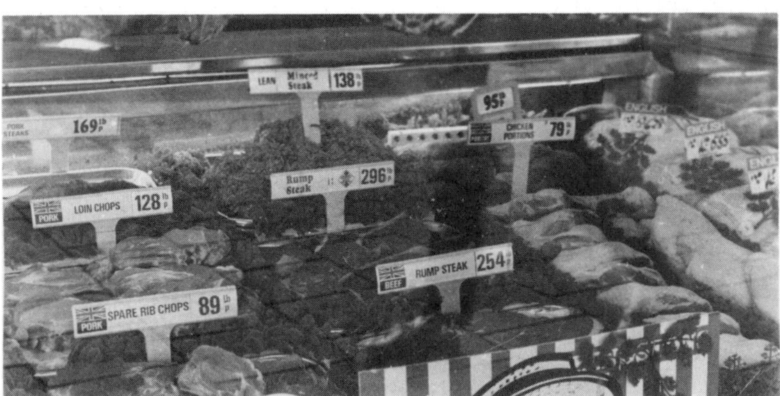

Fig. 2 Fish for sale

Offal

Offal is the name given to the internal organs of an animal. This includes the liver, the heart, the kidneys, the tongue, the sweetbreads, the tripe, the feet, the brains and, in some cases, the heads. The nutrient content of different offal foods varies considerably.

Poultry

The most commonly eaten type of poultry in the UK is chicken. Nowadays, however, turkey is becoming increasingly available. Most of the flesh of these animals is edible. Poultry meat is sometimes used to make low-fat meat products such as sausages and burgers.

Fish

There are two main types of fish. White fish (cod, haddock, sole, etc.) and oily fish (herrings, mackerel, sprats, sardines, etc.). The nutrient qualities of these fish vary. Fish may be bought fresh (Fig. 2), frozen or canned. It can also be found dried and salted and smoked.

Eggs

The most commonly eaten eggs in the UK are hens' eggs. These are usually produced in batteries where large numbers of hens are kept in small cages to lay eggs as often as possible (Fig. 3).

Very occasionally duck eggs may be found. Fish eggs, i.e. roes, are also eaten by some people.

It is now possible to buy free-range eggs although these tend to be more expensive than those produced in batteries. The hens which produce free-range eggs have been kept in barns or yards and not in batteries.

Pulses

Pulses are the seeds of leguminous plants. They include a wide variety of beans and peas such as red kidney beans, soya beans, chick peas, butter beans, pigeon peas, split peas and many more. The pulses most commonly eaten in the UK are canned baked beans, which are made from haricot or navy beans. However, many people from British black and ethnic minority groups regularly eat a variety of different pulses. Pulses are usually bought dried and need to be soaked before they are cooked.

Fig. 3 Battery hens

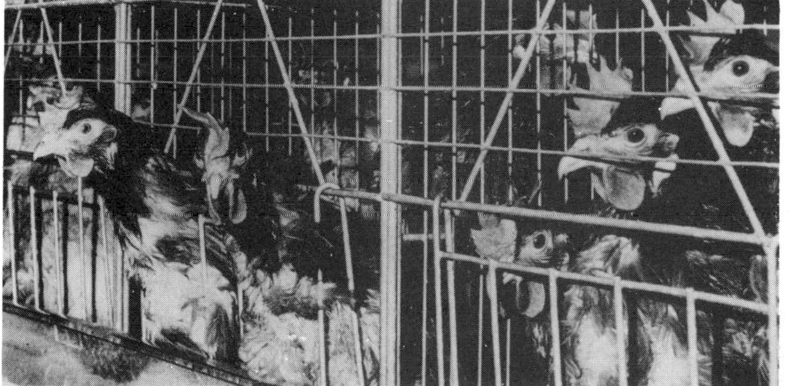

Nuts

There are a variety of nuts available in the UK. They do not form an important part of the diet for most people.

All these foods are classified in the same group because they are all useful sources of protein. They also play a similar role in a balanced diet. Small amounts of these foods are eaten accompanied by larger amounts of vegetables or fruit and cereal foods or starchy vegetables. Cheese may also be used in this way. The nutrient composition of these foods varies widely, so it is important to choose a variety of these foods and not stick to only one.

The consumption of these foods is often affected by social, cultural and religious factors. For example, Muslims, Jews, Rastafarians or Seventh Day Adventists will never eat pork or pig meat. Hindus and Sikhs do not eat beef, and many eat no meat at all. Vegetarians eat none of the animal foods from this group.

Summary

- There are a wide variety of foods in this group – some from animals and some from plants.
- Variety and careful choice is important to get all the nutrients required and to avoid eating too much fat from these foods.
- It is possible to have a balanced diet without eating any animal foods.
- Consumption of the foods in this group is often governed by social, cultural and religious factors.

Questions

1. Which animals are bred for meat production in the UK?
2. What is meant by 'meat products'? What do they usually contain other than meat?
3. What are pulses? Name any six pulses available in your local shops.

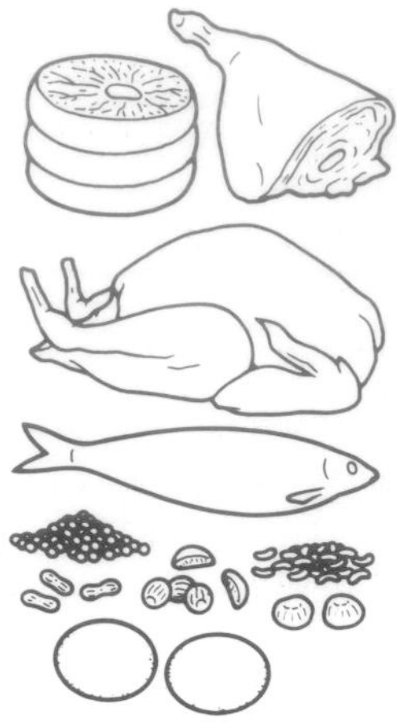

B The place of meat and alternatives in the diet

Although meat is a very useful food it is not absolutely necessary. Fish, pulses (peas, beans and lentils), eggs and nuts are all useful alternatives. Fish and pulses are especially good. They both provide protein and have the advantage of being low in saturated fats. Pulses are also high in dietary fibre. All foods in this group are good sources of **protein**, as well as other vitamins and minerals. Many are valuable sources of **iron**.

There are wide individual variations in the consumption of foods from this group. There are variations both in the amount and in the types of food eaten. Over recent years fresh meat consumption in the UK has been decreasing. At the same time the consumption of poultry has increased dramatically. Fish, eggs, nuts and pulses are all eaten in much smaller quantities. Pulses, apart from baked beans, have not traditionally been used as the main protein food in this country (Fig. 1). However, they are now increasingly eaten in their own right and included in other dishes. They often form a major protein source in the traditional diet of people who come from countries where meat is less available.

Fig. 1 Different pulses

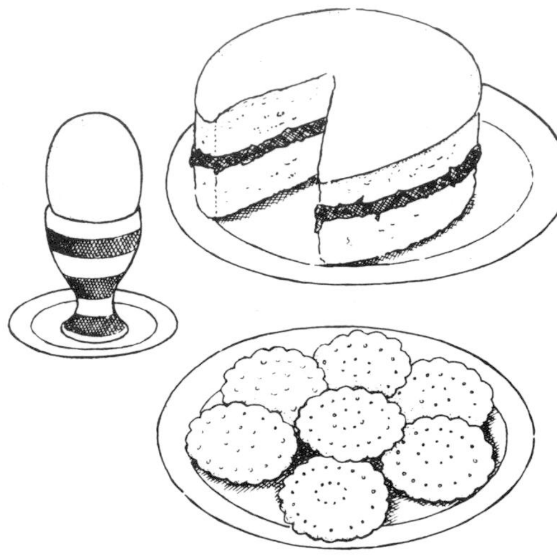

Fig. 2 Eggs are used in many different ways

The average weekly egg consumption is about four eggs per person (Fig. 2). Once again there is very wide variation in this. There has recently been a drop in the consumption of fresh eggs, and more eggs are used in manufactured foods such as cakes and biscuits.

Very careful choice is needed when choosing the foods from this group. Some meat and meat products, for example breast of lamb, minced beef, sausages, pies and tinned meat, can be very high in fat, especially saturated fat, so great care should be taken when choosing, preparing and cooking them (Fig. 3). Care should be taken to cut off as much visible fat as possible. Some cooking methods, for example frying, can actually add extra fat. Others, for example grilling, can help reduce the fat content. Saturated fat is thought to be connected

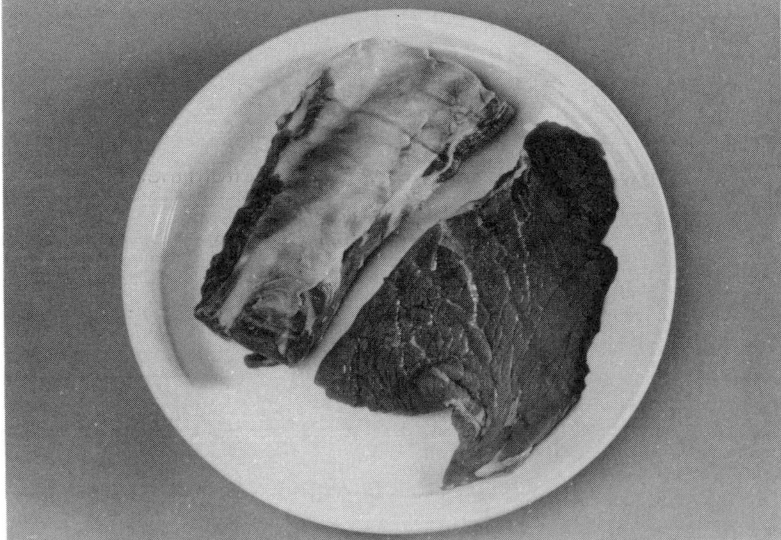

Fig. 3 Lean and fatty meat

with the high incidence of **heart disease** in this country. By replacing some of the meat and meat products we normally eat by smaller amounts of lean meat, and pulses, fish and nuts, we will be not only decreasing the saturated fat in our diet but also increasing the polyunsaturated fat, essential fatty acids and dietary fibre.

Food manufacturing processes have affected the foods in this group considerably. Intensive farming methods have meant that meat and poultry have become much more readily available and cheaper. Freezing and packaging have also led to marketing changes. The market for prepared dishes, frozen, dried or vacuum packed, is a small proportion of total meat consumption but is rapidly growing (Fig. 4).

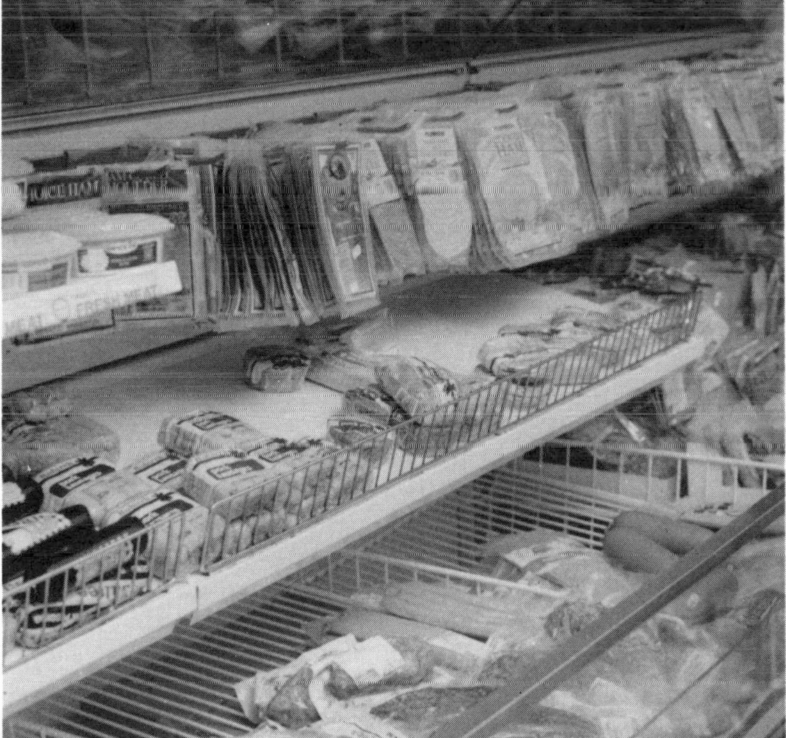

Fig. 4 The market for pre-prepared dishes is growing

Many people, especially women, have to go to work as well as provide meals for their families. For them these convenient, ready prepared foods are very useful. Unfortunately they are usually very expensive or else high in fat and salt.

The type of meat from each animal varies depending on what part of the animal it comes from. Meat which comes from a part of the animal which does not get much exercise is very lean and tender. Meat from parts of the animals that do all the work tends to be much tougher. The nutrient and fat composition of different types of meat vary according to the type of animal and the way in which it is butchered. Generally, the tougher or fattier cuts of meat are cheaper than the leaner, more tender cuts. In the past, meat has been graded according to its fat content. Subsidies and prices have been based on similar criteria. Farmers have got more money for fatty animals than lean ones. This has encouraged the production of fatty meat. Fish and pulses can be very useful alternatives which don't necessarily cost more.

Summary

- A healthy balanced diet includes a variety of foods such as lean meat, fish, pulses, eggs and nuts.
- There is a wide variation in individual intakes of foods from this group.
- As people become richer they tend to eat more of the animal foods in this group.
- Fatty meats and meat products are cheaper than the leaner ones.
- Eating fish and pulses in place of some of the fatty meats and meat products eaten will help to provide a more balanced diet.

Questions

1. What makes fish or pulses healthy alternatives to meat?
2. Some 50 years ago chicken was not eaten often other than at Christmas time, or for other celebrations. Now it is a commonly eaten meat. What do you think might have brought about this change?
3. Why might people on restricted incomes eat fattier, tougher cuts of meat than those with more to spend?

2.5 Milk and milk products (food group 4)

Identifying milk and milk products

Milk and milk products are relatively cheap and nutritious foods which are easily available and convenient to use. However, milk is not essential and some people never consume it. The relative importance of milk in the diet depends on the age and development of the individual. For the first few months of life, all a baby needs is milk. The best milk for a baby is human milk (Fig. 1). For women who do not breastfeed, feeds made from specially modified cows' milk are available.

Milk The most commonly used milk in this country comes from **cows** (Fig. 2). There are strict rules and regulations governing the treatment to ensure its purity. Small amounts of goats' milk and sheep's milk are available, but these are not commonly used. Goats' and sheep's milk are not subject to such strict regulations as cows' milk.

Cows' milk is available in a number of different forms. In liquid form it is available as **whole milk** which contains all the fat, as **semi-skimmed milk** which has had half the fat removed and as **skimmed milk** which has had all of the fat removed. Milk is also dried to produce **powdered milk.** This may either be skimmed or contain fat. Sometimes the milk fat is removed and this is replaced with vegetable fat. Milk can also be **evaporated** or **condensed** and stored in cans. Condensed milk usually has sugar added to it.

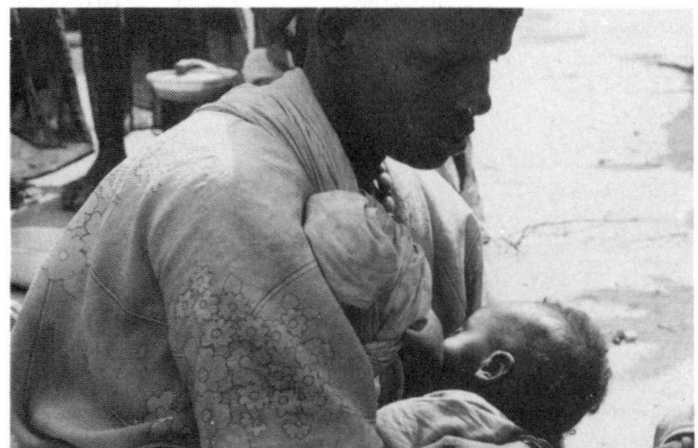
Fig. 1 Breastfeeding a baby

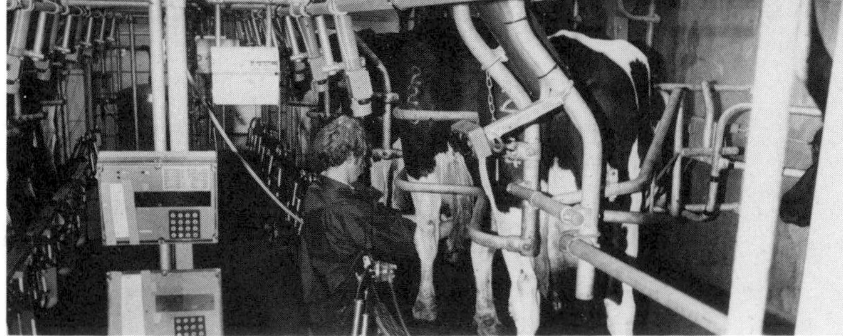
Fig. 2 Cows provide most of our milk

Cheese Cheese is made from milk. It forms when milk proteins **coagulate** to form a **curd**. This curd is then heated in a variety of ways to make cheese of different kinds. Some cheeses are soft and contain a significant amount of water. Others are hard and contain very little water. Hard cheeses include Cheddar, Double Gloucester, Leicester and Wensleydale. Soft cheeses include cottage cheese and cream cheese. There are also medium cheeses, such as Camembert and Brie. The fat content of cheese also depends on the fat content of the milk used to make that cheese. On the whole, hard cheeses tend to be high in fat although, increasingly, reduced fat varieties are becoming available.

Yoghurt is also made from milk. The milk is heated to between 88° and 100° Celsius and is then cooled to between 41° and 45° Celsius. A specially prepared culture of bacteria is then added and this turns the milk into yoghurt. The fat content of yoghurt depends on the fat content of the original milk.

Cream and butter are also milk products but are not included in this group as they consist mainly of fat. They are produced by removing the fat from milk and then eating it as cream or concentrating it even more to form butter.

Plant milk The most common type of plant milk drunk in the UK is **soya milk**. This is produced by boiling soya beans in water and then straining the soya milk that is produced. It is a useful food but is not as nutritionally rich as animal milk. It is often used by people who are allergic to animal milk or vegans who choose not to drink animal milks.

However, soya milk should not be given to young babies unless a special formula is prescribed. Soya milk can be converted into a soft cheese-like substance called **tofu**. This is widely eaten in the Far East.

Milk and milk products in the diet

Milk, cheese and yoghurt are all useful foods. This is especially so for young and growing children, women who are pregnant or breastfeeding and elderly people with small appetites. These foods are relatively cheap and have many uses in cooking. They are especially good sources of protein and riboflavin, and of the minerals calcium and phosphorus. Calcium and phosphorus are needed to build and maintain healthy strong bones.

However milk, cheese and yoghurt can also provide a relatively large amount of saturated fat. Skimmed or semi-skimmed milk and low fat cheese contain less fat but are still valuable for the other nutrients they contain. Reduced fat milks are not suitable for babies and may not be suitable for some young children.

To make sure you're eating a healthy balanced diet try to have either some meat, fish, pulses or eggs, or some milk, cheese or yoghurt at meals or as snacks three times a day. Vary your choice as much as possible.

The average intake of fresh whole milk in the UK is approximately 2 litres per person per week. This varies little according to family size or between different income groups. Cheese intakes vary more widely ranging from 171 g to less than 45 g per person per week.

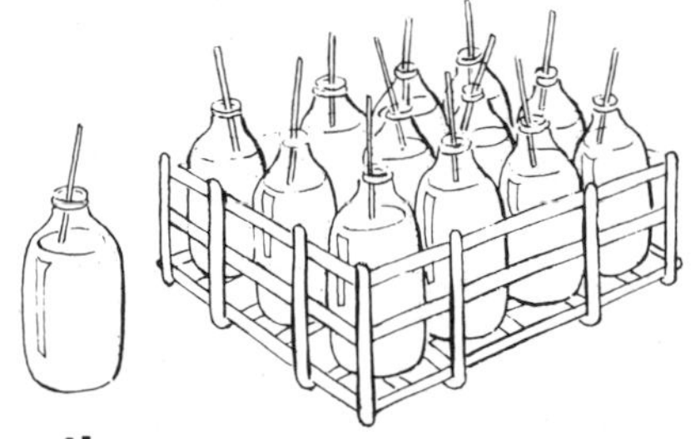

Fig. 3 A crate of milk for a school

Milk consumption in the UK has been stable for many years. Doorstep delivery service is important in maintaining this level. The forms of animal milk available include flavoured milk, milk powders and canned milk. Cows' milk is also available with different fat levels.

Milk, cheese and yoghurt can be useful alternatives to meat and its other alternatives and form an important part of a meal or snack. They are particularly useful for people who are vegetarian.

Milk is the only food which some people receive free of charge. It is available to some people on low incomes or with young children, and is available to children in schools (Fig. 3). Milk is also subsidized by the Government as part of its agricultural policy. This helps to encourage people to maintain a high level of milk consumption.

Summary

- The foods in this group come mainly from animal milk.
- These foods are relatively cheap, accessible and convenient to use.
- A healthy balanced diet contains a variety of dairy produce.
- Milk, cheese and yoghurt can be used as an alternative to meat.
- Milk is the only food which some people receive free of charge.
- For infants, children, pregnant women and women who are breastfeeding, these foods are particularly important because of their high calcium content.
- Some of these foods are particularly high in saturated fats. Low and medium fat alternatives are available.
- Some people use plant milks instead of animal milks. They differ nutritionally.

Questions

1. What kinds of liquid milk are available? How do they differ?
2. What is yoghurt? How is it made?
3. Some kinds of milk are not suitable for babies. Why do you think this is so?
4. Why is it useful to use low fat alternatives to whole milk?
5. What is the effect of the EEC milk subsidy?

2.6 Sugar, sugary foods and drinks (food group 5)

A Identifying sugar, sugary foods and drinks

'Sugars' are the most simple form of carbohydrates. They may be di- or monosaccharides. The three sugars most commonly occurring in our food are **fructose** (a monosaccharide), and **sucrose** and **lactose** (disaccharides). Fructose is found in fruit and lactose in milk. Sucrose is not often consumed in its natural state. It occurs naturally in high concentrations in sugar beet and sugar cane. The sugar from these plants is **refined**. The dietary fibre and water are removed and pure sucrose is extracted. This white crystalline substance is what we know as sugar. It is the type of sugar we are most familiar with. The main use of sugar in the diet is as a sweetener, and it is the only one of the mono- and disaccharides which is consumed in relatively large quantities. It is also used as a preservative, e.g. in jam, and to alter the viscosity of liquids (for example in tomato ketchup) (Fig. 1). Glucose and maltose are produced in food manufacturing by the breakdown of starch molecules. They are used instead of sucrose in many products to provide a sweet flavour. They go under a number of different names which include maltodextrin, corn syrup, invert sugar and liquid glucose.

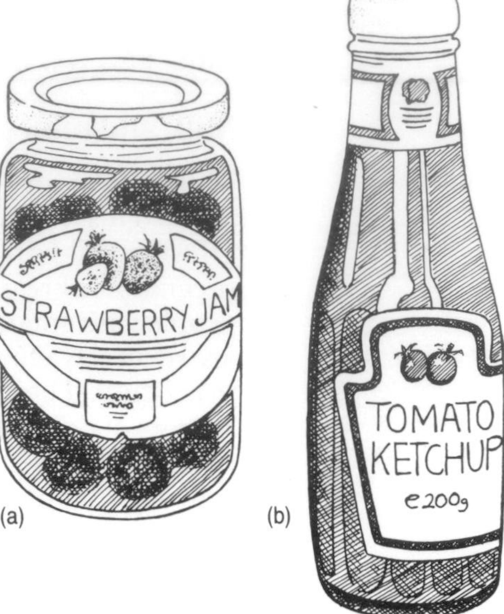

Fig. 1 Sugar used (a) as a preservative, (b) to alter viscosity

The foods in this group all contain appreciable quantities of refined sugars.

Sugar (sucrose) is available in many forms (Fig. 2). These include **raw cane sugar** such as Barbados Muscavado or molasses sugar, jaggery (raw sugar crystallized from coconut or palm sap), soft brown sugar (which is white sugar with added molasses), and demerara (large crystals used mainly in manufacturing). **White sugars** include granulated, caster, icing, cube sugar, coffee crystals and preserving sugar. Molasses and black treacle are produced from the liquid left after raw sugar has been crystallized out. They have a strong bitter taste and contain small amounts of calcium and iron.

Golden syrup is made from liquid white sugar and contains about 20% water.

Honey is about 75% fructose and glucose and contains traces of other minerals.

Biscuits and cakes often contain relatively large amounts of sugar. They also contain flour and some fat.

Fig. 2 Some of the many forms of sugar

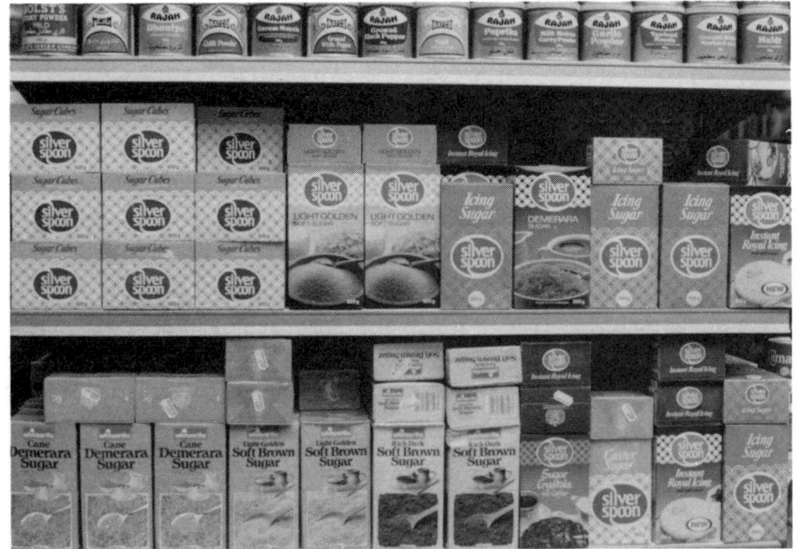

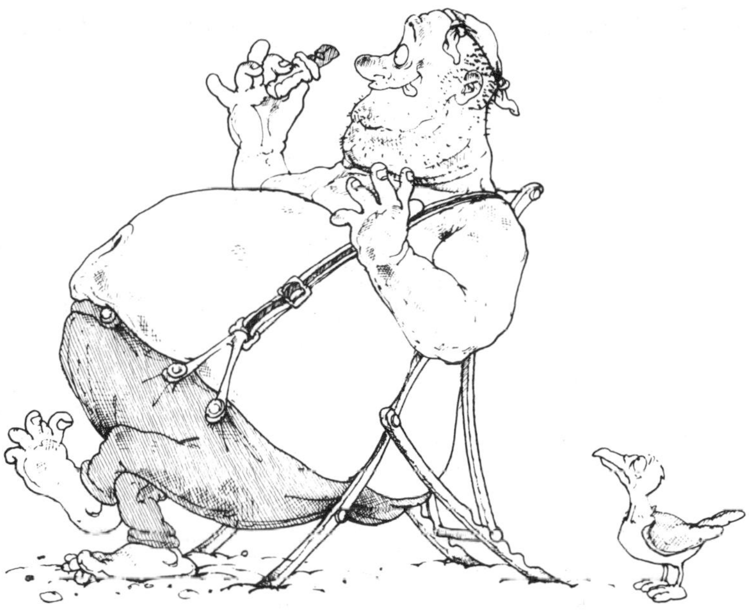

Fig. 3 Sweet foods may be associated with comfort in adult life

Sweets and confectionery One of the main ingredients of all sweets and confectionery is sugar. Glucose is also often used.

Sweets, desserts and jellies are made up largely of sugar. Sometimes modified starch and other chemicals are added.

Soft drinks mostly contain either sucrose or glucose.

Most people enjoy sugar because of its sweet taste. They acquire this taste in early childhood. Babies who are given a choice of food have no particular preference for either sweet or savoury foods. However, if they are frequently given sweet food they develop a taste for sugar. It is then hard to give up this taste. Sugar should not be added to food for children. Sweet foods are often used as rewards or withdrawn as forms of punishment. These associations may persist into adult life so that sweet foods become associated with comfort and solace (Fig. 3).

Sugary foods often play an important cultural role. They are often offered at festivals and parties as gifts or as a form of hospitality. They also play an important role as a form of currency for many young children. They are cheap and easily accessible and can be swapped with friends very easily.

Sugar and sugary foods do not have an important nutritional role. They tend to dilute the nutrient density of the diet and should only be eaten in small quantities. They also have a very damaging effect on teeth.

Summary

- All foods in this group contain significant amounts of refined simple sugars.
- The most commonly used simple sugar in the UK is sucrose. This is what everyone calls 'sugar'.
- These foods provide very little in the way of useful nutrients.
- These foods should only form a very small part of the diet.

Questions

1. What are the commonest kinds of sugar, and where do they occur naturally?
2. Make a list of the names under which sucrose is marketed.
3. What is (a) molasses, (b) honey?
4. Why is it important to limit your intake of foods from this group?

B The place of sugar, sugary foods and drinks in the diet

The NACNE committee recommended that by the year 2000 sugar intakes in the UK should be halved. Most people enjoy the taste of sugar but our bodies do not need it and it damages our teeth. Sugar is digested to form **glucose** which gives us energy, but it provides no other useful nutrients. Starchy foods, which contain other nutrients, are also digested to form glucose.

There is no need to avoid sugar completely. Just try to eat foods containing it only occasionally at meal times. Be careful not to eat sticky sweets or cakes or drink sugary drinks between meals. These are the worst things for your teeth.

Looking for alternative snack foods

Sweets and confectionery are readily available, relatively cheap snack foods. Manufacturers need to produce alternative snack foods which have lower sugar content and that are available at similar prices. The consumption of sugary foods and drinks between meals should be strictly limited. There is a variety of alternatives available (Fig. 1). These include fresh fruits, some dried fruits, nuts, breads and sandwiches, some fruit breads, scones and yoghurts. Milk, unsweetened fruit juice and mineral water make useful alternatives to sugary drinks.

Altering recipes and cooking methods

Cooking methods can be altered to reduce the sugar content of foods. Many traditional recipes still work when sugar is reduced by as much as a half. Dried fruits in small quantities can be used to sweeten breads, cakes and stewed fruit in place of sugar.

Alternative sweeteners

There are increasing numbers of sugar substitutes now available in the UK. These are used mostly in food manufacture and include **saccharine** and **aspartame** (Fig. 2).

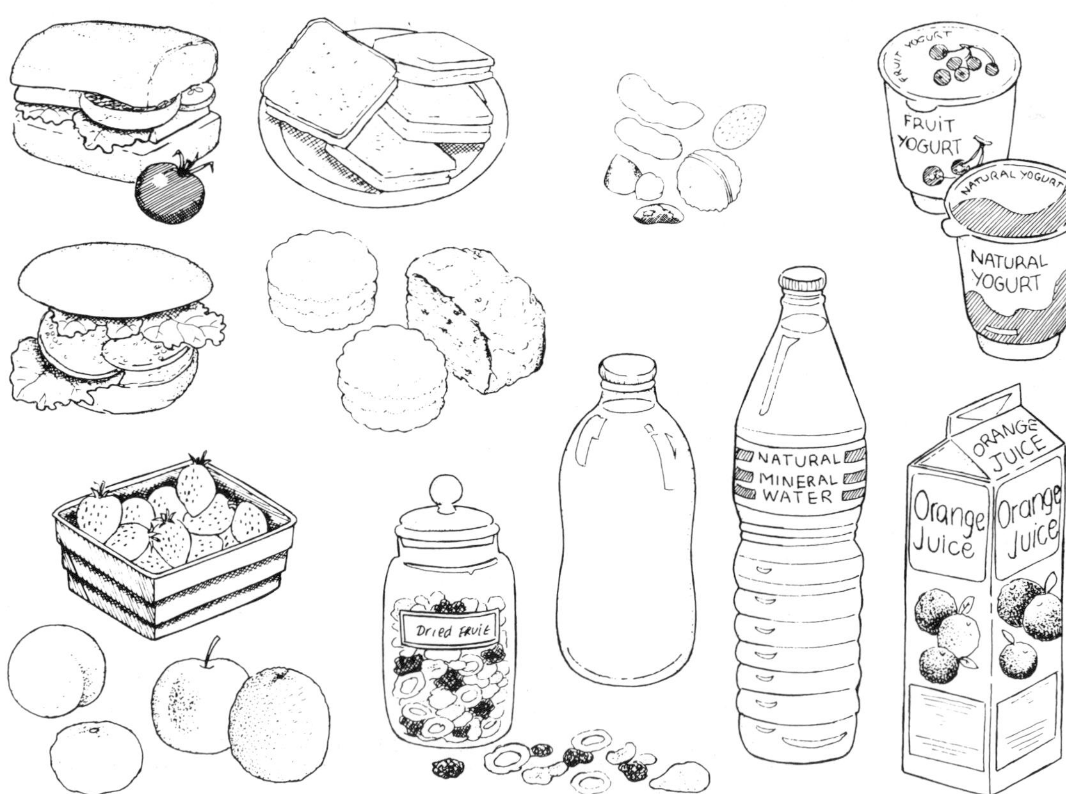

Fig. 1 Some of the alternatives to sugary foods and drinks

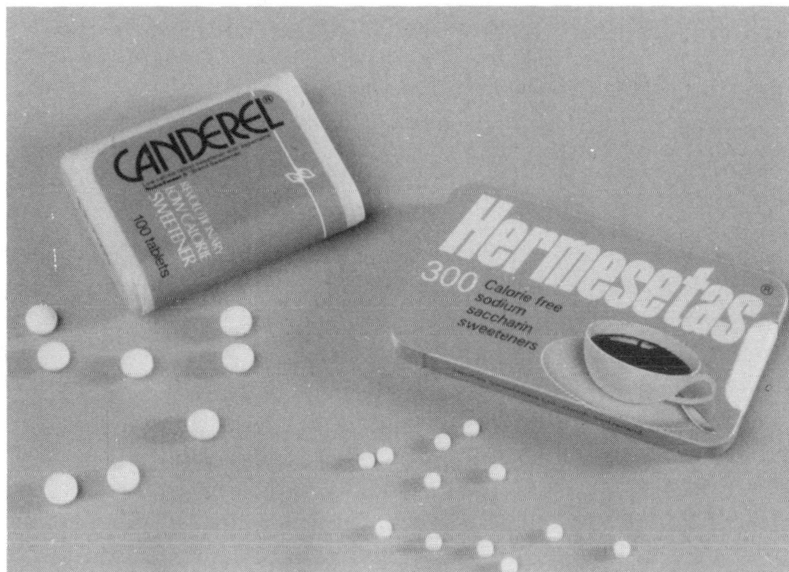

Fig. 2 Alternative sweeteners

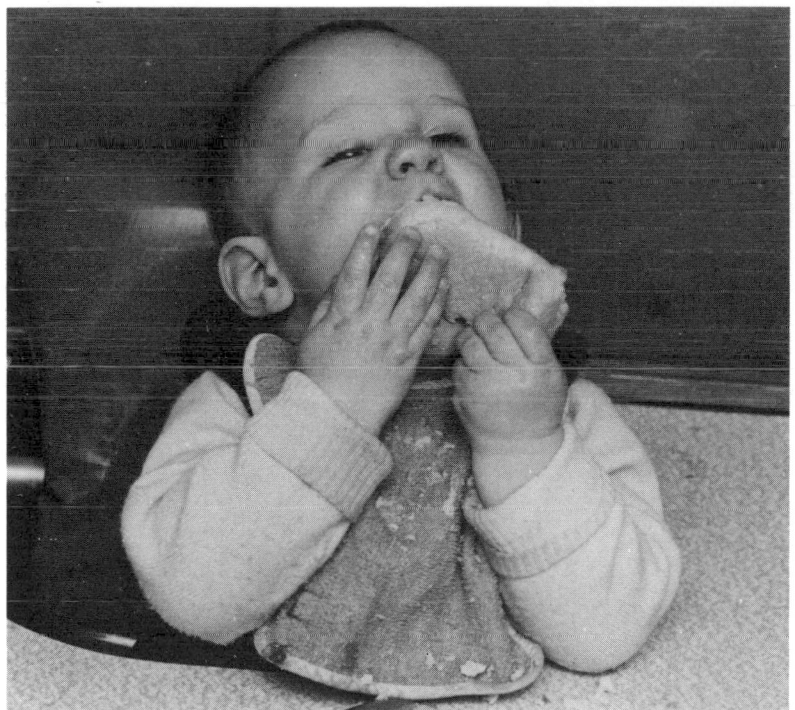

Fig. 3 This baby is enjoying a sugarless crust

Combating a sweet tooth

The best way to cut down sugar and sugary foods intake is to try to get rid of your 'sweet tooth'. The only way to do this is to cut down gradually on the amount of sugar and sugary foods that you use. By gradually cutting down it is hard to notice the difference. However, when you have cut down the amount of sugar you use and you suddenly taste a sweetened drink you will be very surprised at how sweet it tastes. Babies and young children should not be given sugar or sugary foods as this only helps them to develop a sweet tooth (Fig. 3). The use of these foods should be only occasional and as part of a normal diet.

Summary

- There are other foods available which are as good for snacks as sweets but are nutritionally more useful.
- Recipes can be adapted to use less sugar
- Alternative sweeteners are available.
- Children should be discouraged from developing a sweet tooth.

Questions

1. What snacks might be sold in a school tuck shop instead of sweet sticky things which are bad for the teeth?
2. How could you reduce the amount of sugar you consume?
3. Explain how sugar is reduced in cooking.
4. Why is it inadvisable to add sugar to babies' food?

2.7 Fats and oils (food group 6)

A Identifying fats and oils

Fats and oils are highly refined extracted foods. They may be of either plant or animal origin (Fig. 1). They are the major source of fat in most UK diets. Many other foods, including milk, cheese, meat and meat products, are also major sources of fat in the diet. They are not included in this group because they are not highly refined extracted foods.

Fats of plant origin come mainly from nuts and seeds, which contain relatively high proportions of fat. This fat is extracted and purified to make vegetable fats and oils used in cooking and food manufacture. Plant seeds used for producing oil include soya beans, safflower seeds, ground nuts, cotton seeds, rape seeds, coconuts, palm kernels, olives, sesame seeds, maize (corn) and sunflower seeds. Some of these oils are used to produce margarine and other solid fats.

Animal fats include cream, butter, lard, suet, dripping, fish and whale oils. Many processed foods contain these fats.

Sauces containing large amounts of fat, for example mayonnaise, salad cream and French dressing, are included in this group.

Fats and oils are used in cooking and food manufacture to alter the taste and texture of foods. They add variety and palatability to many people's diets. But the production of fat and oils is relatively expensive compared with other foods, for example cereal foods and starchy vegetables. In poor countries where there is not enough food, fat is usually one of the foods hardest to buy. For children whose appetites and stomachs may be too small to consume large amounts of low energy dense foods, fats can be very important. By adding small amounts of fat to the cereal foods and starchy vegetables, adequate dietary energy supplies can be provided.

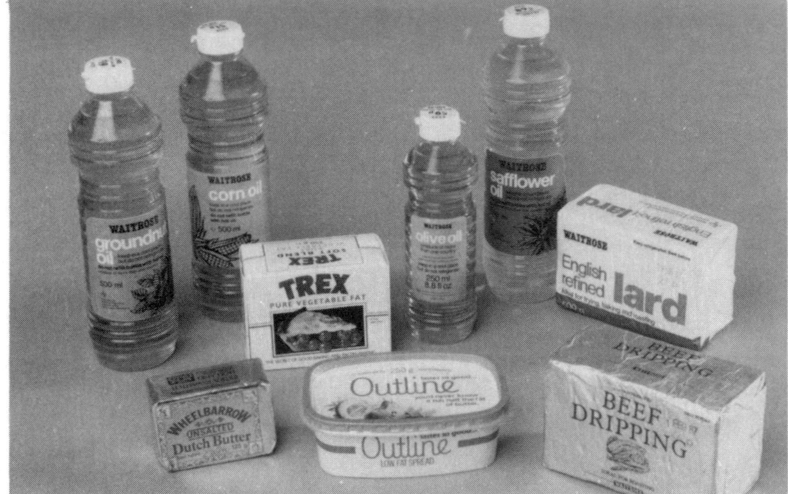

Fig. 1 Some of the different fats and oils that may be bought

B The place of fats and oils in the diet

Fats and oils are used in the home for cooking, spreading and for salad dressing. The average consumption is about 35 g per person per day (Fig. 2). Although we do need some types of fat we do not need very much. We must be careful to look out for fat content, not only when choosing food, but also when choosing cooking methods. Use methods which add as little fat as possible, such as grilling, baking, boiling or steaming (see pages 144–5). When fat is used in cooking it is better to use polyunsaturated fats.

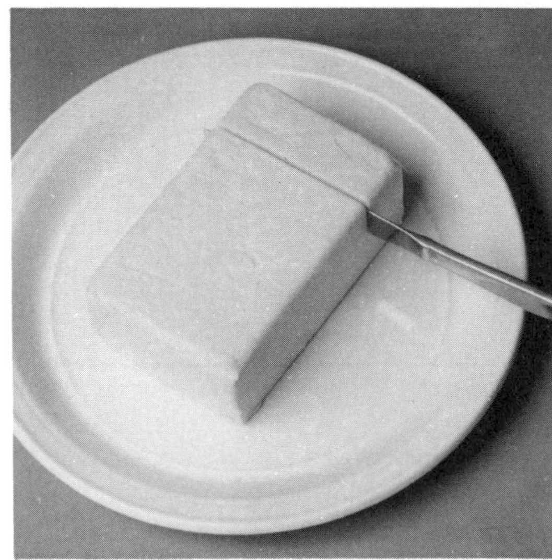

Fig. 2 The small portion is equivalent to the daily average consumption of fat

Fats play an important part in determining the taste, texture and palatability of food. Dry bread has less flavour, a drier texture and is harder to swallow than that which has got butter or margarine spread on it. Low fat cheeses tend to have blander flavours than high fat cheeses. Meat products, for example sausages and beefburgers, have distinctive flavours partly because of the fat in them. Gradual decreases in fat content of such foods would not be very noticeable. This is one way that fat can be cut down.

Many meat products contain relatively large amounts of saturated fat. This is because when meat is produced and cut off the carcass, the fat is trimmed away. Nobody wants to buy this fat and so it is used in products where it will not be seen. It is hidden in many processed foods. It is therefore very easy to eat a lot of fat without realizing it.

We receive a lot of confused information about fat and the fats in our diet. This information comes mainly through advertisements and propaganda put about by people who manufacture one or other type of fat (Fig. 3). They claim that there is little evidence to link the consumption of fat with ill health. It is currently felt by most nutritionists and doctors in the UK, however, that the high amounts of fat, particularly saturated fat, we eat are related to **heart disease** and overweight. Research is continually looking at this question and trying to discover the exact relationship. There is no known harm in cutting down fat consumption to the levels recommended by the NACNE and COMA committees, and it is very likely the best thing for our health (Fig. 4).

Wholefood Cream
Wholefood cream: thick, rich yellow cream from naturally raised Jersey cows, with all of the goodness of full cream milk.

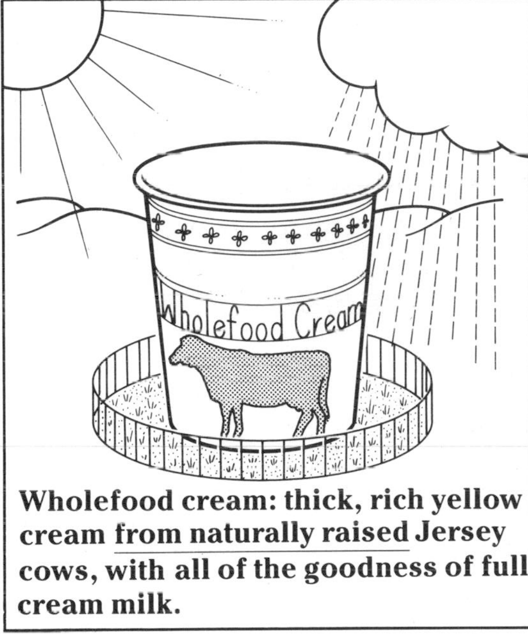

Fig. 3 The information we receive about the fats in our diet can be confusing.

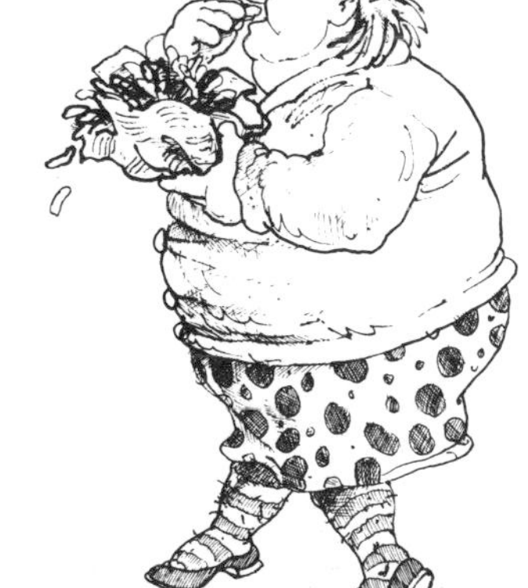

Fig. 4 Chips will not help this woman's obesity

Summary

- Fats and oils come from animal sources and from the seeds of plants.
- The amount of fats and oils in the diet can be controlled by the people preparing and eating the food.
- Fats and oils alter the palatability of foods.
- Many foods contain invisible fat.
- In the UK people need to eat less fat. In poor countries they need to eat more.

Questions

1. Where does most of the fat in our diets come from?
2. Why is fat important in the diet of children in poor countries who might be malnourished?
3. Why do most nutritionists advise a reduction in fat in the UK diet?
4. How might you go about reducing your fat intake?

2.8 Salt in the diet

The substance we call **salt** is the chemical compound **sodium chloride**. Salt also contains small amounts of other trace elements including calcium, magnesium and iodine.

Salt in the diet comes mainly from processed foods such as crisps, nuts, cheese, pickled vegetables, sauces and smoked foods (Fig. 1). It is also added to food during preparation, cooking and at the table. Small quantities occur naturally in some foods (Fig. 2). Nobody is quite sure exactly how much salt we need to eat, but it is a relatively small amount.

In the past salt has been a highly valued commodity. It has often held an economic and social value. It has been used as a form of purification, as a medicine and for embalming.

Fig. 1 Salt is contained in many foods

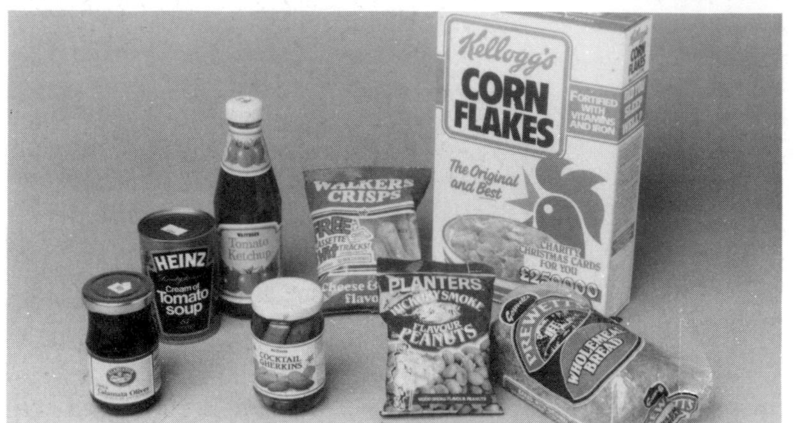

Children's diets

Babies need very little salt. Their **kidneys** are not well enough developed to get rid of extra salt. If they have too much it can cause problems. The main problem is hypernatraemia, which causes dehydration with symptoms of irritability, poor appetite and sometimes convulsions. If hypernatraemia is not treated it can cause permanent brain damage and can be fatal. Children who have high salt intakes also develop a taste for salty foods which is hard to shake off in later life.

Fig. 2 Comparison between sodium content of some fresh and processed foods

Fresh	*mg/100 g*
Flour (wholemeal)	3
Boiled spaghetti	2
Boiled potatoes	3
Boiled new carrots	23
Boiled fresh peas	Trace
Beef	55
Pork	65
Liver	80
Oily fish (salmon)	98
Boiled haricot beans	15
Peanuts (fresh)	6
Milk (fresh, cows')	50

Processed	*mg/100 g*
Bread (wholemeal)	540
Canned spaghetti in tomato sauce	500
Instant mash (made-up) Crisps	260 550
Canned carrots	280
Canned garden peas Processed peas	230 330
Corned beef Beefburgers	950 600
Ham Luncheon meat	1250 1050
Liver sausage	860
Canned salmon	570
Baked beans (canned in tomato sauce)	480
Roasted and salted peanuts Peanut butter	440 350
Cheese	300–1420

Salt and health

There is some weak evidence that eating too much salt is connected with **high blood pressure** (Fig. 3). In countries where people eat a lot of salt there is high blood pressure, and where they do not eat a lot of salt high blood pressure is not a problem. This has not, however, been shown within countries. For example, in the UK it has never been shown that people who eat a lot of salt are more likely to have high blood pressure than those who do not. The mechanism by which salt might cause high blood pressure is not understood either, although some evidence suggests that it is the sodium component which people react to. If this is so, care may need to be taken over the consumption of other sodium salts in food. These include sodium nitrate, sodium caseinate, monosodium glutamate and a number of others. There is, however, no evidence to suggest that these salts are connected with high blood pressure.

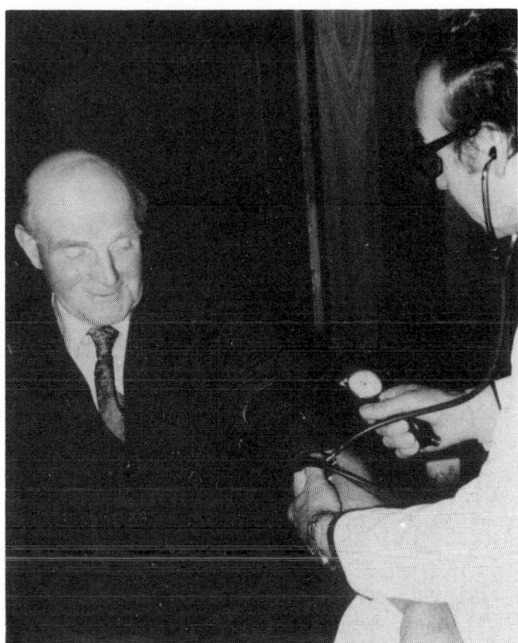

Fig. 3 This man is having his blood pressure taken

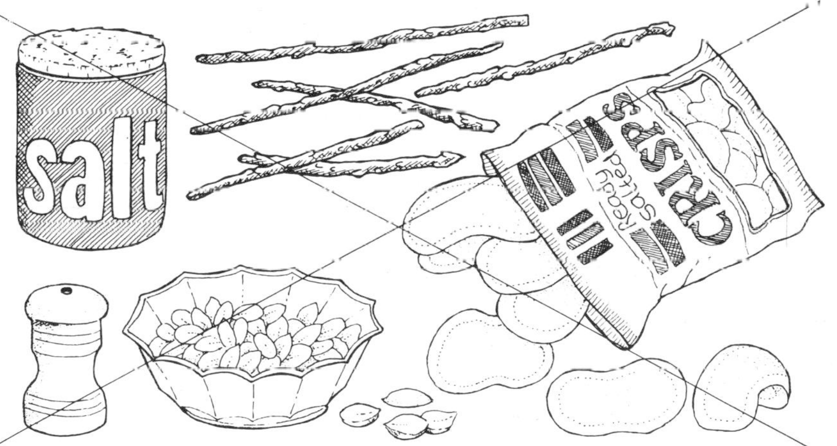

Fig. 4 Choose fewer salty foods

Ways of cutting down on salt

Even though the evidence for the link between salt and high blood pressure is not clear, we do know that in the UK we eat much more salt than is needed. Ways of cutting down salt in food include using less salt in cooking, not adding salt at the table and choosing fewer highly processed and salty snacks and foods (Fig. 4).

Summary

- Salt is used in cooking and in preserving food.
- In the UK many people eat more salt than they need to.
- Infants and young children should not be given salt in their food.

Questions

1. Look at Fig. 2. Do you normally eat any of the foods containing a high level of salt? Say which they are and how much salt they contain.
2. Where do most people obtain the majority of the salt in their diet?
3. Why are most people advised to reduce salt in their diet?
4. Why should infant foods contain no salt?
5. Give three ways of reducing salt in your diet.
6. Make a list of the salts other than common salt (sodium chloride) found in processed foods.

2.9 Water and fluids in the diet

About two thirds of the body's weight is water. Almost every process in the body needs water in order to work. People can live for up to six weeks without food but only for a few days without water. For example, in the early 1980s Bobby Sands, a political prisoner in Northern Ireland, lived for over six weeks on water alone before he died as a result of his hunger strike.

Water comes mainly from drink but is also found in many solid foods, for example fruit, vegetables, foods cooked in water which absorb it, meat, fish, eggs and so on (Fig. 1).

It is lost from the body by **evaporation** of sweat from the skin, which regulates body temperature, in **exhaled breath** from the lungs and via the **kidneys**. The kidneys use water as a vehicle for getting rid of the soluble waste products of the body (Fig. 2).

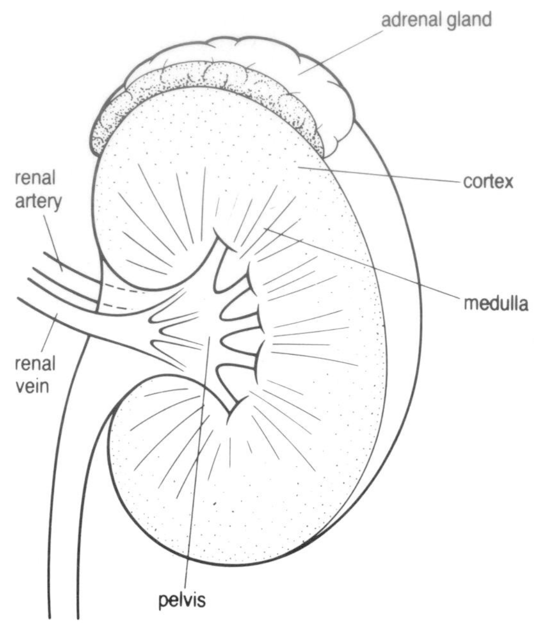

Fig. 2 (a) Human kidney

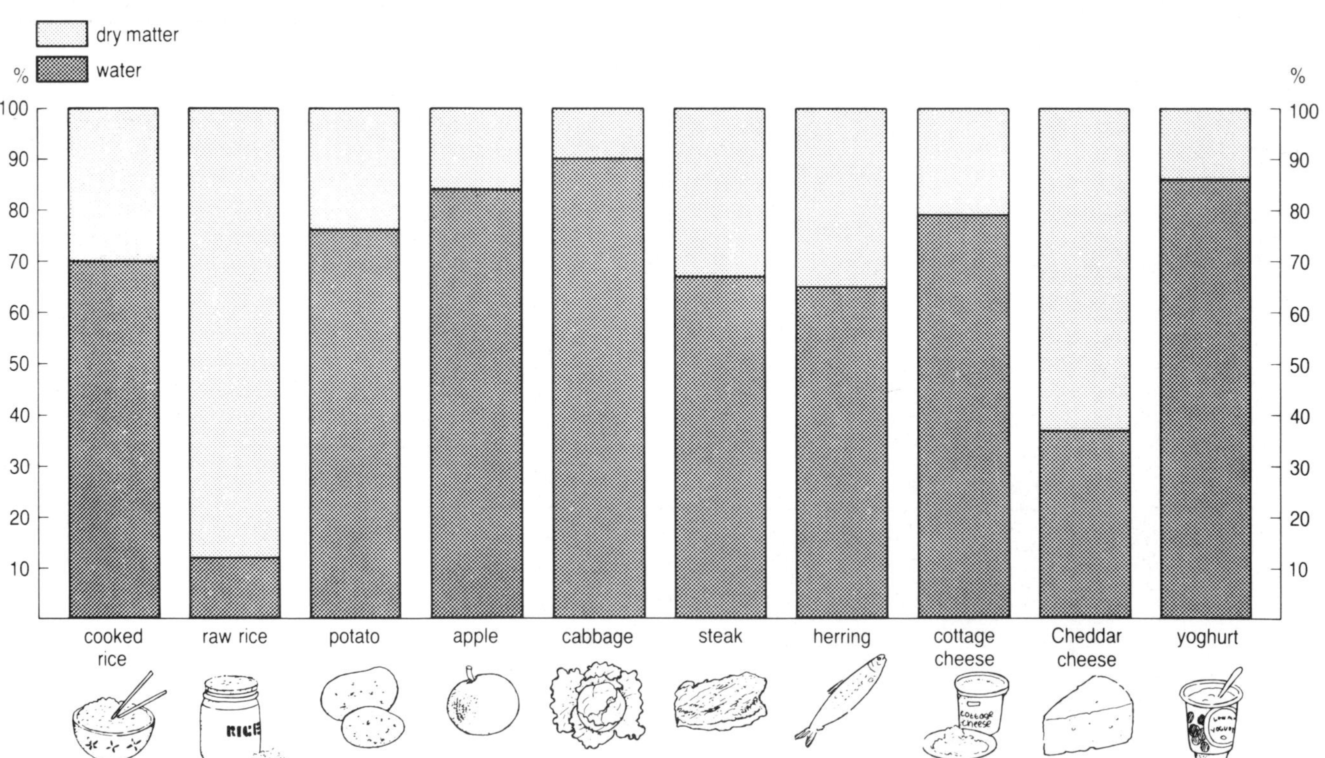

Fig. 1 Diagram showing the water content of different foods

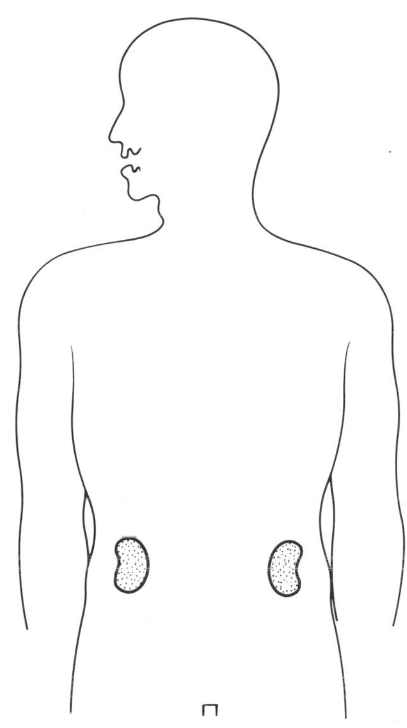

Fig. 2 (b) The position of the kidneys in the body

If more water than is needed is taken in it is got rid of through the kidneys in the **urine**. If insufficient water is taken in the body compensates for a short time by concentrating the urine and getting rid of less water. However, if water intake is not increased **dehydration** may result.

Fluid intakes are affected by a number of factors. These include heavy sweating when doing strenuous activity (Fig. 3) or in a hot climate, and illnesses which cause vomiting or diarrhoea. In temperate climates such as ours at least one litre of water or other fluid should be drunk each day. More may be needed if heavy work is being done.

Water can be an important dietary source of fluoride and calcium. This depends on the local soil conditions and policies regarding **fluoridation** of water supply. Fluoride is important in protecting teeth from decay.

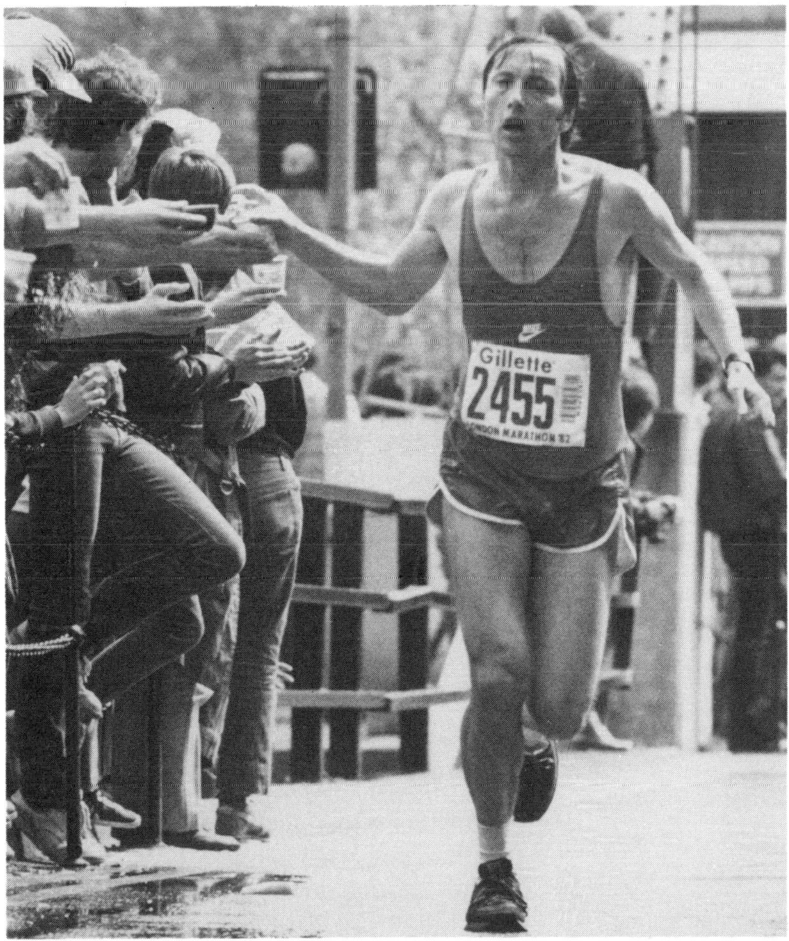

Fig. 3 This man will need extra fluid intake to compensate for heavy sweating

Summary

- Water is vital for life.
- Water comes from both drinks and food.
- The amount of water needed daily depends on exercise and the climate.

Questions

1. What effect does cooking have on the water content of rice?
2. Why do we need water in our diet?
3. How is excess water lost from the body?
4. Which important minerals are found in water?
5. Why is it necessary to drink more water in a hotter climate or when doing manual work?

2.10 Alcohol in the diet

Alcohol is not a necessary food but can contribute to dietary energy. It is a poison, but in small quantities is not harmful (Fig. 1). Alcohol is quickly absorbed into the blood after it has been drunk. It is then carried to the liver where it is turned into harmless products. However, excess alcohol consumption can lead to a loss of appetite and malnutrition. It can also lead to liver damage and can be **addictive**.

Fig. 1 Alcoholic and energy content of different drinks

	Volume of alcohol	Normal English measure	Quantity of alcohol	kJ 100 ml
Beer or cider – ordinary	4%	½pt (284 ml)	11ml	132 (Draught bitter) 176 (Sweet cider)
Beer or cider – strong	6%	½pt (284 ml)	17ml	
Table wine	10%	125 ml	12ml	275 (Dry white wine)
Port, sherry, vermouth	20%	50 ml	10ml	481 (Dry sherry)
Spirits	40%	25 ml	10ml	919

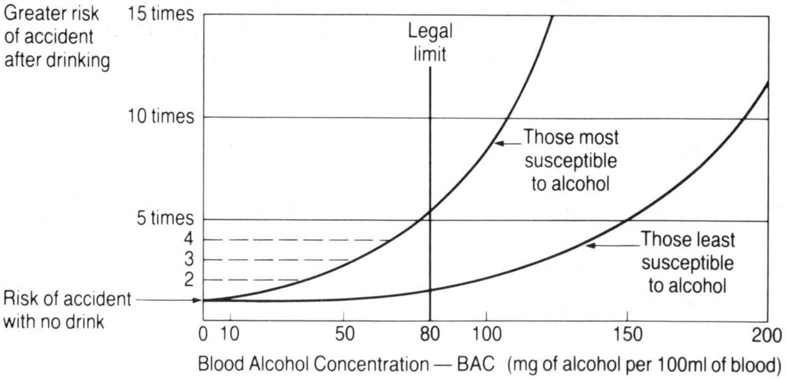

Fig. 2 The effect of alcohol on accident risk

Drinking too much alcohol is the cause of many accidents, social problems and violent attacks. Although initially it seems to make you feel more lively and cheerful, it is in fact a **depressant**. It has very strong after-effects.

The single biggest factor in all road deaths and injuries is alcohol, particularly amongst young people. In the UK:

- 1 in 3 drivers killed have a blood/alcohol content above the legal limit.
- 2 in 3 drivers killed at night are above the legal limit.
- 1 in 3 drivers tested as the result of an accident fails the breath test.
- 1 in 4 young motorcyclists killed has a blood/alcohol content above the legal limit.
- Half the motorcyclists killed at night are above the legal limit.
- 2 in 5 drivers and motorcyclists killed have consumed some alcohol prior to their deaths.

We know this because, following a road death, blood from the body is analysed to determine the alcohol content.

Many people have the wrong idea about alcohol because of the way in which it is advertised. Drinking is usually shown as grown-up and glamorous. In reality overdoing it is quite the reverse. Alcohol may give you a feeling of wellbeing; actually it is a depressant, slowing down the processes in the brain.

- It lessens co-ordination of movement and lengthens reaction time.
- It blurs vision and decreases awareness.
- It impairs ability to judge speed and distance.

All of these affect driving performance.

- It also impairs your judgement of how fit you are to drive, so that under the influence of alcohol you may genuinely believe yourself to be driving better than you really are.

The consequence is a higher risk of accident (Fig. 2).

Alcohol in the blood is measured in milligrams (mg) of alcohol per 100 millilitres (ml) of blood (Fig. 3). The legal limit is 80 mg/100 ml.
Alcohol levels can be measured in urine and breath as well as in blood (Fig. 4).

Summary

- Alcohol taken in excess can cause nutritional, mental, social and physical problems.
- Alcohol is the biggest single factor in all road deaths.

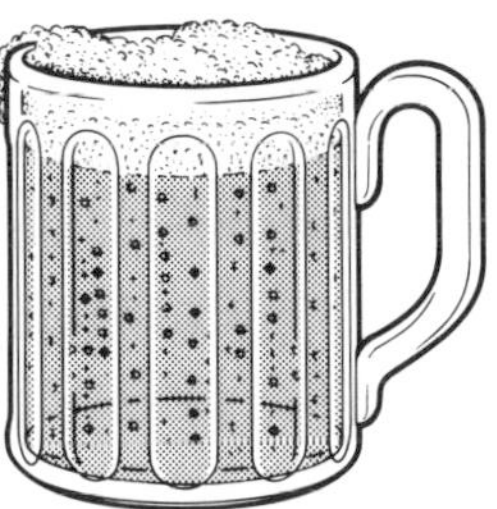
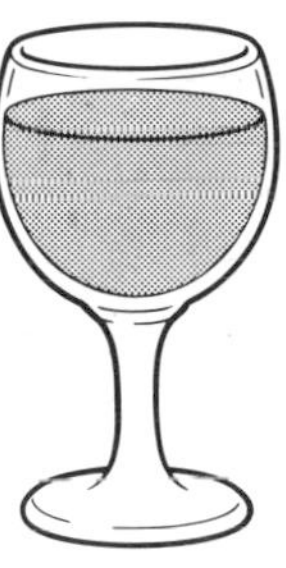
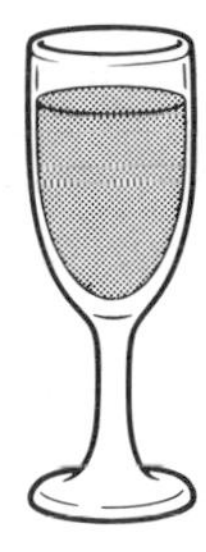
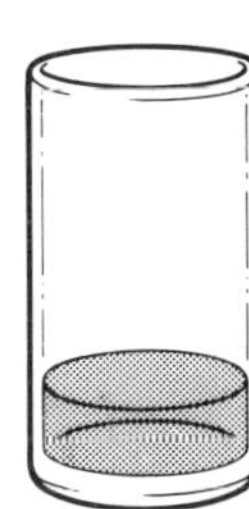

Fig. 3 Equivalent measures of alcohol

1 unit of alcohol = ½ pint beer = 1 glass table wine = 1 glass sherry = 1 measure spirit

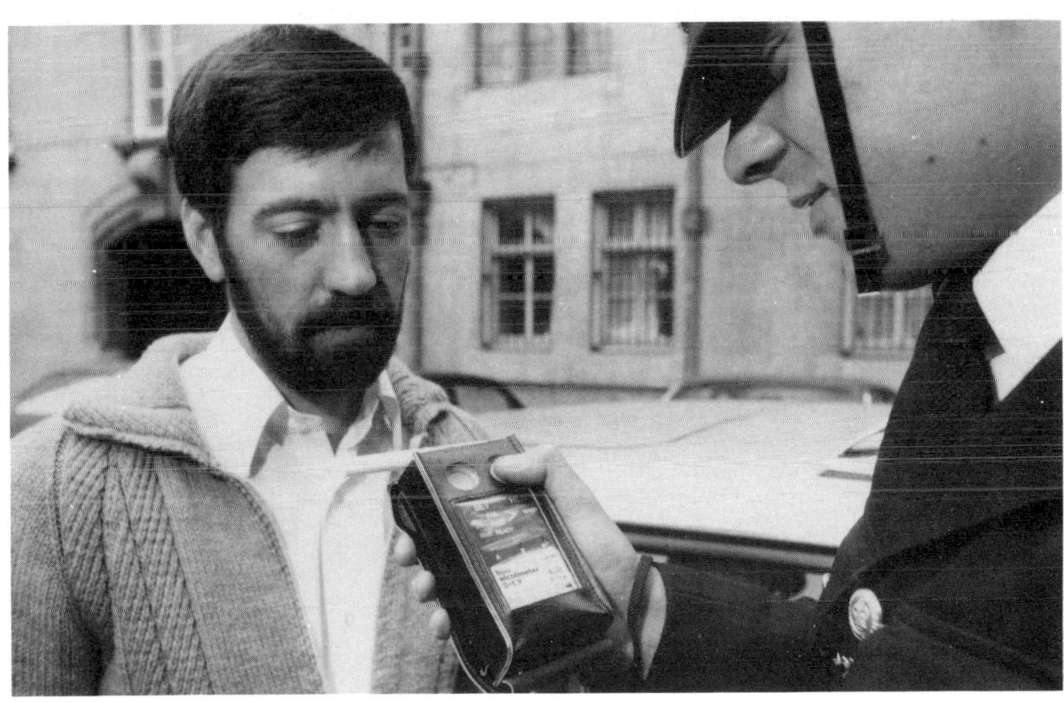

Fig. 4 Measuring alcohol in the breath

Questions

1. What are the effects of excess alcohol?
2. A glass of wine contains 1 unit of alcohol. How much (a) beer, (b) sherry and (c) spirits contain the same quantity?
3. What is the legal limit of alcohol in the blood?
4. How does a blood alcohol concentration five times the legal limit affect the chances of having an accident for those (a) most susceptible and (b) least susceptible to alcohol?
5. What are the connections between drinking alcohol and accidents involving motorcycles?

2.11 Food additives in the diet

Food additives are not a new phenomenon. For generations foods have been preserved by the addition of sodium chloride (salt), acetic acid (vinegar), ethyl alcohol (alcohols) or sucrose (sugar) (Fig. 1).

Rapid expansion of **food technology** has led to a tremendous increase in the number of chemical additives available to the food industry. Additives are now used for **colouring** and **flavouring** foods, as well as for **preserving** it. Most processed foods contain additives. The information given to consumers about additives contained in the food they eat is far from complete. New regulations came into force on 1 January 1986. These require manufacturers to list E numbers or names of additives except flavourings. The E numbers refer to published lists of additives generally regarded as safe, drawn up by the **EEC**. However, there is a debate about the safety of some tested additives, and not all scientists agree at present. The fact that all EEC countries recognize this code makes for easier legislation within Europe.

The following are the main groups of food additives in use (Fig. 2).

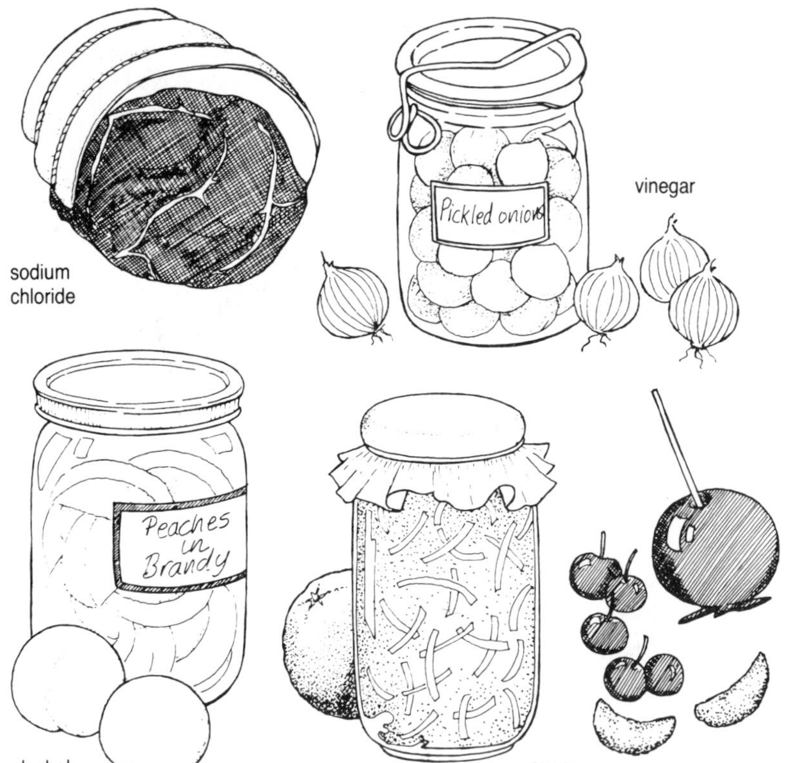

Fig. 1 Some food additives are not new

Permitted colours (E100–E180)

A number of permitted colours are natural in origin (E100 comes from turmeric root, E120 is cochineal). Colour is used in food for **cosmetic** reasons and is therefore unnecessary. The food industry believes that consumers do not want 'natural' colours, some of which are not particularly attractive. Homemade strawberry jam, for example, is browny red, not the brilliant colour of the commercial product.

Preservatives (E200–E290)

These prevent the growth of **micro-organisms** and therefore have considerable value in safeguarding health. In our society it is impossible to obtain enough fresh food to avoid that which has been preserved by various means.

Antioxidants (E300–E321)

Oils and fats become **rancid** in the presence of oxygen. Some antioxidants are natural, e.g. vitamin C (E300), vitamin E (E306). Antioxidants are necessary in many oil and fat containing foods to prevent the food becoming inedible.

Emulsifiers and stabilizers (E322–E494)

These stop fat and water separating. Many are natural (e.g. Lecithin E322 which is found in eggs and 'binds' mayonnaise). Some are used to allow the addition of water in chicken or ham. These are the polyphosphates (E450). By increasing the water content of meat and meat products, manufactures are able to increase the weight and therefore the

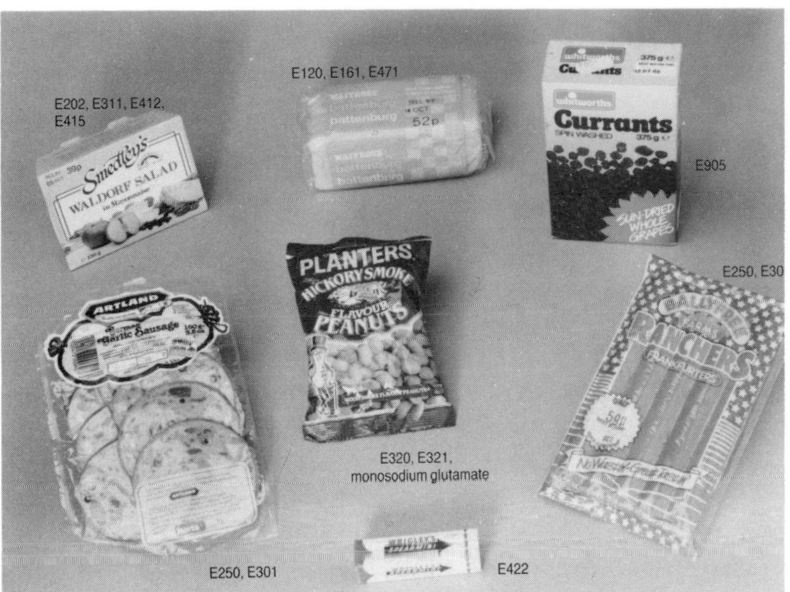

Fig. 2 The chemical additives generally regarded as safe are widely used in the food industry

price of their products. Much of this water is lost in cooking and as customers we are inadvertently paying money for water. Others allow the incorporation of a good deal of fat in processed meat.

Sweeteners (E420–E421)

Sorbitol and mannitol have E numbers. The others, like glucose, lactose and fructose, have no E numbers because they are classed as foods.

Mineral hydrocarbons (E905–E907)

These are used to prevent drying out and make food shine (e.g. chewy sweets, dried fruit, cheese rind and eggs).

Others

There are many other additives which are used for a variety of reasons. Monosodium glutamate is a flavour enhancer, some substances are used to prevent foaming, to glaze, to sweeten or as a propellant for food aerosols.

Additives are often used by food manufacturers to make cheap, refined ingredients such as sugar, refined starch and fat into 'foods', which are often high in fat and sugar. For example, packet fruit juice, instant soup and dessert mix basically contain similar ingredients. These are turned into what seem to be three quite different foods by the use of artificial flavours, colours, emulsifiers and preservatives.

There is considerable doubt about the safety of many food additives. Many additives in use in the UK are banned in other European countries, and some are thought to be capable of causing **cancer**. Safety testing of additives takes place on individual chemicals and not on combinations. They are almost always eaten in combinations. There are growing concerns regarding the links between **hyperactivity** in children and additives, and many people believe that some additives result in **allergic** problems in sensitive people.

The additives which prevent spoilage (preservatives, antioxidants) are valuable although their safety must be assured. Many people would like to see the abolition of colourants, flavouring agents and other additives which are not necessary for the production of safe food.

Summary

- Most processed food contains chemical additives.
- Not all the additives in use in the UK are necessary for the production of safe food.
- Not all additives used in the UK are considered safe in other countries.
- Additives are used to turn cheap, refined ingredients into 'foods' which are often high in fat and sugar.

Questions

1. What is an E number?
2. What are the main groups of additives and for what reasons are they added to foods?
3. How would you recognize each group merely by its E number?
4. Which health problems have been linked with additives?
5. Which additives are used for 'cosmetic' reasons?

SECTION 3 Eating patterns and special needs

3.1 | Eating patterns in the UK

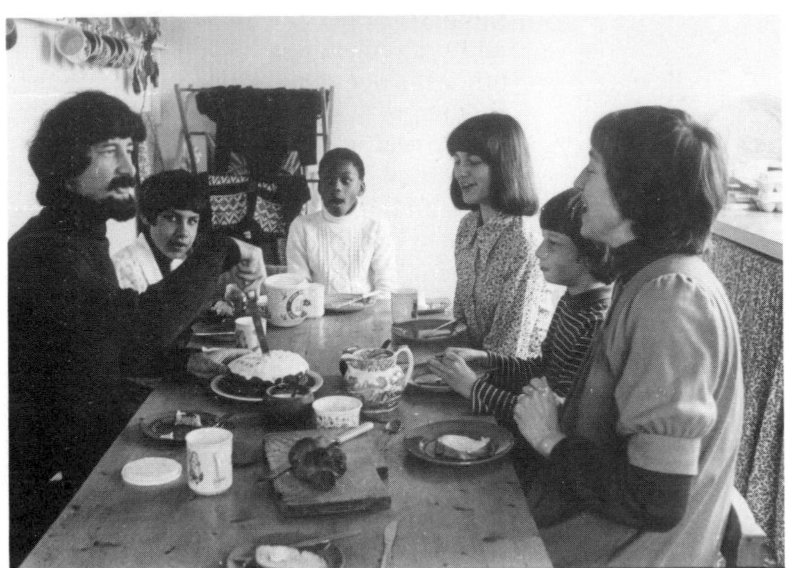

Fig. 1 Family and guests sharing a meal together

Fig. 2 Eating in front of the television

Most people in this country eat between two and five times a day. One of these times is usually more important than the others. This **main meal** happens when most of the household is together. Guests are sometimes invited as well (Fig. 1). The other meals of the day are usually breakfast and lighter meals or snacks.

Changing eating patterns

The way people eat changes over time and now tends to be much less formal. Many people eat their meals away from home. A lot of meals are eaten sitting in front of the television rather than at the table (Fig. 2). In some households, each member of the household has her or his meal at a different time depending on when they come in, and the whole household are together rarely. In many parts of the country the only time when the whole household eats together is a Sunday lunchtime, or if there is a regular religious festival on a Friday or Saturday. There is usually a full **traditional meal** at this time.

A survey carried out in 1981 by the National Dairy Council ('What are children eating these days?') showed that of the 1446 children they surveyed, many were at risk of eating poor diets. For example, 5% had no breakfast and only one 'meal', while 3% had only a cereal breakfast and no meals throughout the day. They were mainly eating snacks. These eating patterns are very unlikely to provide a healthy balanced diet. A more recent survey carried out by the Department of Health and Social Security also showed that, in general, teenagers are eating very poor diets (*The Diets of British School Children*, DHSS 1986).

Effects of the changes on nutrition

Many people hardly ever sit down to a meal round a table (Fig. 3). This can make it harder to choose a **balanced diet**. Traditional meals, whatever the culture, tend to be nutritionally balanced. They contain a variety of foods from the four main food groups: for example rice, dahl and salad; roast meat, potatoes and vegetables; noodles, fish and stir fry vegetables. Eating mainly snacks and quick meals which have not been planned is less likely to provide a balanced diet.

Breakfast is an important meal which is often forgotten. The foods most people eat at breakfast, such as bread and breakfast cereals, are good sources of vitamins, particularly the B vitamins. Although there are B vitamins in some of the foods they will eat during the rest of the day, it has been shown that not eating breakfast reduces the daily intake of the vitamins, usually eaten at breakfast.

Fig. 3 Eating in the street

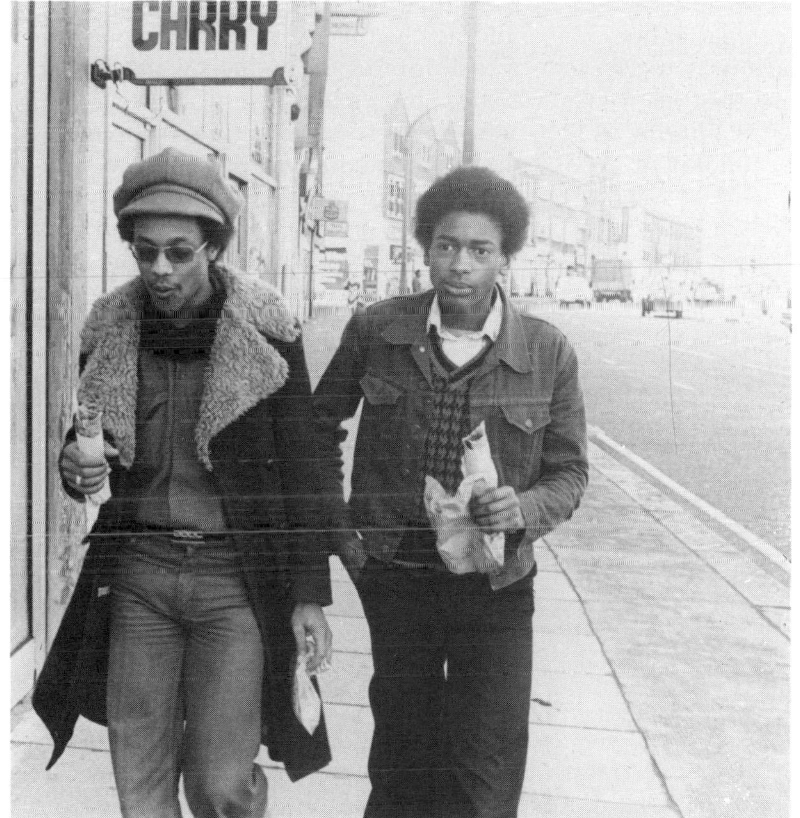

Choosing a balanced diet

Because eating has become less formal, it is important to take even greater care when choosing a balanced diet. It is important to eat regularly, whether you are eating main meals or snacks. This is because the casual eating of snack foods which contain relatively few nutrients does not lead to a balanced diet. It is important to know more about what is in the food. To make sure you are eating a balanced diet, eat regularly at least three times a day. Make sure that you are including foods from the main food groups. Irregular snacking on individual foods such as sweets and confectionery, biscuits, cheese or crisps is not likely to give you a balanced diet.

Summary

- People are changing to less formal eating patterns.
- More food is being eaten outside the home.
- More pre-prepared food is being eaten.
- Eating regularly is important.
- Knowing about what is in food is important.

Questions

1. Why is it important to eat breakfast? Plan a balanced meal for breakfast which can be prepared and eaten quickly.
2. List three simple rules for ensuring that you eat a balanced diet.
3. Write a menu for a meal you might eat at home with other people. Note which food groups you choose from and say if you think the meal was a balanced one.
4. Eating patterns have changed recently. Describe any three of these changes.
5. Why is regular 'snack' eating not a good idea?

3.2 Availability of food

In the UK, agricultural policy is determined very much by the **Common Agricultural Policy** of the EEC. The main aims of this policy are to make sure that there is always enough food for everybody, to fix prices so they do not vary too much and to see that small farmers in particular can always earn a good living. Although these may seem to be good aims, they have caused too much food to be produced. The farmer is paid for the food, even if we do not need it. The extra produced is stored, hence the **food mountains** and **wine lakes** (Figs 1 and 2).

Government policy can also influence the amount of **information** we receive about food. For example, the Government makes laws about the labelling of food and the amount of information given to us on the packet. They are also responsible for the laws relating to food hygiene and food handling, and for ensuring that the food we receive is of good quality and not going to poison us.

Fig. 1 The food story

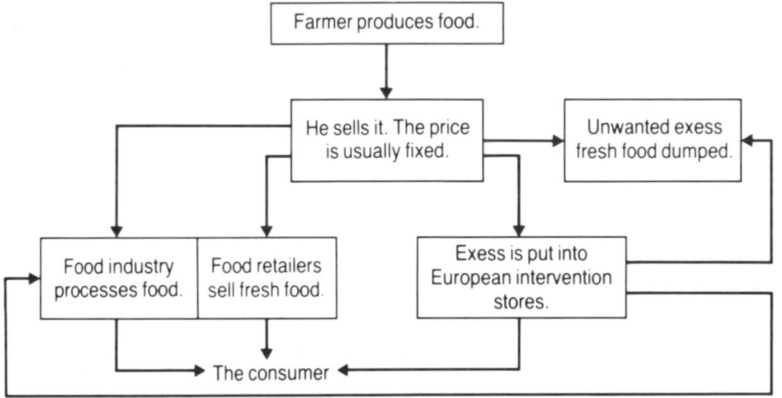

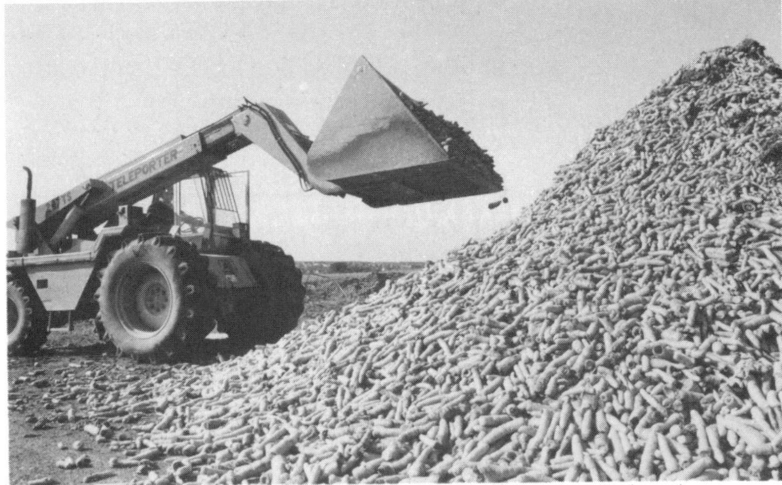

Fig. 2 After a good harvest, food may be dumped. This prevents the prices from dropping

Agriculture in the UK has changed a lot in the last 40 years (since World War II). Changes in methods as well as policy have affected food availability. The same farms and land now produce more food.

In recent years a very wide range of **processed foods** has become available in the UK. Food companies take basic foodstuffs and by processing them and adding chemicals, they manage to make a vast number of products which appear to be completely different. These foods need very little preparation before they are eaten and include full meals as well as individual items. The food industry needs to go on developing these products in order to keep its profits up. Sometimes this is done by using cheaper ingredients, which are not necessarily nutritionally desirable. The food manufacturing industry has a lot of influence on the foods that are available for us to buy in the shops.

The **distribution** of food throughout the world depends on a number of very complicated economic and political factors. One of the most important of these is the development of good **transport systems**. Because transport systems are now so well developed, it is possible for us in the UK to get fruit, vegetables and other foods which have been flown in from all parts of the world. Bulky items still travel by sea. Once it arrives in the UK, food is sent by both road and rail to its destination. Transporting food in this way adds to its cost. If there are strikes in these transport systems or hold-ups of any other sort, then food becomes less available.

Fruit and vegetables in particular are subject to **climate** and **seasonal variations**. If for any reason there are small harvests and foods become less available, the prices go up immediately.

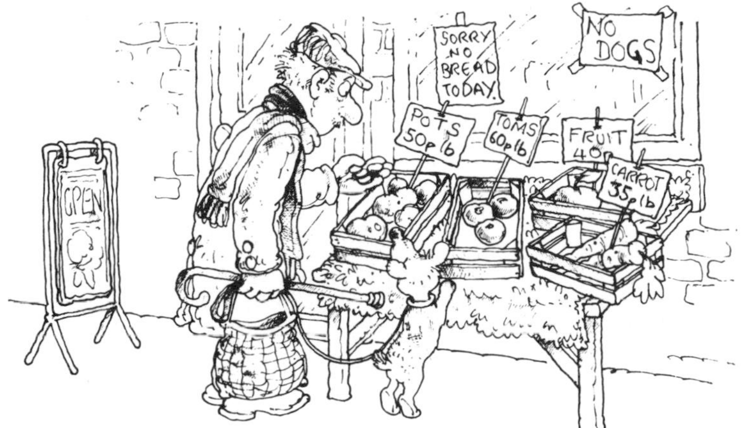

Fig. 3 Elderly people often have to use expensive local shops

This is often seen in the price of vegetables.

In the UK most of the **supermarkets** are owned by a few **retailing** companies. These actually determine to a large extent foods that will be on sale there. You have very little choice about what is available in a shop.

The effect of access to food on availability

There are three important factors which affect access to food. These are the **location** of the shops in relation to where you live, local **transport** facilities and individual **mobility**.

Quite often, the large supermarket chains set up **superstores** on the outskirts of big cities or in areas where there are not a lot of people living. This means that to reach these shops you really need to have a car. At the same time, because a lot of people now go to these big shops, smaller shops in city centres and local shopping areas are having to close down. They can no longer get all the business they need. The result is that the shops left in these areas tend to be small, with little choice, and more expensive than the big superstores. The superstores are very handy for people who have transport and enough money to buy large quantities of food all at once. But those people who do not live nearby and have difficulty getting there are forced to shop in the local more expensive shops (Fig. 3). In large supermarkets it is also often difficult to buy food in small quantities, suitable for people living alone or without sufficient money to buy in bulk.

If you do not live very near to the shops and do not have a car or cannot drive, then the local transport facilities will affect you whether or not you can get to the best shops or the shops that you want to. If these are good and make it easy for people travelling with young children, then there is no problem. Unfortunately, local transport facilities are not always very good and cause these people to have difficulty getting to the shops.

Some people also have difficulty in walking long distances, getting on and off buses and generally moving around. For them too it becomes difficult to go to the best shops in order to buy the foods that they want to stay healthy.

Although we are often told that we are free to choose exactly what we want to eat and that our health depends on our own choice of food, we see that it is not always easy. For many people, improving their nutrition means looking at ways of solving all the problems outlined above.

Summary

- People have to choose from what is available at a price they can afford.
- Availability is determined by many factors outside the control of consumers.
- Availability depends on the siting of shops, local transport facilities and individual mobility.

Questions

1. Describe the aims of the Common Agricultural Policy. What is the main disadvantage of these aims and what are the results?
2. What changes have occurred in UK agriculture over the past 40 years?.
3. Make a list of things (factors) which can affect food distribution and availability.
4. Explain how the siting of shops, local transport facilities and individual mobility can affect food choices.

3.3 Individual choice

Even if healthy food were available to everyone at a price they could afford, there are still other important things which affect what we choose to eat. Some of these we decide for ourselves, some we do not.

Individual needs

We all have our own likes and dislikes for food as well as for many other things. Where food is concerned these are called our **taste preferences**. Taste preferences and food habits are laid down when we are very young children (Fig. 1).

The way we live our lives, the amount of time we have to do different things and the things we like to do best will also affect what we eat. For example, if you are busy working or out in the street all day you do not have time to go home and cook or eat a proper meal. There is a need for quick, cheap, convenient food which will give all the members of a household a **well balanced diet**.

Knowledge and information

It is very important that we understand how to **assess information** we receive about food and health. We get information from many different sources. These include friends and relatives, advertisements, magazines and newspapers, the television and radio, and teachers and people who work in the medical field, for example doctors, dietitians, nurses and nutritionists. It is important to remember that in advertisements the main aim is to persuade you to buy the product. The information usually has some truth in it but it is not necessarily the whole truth. For example, some yoghurts are advertised as being low in fat while they also have a relatively high sugar content. Advertisements stress the good points about the food (Fig. 2).

Another important source of information can be **food labels**. It is likely that by the end of the 1980s the fat content of most foods will have to be displayed on the label. There may also be other nutrient information given, but this is likely to be voluntary. At the moment, a label has to give the ingredients (listed in the order of the amount they occur in the food), the weight of the food, the date until which it will keep, the country of origin and the name and address of the manufacturer or packager. **Nutritional labelling** will be in addition to this.

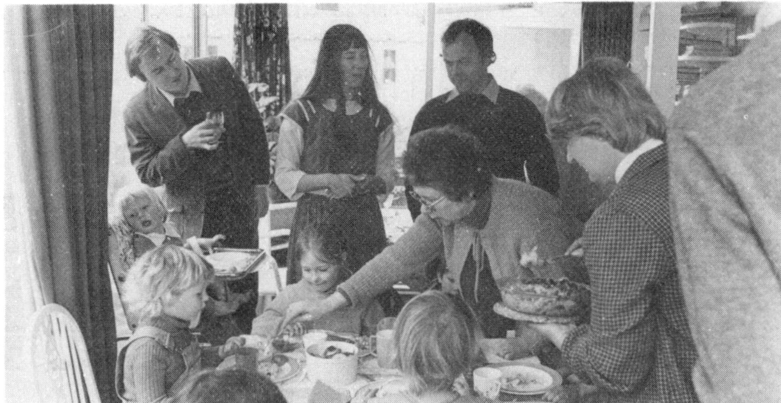

Fig. 1 Babies learn their food habits from their families

Social and cultural factors

Every society has different rules and ideas about food and drink. These grow up over long periods of time and develop as traditions within the culture. The foods eaten, the cooking methods used and meal patterns all contribute to a person's **cultural identity**. Food and drink are often associated with hospitality and friendship. At the same time all cultures have **taboo** foods. In this country, few people would consider eating insects or dogs. However, in other countries these are considered as delicacies. Sometimes specific foods are forbidden at certain times in a person's life. For example, alcohol is not recommended during pregnancy. In some cultures foods are eaten in certain combinations to balance each other. For example, in many Asian communities there are the principles of 'hot' and 'cold' foods.

In the UK, sweet foods are often used as bribes and rewards, particularly for young children. One of the effects of this is that people tend to turn to these foods for comfort and reward. Foods often have special associations connected with them which have nothing to do with nutrition. For example, eating large amounts of bread and potatoes tends to be associated with poverty.

Religious, **moral** and **ethical** beliefs can play a very important part in determining an individual's food choice. For example, in the Hindu religion the cow is sacred. It is therefore symbolic and its products, milk and clarified butter, are sacred. Therefore no Hindu will ever eat beef. People from other religions, such as Muslims, Jews and Rastafarians, consider pig meat unclean because of the scavenging habits of the pig. Their dietary laws forbid the eating of pork or any pork products. Many people do not eat meat or animal products because they disagree with the killing of animals for food as a general principle. Some do not even eat dairy products, as they see this as the taking of life from young animals who would normally drink the milk. These people are **vegetarians** and **vegans**.

Some people also prefer not to buy products which originate where they disagree with the **political** situation. For example, many people in the UK disagree with the apartheid regime in South Africa and therefore avoid buying any products from that country.

Perhaps some of these food habits come from our **peer group** and **family pressure**. It is not very easy to go against the habits of our group of friends. It is important for most of us to be part of that group and to stick to the rules of the group (Fig. 3). Breaking away can be very difficult and upsetting.

Fig. 2 Advertisements stress the good points about the products they describe

No additives, no preservatives, just the pure taste of duckling. . .
Perfect on its own or with a rich, fruity sauce, Cherry Duckling is a completely natural product with plenty of lean meat.
Nothing could be simpler to cook either. Simply prick the skin with a fork, rub with salt and roast on a trivet.
Its unique taste gives it a special quality that

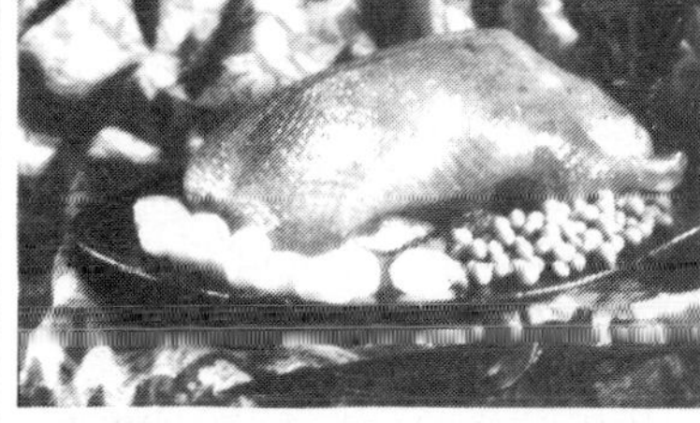

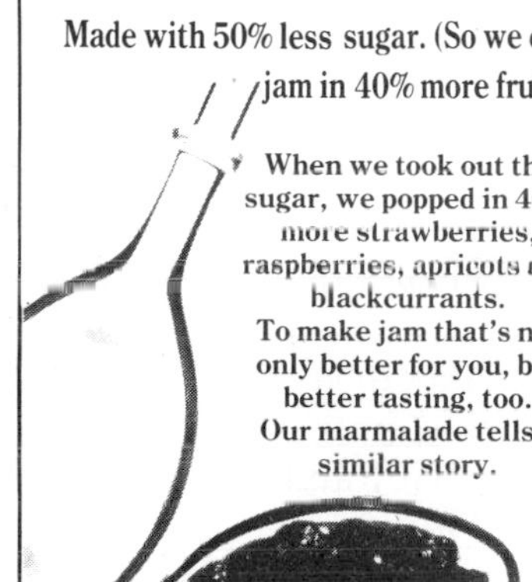

DRINKS

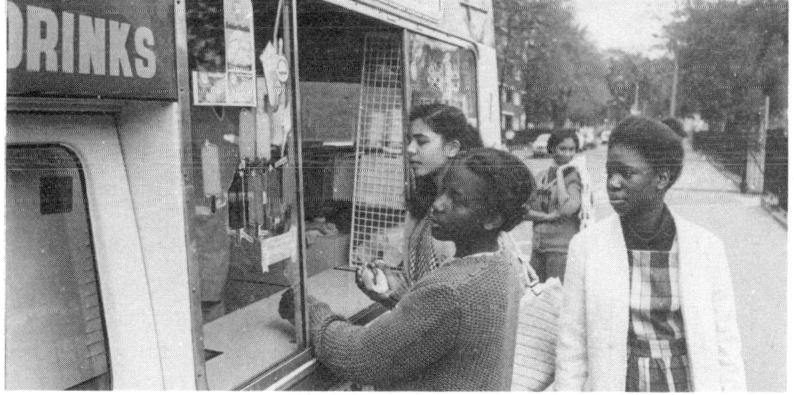

Fig. 3 This group always meets outside this take-away

Summary

- Many factors influence individual choice from what is available.
- Some of these factors are under the control of individuals, some are not.

Questions

1. Look at Figure 2. Describe one advertisement and say
   (a) what the advertisement tells you about the food, in words,
   (b) what the advertisement tells you about the food, in pictures,
   (c) what age and sex you think the advertisement is aimed at.
   (d) Do you buy this food? Does the advertisement make you want to try it? Explain why it does or does not.
   (e) Write what you know about this food that is not in the advertisement. Say where you think you got this information.
   (f) Explain why you chose that particular advertisement.
2. Name four things (factors) which influence individual food choice. Describe the way in which these factors affect food choice.

3.4 The special needs of infants and toddlers

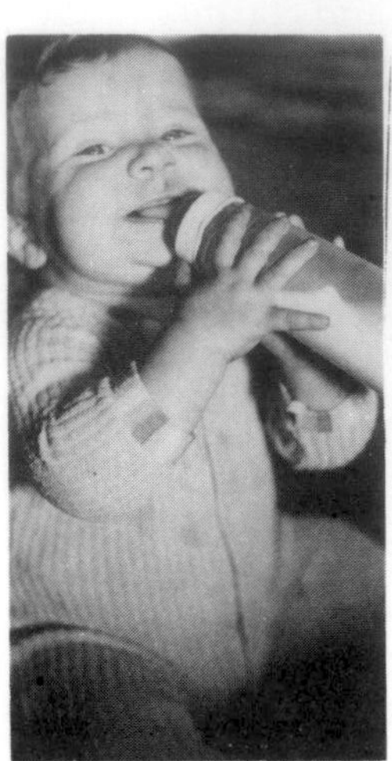

Fig. 1 Bottlefeeding is the alternative to breastfeeding

Infant feeding

For the first three months of life an infant needs only milk and nothing else. The best milk is **breast milk** from the mother. Breast milk provides all the nutrients the baby needs in the right amounts. It is easily digested and absorbed, and it contains special **antibodies**. These protect the baby from illness and infection. Breastfeeding also helps to make the mother and baby feel very close to each other. This is called **bonding**.

Breastfeeding is much cheaper than the alternative, bottle feeding. The only cost is the small amount of extra food the mother needs to eat. The breast milk is at the right temperature for the baby and comes in the right amount. The baby decides how much milk it will have by the amount of time it suckles. The risk of contaminating breast milk is lower than that for bottle milk. The milk goes directly from the breast to the baby's mouth, so there are no bottles and teats to be cleaned.

If the mother is upset or tense about something, however, the milk does not come through properly. Also, if she does not take care, the milk begins to dry up. If a woman wants to go out or return to work then again breastfeeding can be very difficult.

The alternative to breastfeeding is **bottle-feeding** (Fig. 1). Special baby milks are made which are very similar in composition to breast milk (Fig. 2). These baby milks do not, however, have the same antibodies, and so the babies do not have the initial form of protection. Bottles and teats and sterilizing solutions can be expensive. Unless the bottlefed baby is being demand fed it is harder to make sure the baby is getting exactly the right amount of feed.

Fig. 2 Comparison of the nutrient composition of human and other milks per 100 g

	Human milk		Infant formula 1	Infant formula 2	Cows' milk (silver/red top)	Goats' milk
	mature	transitional				
megajoules	0.29	0.28	0.27	0.29	0.27	0.30
protein (mg)	1.3	2.0	1.5	1.9	3.3	3.3
fat (mg)	4.1	3.7	3.6	3.1	3.8	4.5
carbohydrate (mg)	7.2	6.9	7.2	8.4	4.7	4.6
sodium (mg)	14	4.8	18	27	50	40
potassium (mg)	58	68	n/a	n/a	150	180
calcium (mg)	34	25	57	71	120	130
iron (mg)	0.07	0.04	0.7	0.7	0.05	0.04
zinc (mg)	0.28	n/a	0.3	n/a	0.35	0.30
vitamin A (μg)	60	n/a	61	61	28	40
vitamin D (μg)	0.025	n/a	1.0	1.0	0.013	0.060
thiamin (mg)	0.02	n/a	0.04	0.04	0.04	0.04
riboflavin (mg)	0.03	n/a	0.05	0.05	0.19	0.15
nicotinic acid (mg)	0.22	n/a	0.4	0.4	0.09	0.20
vitamin C (mg)	3.7	n/a	6.0	6.0	1.5	1.78
vitamin E (mg)	0.34	n/a	0.6	0.6	0.1	1.5
vitamin B (mg)	0.01	n/a	0.03	0.03	0.04	n/a
vitamin B^6 (μg)	Tr	n/a	0.15	0.15	0.3	0.04
folic acid^{12} (μg)	5	n/a	10.0	10.0	5	Tr
pantothenic acid (mg)	0.25	n/a	0.4	0.4	0.35	0.34
biotin (μg)	0.7	n/a	1.1	1.1	2.0	2.0

n/a = figure not available
Tr = trace

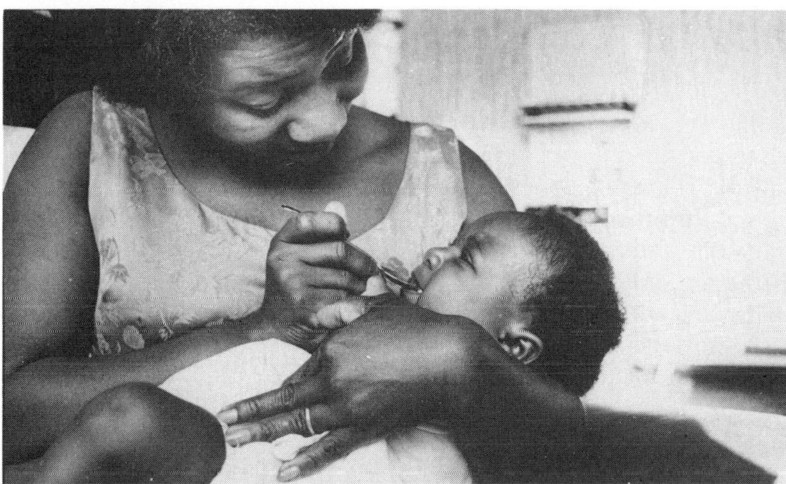

Fig. 3 A baby being fed puréed food – the first 'solids'

Weaning

Between three and six months the baby will not be satisfied by breast or bottle milk alone. At this time she/he needs to be given some extra food. The first foods are puréed vegetables, fruits and smooth cereal porridges (Fig. 3). As the baby gets older other foods can be introduced. By nine months to one year the baby can be eating the same foods as the rest of the household. The consistency of the baby's food should be changed as it is able to learn to chew, and by the age of a year the food may just be cut up.

The best milk for all babies up to one year is either breast milk or the special infant formulae. If ordinary cows' milk is to be given it should not be introduced before 6 months.

The Government report *Present Day Practice in Infant Feeding* published in 1980 recommends that 'mothers be advised not to add sugar (sucrose) or salt (sodium chloride) to the solid foods in an infant's diet, and that caution should be exercised by manufacturers in the addition of sucrose and of sodium chloride to their infant food products'.

Toddlers and children

Like everyone else, toddlers and children need a balanced diet. Milk is still a very important part of the diet, but as the range of food that the child eats increases, the amount of milk it needs will decrease. Milk and milk products are important because of the **protein**, **calcium** and **dietary energy** they provide. For children who are faddy eaters and have small appetites, milk and milk products may be particularly important. During this time of life, likes and dislikes emerge. It is therefore very important to make sure that if a child dislikes one sort of food from one of the food groups, it has one of the other foods in that group. For example, if the child eats no vegetables then it should have some fruit each day.

If a child has a good appetite and eats a wide variety of food then the type of milk used may not be important although skimmed milk is not recommended. However, if the child has a poor appetite and is a faddy eater it is best to use whole milk rather than reduced fat milks. Not more than half to three quarters of a litre of milk a day is necessary. If a child drinks more than this then it can spoil its appetite for other foods needed to balance the diet.

Summary

- Breastfeeding is best for young babies.
- Infants and toddlers do not need sugar or salt added to their food, and it can cause problems.
- Toddlers and children need a balanced diet, just like anyone else.
- Dairy foods are particularly important for growing children for the calcium they provide.

Questions

1. There are many reasons for mothers to breastfeed babies. Describe four of them.
2. How does human, cow and goat milk vary in the content of the following nutrients: protein, carbohydrate, calcium, iron?
3. Plan a day's meals suitable for weaning a child.
4. Why is milk a good food for young children?

3.5 The special needs of teenagers

Teenagers are growing and developing fast. To keep up with this they need to eat more food than many adults. They therefore have much bigger **appetites** (Fig. 1). This means quite often that as a teenager you will be eating not only your three meals or snacks a day but often between meals. It is really important to look at what you are eating and make sure that you are getting the right balance of nutrients. If you are doing a lot of sport or physical activity then you may need more food than other people.

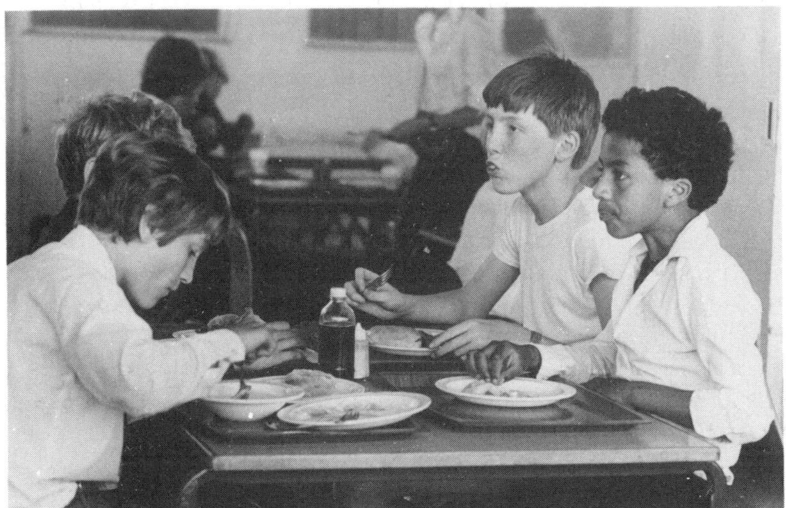

Fig. 1 Teenagers need to eat well

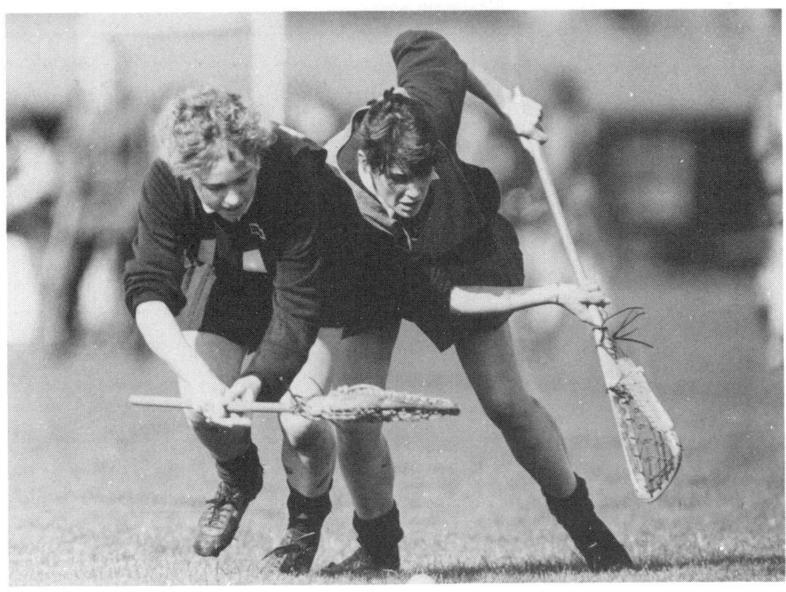

Fig. 2 Young women must eat a lot of iron-containing foods

The specific needs of young women

In their early teens most women begin to **menstruate**. This means that regularly each month they lose blood. Blood contains iron, so the blood loss also results in an **iron loss** from the body. This iron needs replacing in the diet and if it is not then they will become anaemic. It is important therefore for young women who are menstruating to make sure that they eat plenty of foods which are rich in iron (see pages 80–1), particularly if they are active (Fig. 2).

Many young women are also taking the **contraceptive pill**. This pill may increase their requirements for vitamin B6 (pyridoxine) and vitamin C. Young women taking the pill should make sure that their diet contains plenty of these nutrients (see pages 90–1, 100).

It is also particularly important for young women who are thinking of becoming pregnant to take special care of their diets. A poor diet before or at the time of conception may have an effect on the baby when it is born. Women who are in a poor nutritional state at the time of conception are more likely to have small or sick babies.

Obesity and anorexia nervosa

Many teenagers are concerned about the way they look. They are also often under pressure from exams, want to do well and are worried generally about the way they fit in with their friends and how they are getting on. The result of this **emotional stress** can often be either over or under eating.

Many people who are under pressure, worried or depressed turn to food for comfort. They feel they get some satisfaction from food and often eat relatively large amounts of sugary or fatty foods. Eventually they become **obese** (overweight) and it can be very hard to get back to normal healthy eating habits.

Some people go the other way and stop

eating almost completely. They may be suffering from **anorexia nervosa**. Anorexia nervosa is often connected with self-image. However thin the sufferers get, they imagine they are fat and continue dieting. Anorexics may eat a lot of food and then force themselves to be sick, or they may take laxatives or purgatives to ensure their gut does not absorb the food. Anorexia nervosa is a very serious psychological condition and it needs professional help. It can be fatal and sufferers have been known to literally starve themselves to death.

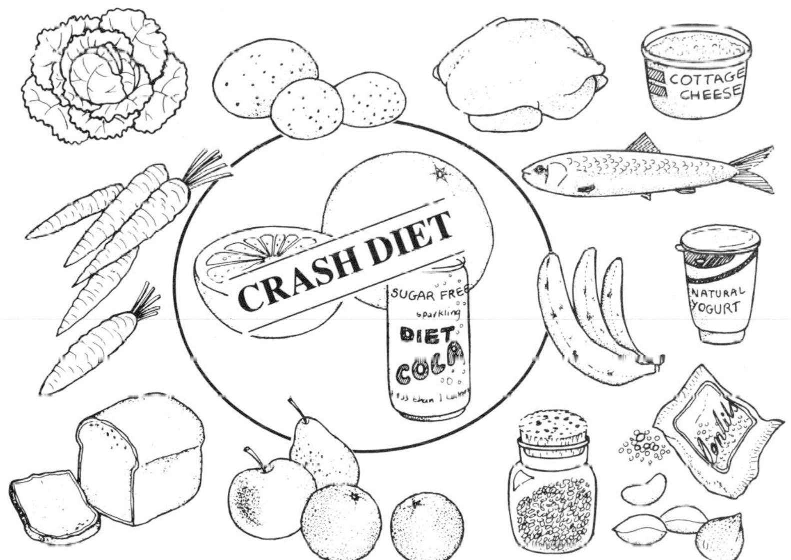

Fig. 3 Crash diets are not a good idea

Teenagers who are trying to lose weight often cut down on their diets quite considerably. They tend to go on **crash diets** (Fig. 3). These mean that they cut out not only the unimportant foods but the important foods as well. The amount of nutrients in the diet is severely decreased and anaemia and other problems can result. Crash diets are not a good idea. If you want to lose weight, then try to eat a healthy balanced diet containing plenty of low energy density foods which also have a high nutrient density (see page 124). Weight which is lost quickly is usually put back on again quickly. The most successful way of losing weight, and keeping it off, is by gradual but permanent dietary changes.

Summary

- Teenagers who are growing fast need to eat plenty to satisfy their appetites.
- Teenagers need a well balanced diet just like anyone else.
- Young women need more iron containing foods after they have started menstruating.
- Young women on the contraceptive pill may have higher requirements of some of the B vitamins and vitamin C.
- Obesity and anorexia nervosa may be problems for teenagers.

Questions

1. Which nutrients may be eaten in insufficient quantities by the following groups of people?
   (a) young women
   (b) some women using the contraceptive pill
2. Write a few sentences about (a) anorexia nervosa, (b) obesity.
3. Why are crash diets not a good idea?
4. What is the best way to lose some weight and maintain this lower weight?

3.6 The special needs of women who are pregnant or breastfeeding

It is important that at the time of conception a woman's body is in a good nutritional state. Diet before conception is therefore very important if the baby is to be healthy.

Pregnancy

During pregnancy a woman's needs for **dietary energy** and most **nutrients** are increased. Small increases in the amount of protein and B group vitamins are required. Larger increases in the amount of folic acid (one of the B group vitamins), vitamin C, iron, vitamin D and calcium are also required. Usually by satisfying her increased appetite a woman will have sufficient of most of the nutrients. However, the increased dietary energy needs are not as great as the increased need for some of the nutrients. Therefore it is important that a **nutrient dense diet** is consumed. Special care should be taken to include plenty of fruit and vegetables, foods providing calcium, vitamin D and iron. Iron and folate tablets are usually given to pregnant women.

The amount of weight women put on when they are pregnant varies from one woman to another (Fig. 1). Average weight gain is around 12.5 kilograms. Extra weight gain resulting from eating more food than is really needed should be avoided. If a woman feels she is putting on too much weight she should be particularly careful not to eat many foods which are high in fat or sugar. She should not go on a strict slimming diet. This can make her feel tired and lethargic and is not a good thing for the baby.

Most women while they are pregnant are also advised to give up smoking and drinking alcohol. It is the first few months of pregnancy which are the most

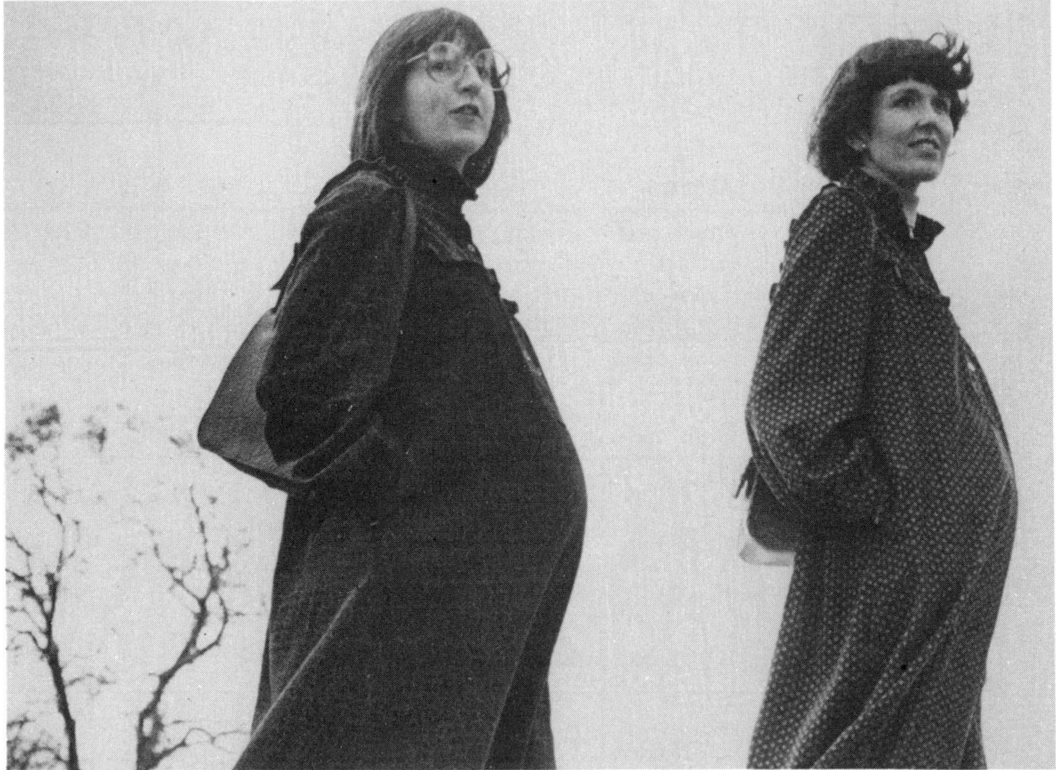

Fig. 1 These pregnant women will put on different amounts of weight

important and this is the time when women do not necessarily know that they are pregnant. If a women is trying to get pregnant then she should take special care not only over her diet but also over her consumption of alcohol and cigarettes (Fig. 2).

No wonder smokers cough
The tar and discharge that collects in the lung of an average smoker.
HEALTH EDUCATION COUNCIL

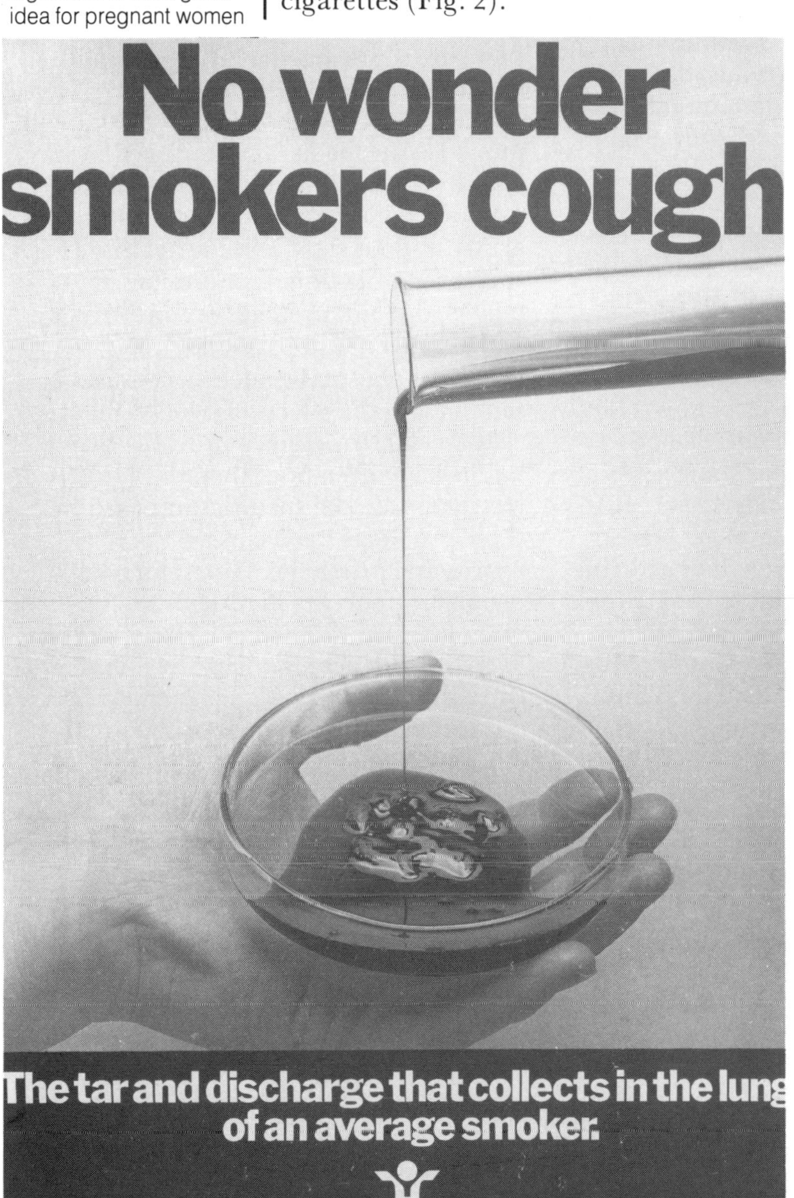

Fig. 2 Smoking cigarettes is not a good idea for pregnant women

Nutritional needs of women while they are breastfeeding

The production of milk by women for breastfeeding is also called **lactation**. When a woman is breastfeeding a baby, her diet is particularly important. Her requirements for dietary energy, calcium, protein, iron, folates (a B vitamin), nicotinic acid, vitamins A, C and D and water are all increased. She needs to eat plenty of fruit and vegetables with a good variety of foods from each of the food groups. Sugary and fatty foods should only be eaten if plenty of foods from the other four groups have been included. It is important that women who are breastfeeding drink plenty of fluid – more than normal. If there is any doubt about the diet it might be necessary for the woman to take vitamin supplements or for the baby to be given vitamin drops.

Many women do put on extra weight when they have been pregnant or have been previously overweight. They may decide to try and lose weight while they are breastfeeding. This can cause problems. Tiredness and a reduced milk supply can result. It is not a good idea. Much of the extra weight put on during pregnancy will be lost while breastfeeding anyway. The fat stored during pregnancy is there specifically for providing milk during breastfeeding.

Summary

- The nutritional state of a woman at the time of conception may be very important to the health of her baby.
- Diets during pregnancy and breastfeeding need to be more nutrient dense than at other times.
- Going on a slimming diet during pregnancy or when breastfeeding is not advisable.

Questions

1. Which nutrients are particularly important during pregnancy?
2. How much weight (roughly) should a woman gain during pregnancy?
3. What should be avoided during pregnancy?
4. What is meant by lactation?
5. Which nutrients are important during breastfeeding?

3.7 | *The special needs of the elderly*

As people get older they generally become less physically active. At the same time, their appetites become smaller and they eat less food. However, despite the fact that their requirements for dietary energy have reduced, their needs for all vitamins and minerals stay the same and in some cases they even increase. Elderly people need therefore to make sure that they have a diet which is relatively nutrient dense.

The nutritional needs of the elderly

A healthy balanced diet chosen from the four main food groups (see page 21) will meet the nutritional needs of most elderly people. However, the choice of foods must be made carefully as some foods are more difficult for some elderly people to eat than others. For example, a person with poorly fitting false teeth or arthritis might find it very difficult to eat an apple or to peel an orange. Fruit juice may therefore be a suitable alternative. Milk is also a very important food for many elderly people. Its relative cheapness, ease of use and high nutrient density are all useful.

Problems which might arise

Most elderly people are able to eat normal well balanced diets. However there are some, particularly those with low incomes, who are more likely to have difficulties. It may be difficult actually to purchase the foods that they need to stay healthy. Other difficulties may include isolation and physical disabilities such as arthritis, poor sight and immobility (Fig.1). Increased nutritional requirements may be due to the effects of some drugs and laxatives, and psychological problems may arise, such as confusion, senility and the effects of bereavement.

If an elderly person's previous eating habits have been poor then the restrictions and difficulties imposed by these problems may cause greater nutritional problems. Once elderly people begin to get slightly malnourished, they then have less energy to go out and get food and a vicious circle can result.

Most of the nutritional problems of elderly people arise as a result of social problems. Elderly people living in their

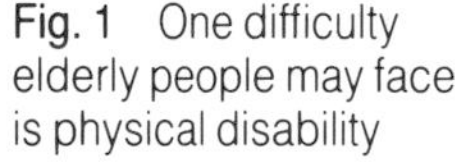

Fig. 1 One difficulty elderly people may face is physical disability

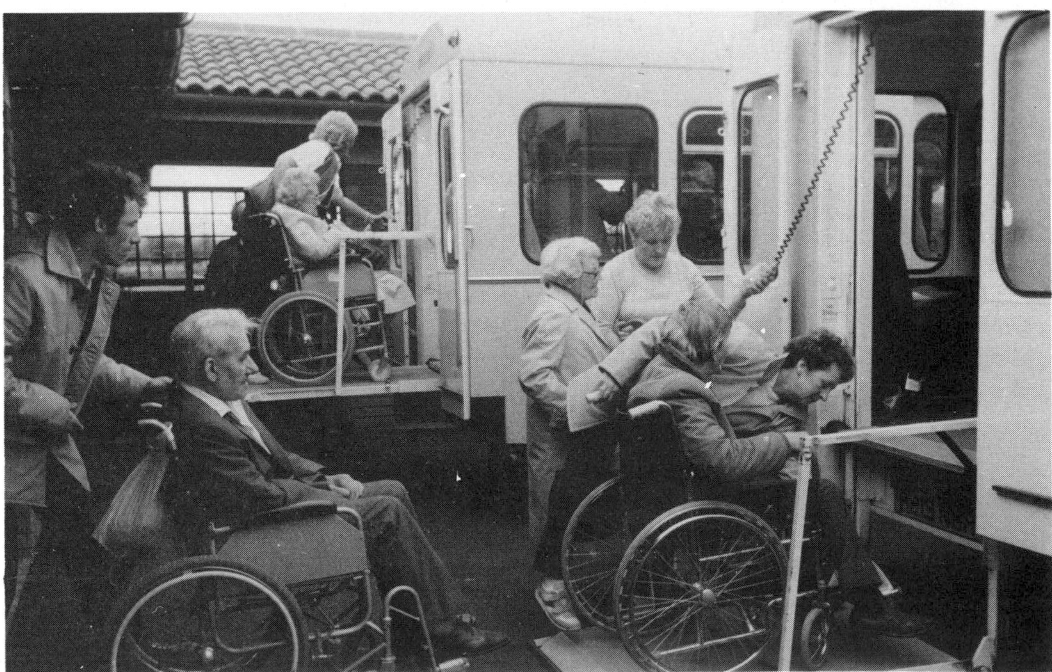

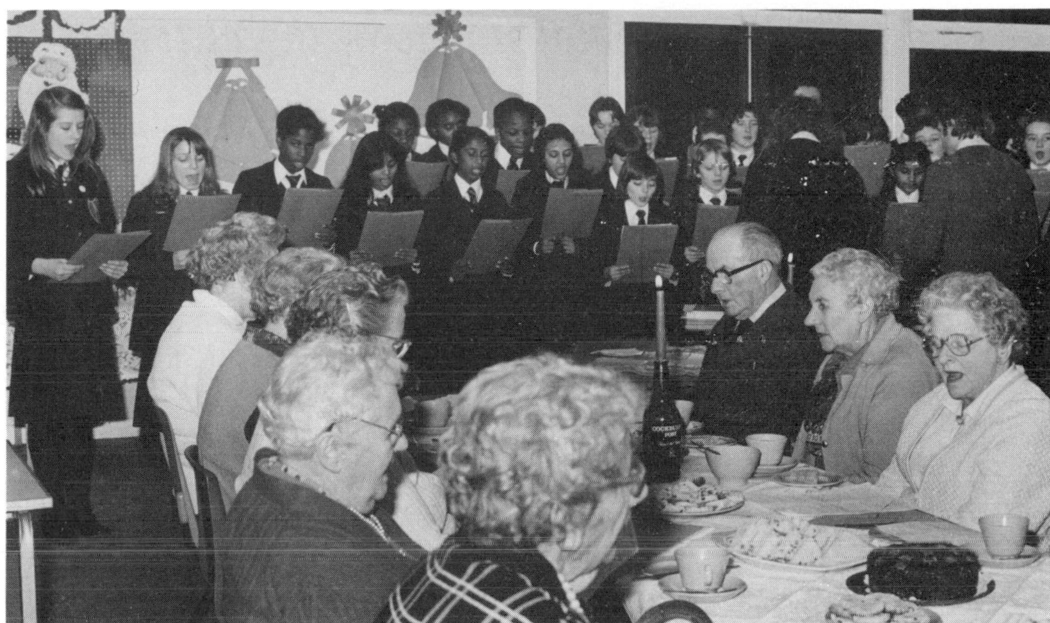

Fig. 2 A luncheon club

own homes are often on restricted incomes and reluctant to spend a good deal on food. They may also neglect their diet due to loneliness and lack of interest. Luncheon clubs help overcome some of these problems (Fig. 2).

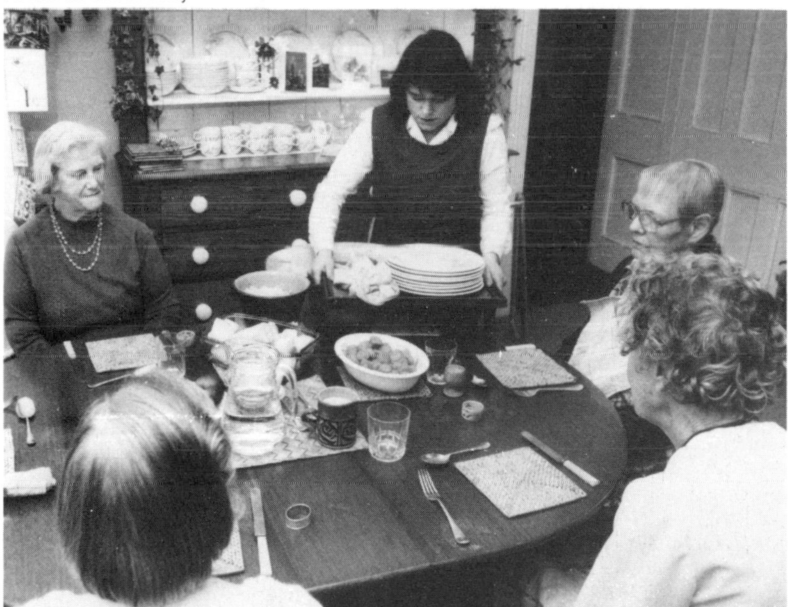

Fig. 3 A residential home for the elderly

Residential homes for the elderly vary in the quality of food they provide (Fig. 3). Food may well be prepared and cooked in large quantities. Such institutional catering may not provide ideal food for people with small appetites and particular dietary needs.

There are some particular nutritional hazards for older people: **scurvy** resulting from lack of vitamin C, **osteomalacia** resulting from lack of vitamin D and **anaemia** resulting from the lack of folates and iron. These are all nutritional problems found amongst elderly people in the UK.

Summary

- Elderly people tend to have small appetites but need the same amounts or possibly more of some nutrients.
- Their diets need to be more nutrient dense.
- Physical difficulties and social isolation can affect the diets of many elderly people.

Questions

1. Why is it important for elderly people to have a nutrient dense diet?
2. What conditions might make it difficult for the elderly to eat a good diet?
3. Which nutrients are specially important for elderly people?
4. Plan a suitable balanced meal for an elderly person with a poor appetite.

3.8 | The special needs of vegetarians and vegans

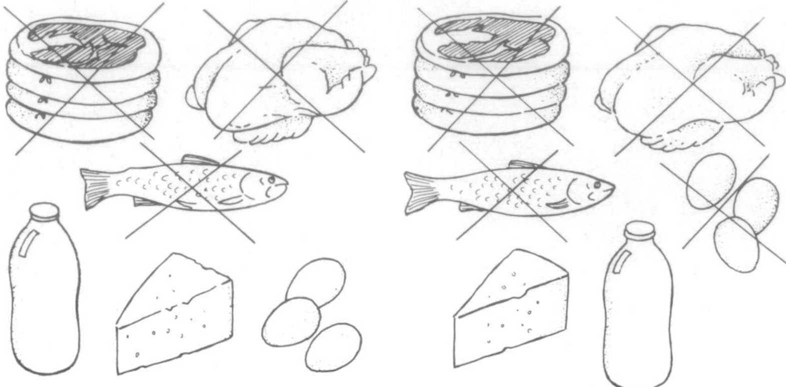

Fig. 1 Lacto-ovo-vegetarianism

Fig. 2 Lacto-vegetarianism

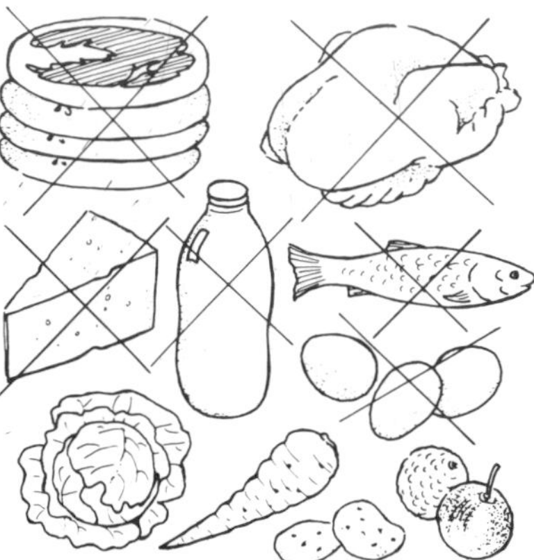

Fig. 3 Veganism

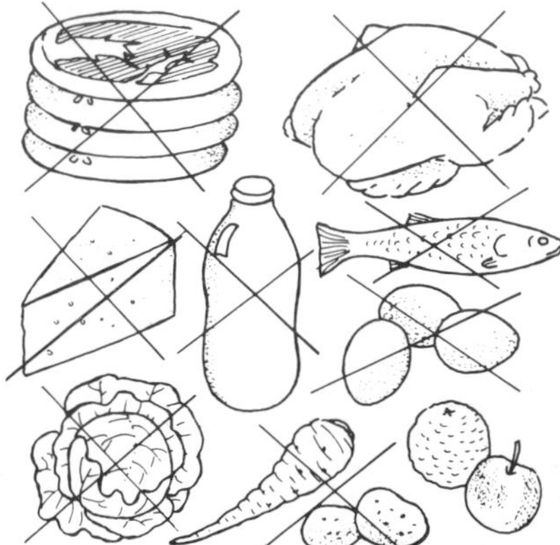

Fig. 4 Fruitarianism

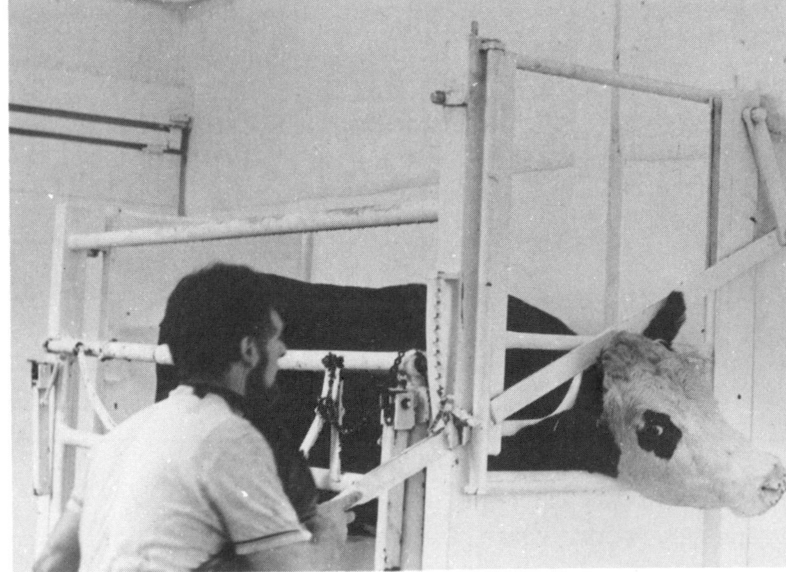

Fig. 5 This cow will be slaughtered to provide meat

There are many different types of vegetarians. Some only avoid red meat, while others eat no animal products whatsoever. **Lacto-ovo-vegetarians** eat no meat, fish or poultry, but they do include milk, milk products and eggs in their diets (Fig. 1). **Lacto-vegetarians** do not include meat, fish, poultry or eggs, but they will include milk and milk products (Fig. 2). **Vegans** eat no foods from animal sources whatsoever. Their complete diet consists of foods from plant sources (Fig. 3). **Fruitarians** are people who eat no vegetables, cereals or pulses and only fruits. These are the most extreme types of vegetarian (Fig. 4).

Reasons for being vegetarian

People have many different reasons for being vegetarian. Usually it is because they do not want to eat foods which have caused suffering or death to animals (Fig. 5). Others are vegetarian because they feel that meat consumption is more costly in terms of land use and the environment than vegetable consumption. For example, to produce large quantities of meat, grains and pulses are often used to feed the animals (Fig. 6). This is a very inefficient way of using food which could be eaten directly by humans. A few people feel that being vegetarian is more healthy than not. Some studies show that people who are vegan are more healthy than meat-eaters. Fruitarians are the type of vegetarian most likely to run into nutritional problems, as their diet is very limited.

The nutritional needs of vegetarians

The more foods that are cut out, the more important the **combinations** of those foods that are eaten become. It is possible for vegetarians to fulfil all their nutritional requirements, but great care needs to be taken in choosing the foods.

When all animal foods are excluded, as with vegans, it is usually necessary to take a **supplement** of vitamin B12.

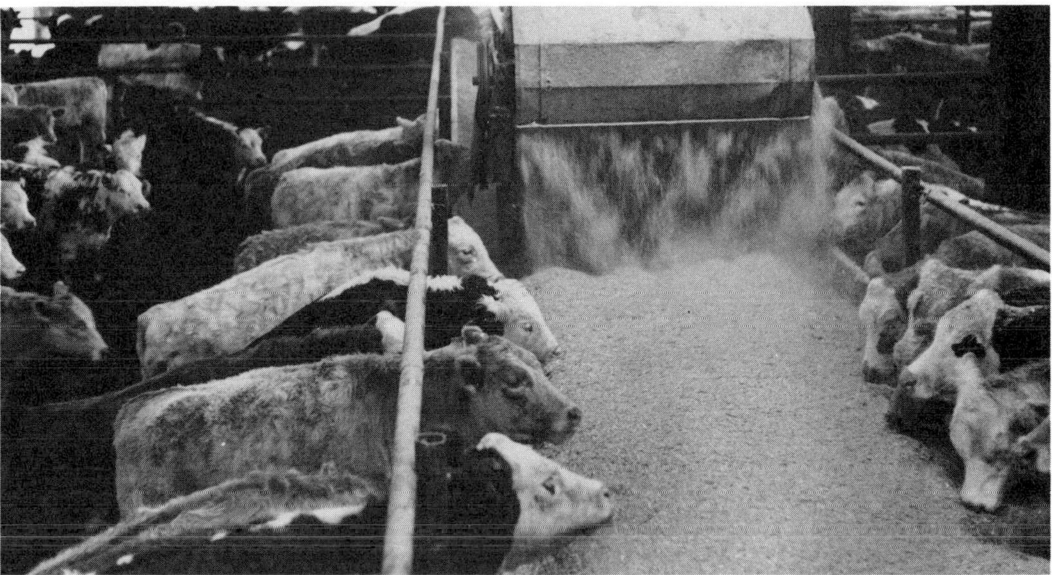

Fig. 6 Cattle are fed large quantities of grain and pulses

Vitamin B12 is not generally found in plant foods, although a few plant foods from the Far East made from fermented soya beans may contain some vitamin B12. These foods are not easily available in the UK and are unreliable sources. Vegans should therefore take a regular supplement of vitamin B12. If very few or no animal foods are eaten then care has to be taken to get the right combinations of plant foods to get the best nutrients. The protein in cereal foods complements the protein found in pulses to give protein similar to that found in meat. If the cereal and pulses are eaten at different times, however, this does not occur.

People on fruitarian diets are likely to run into nutritional problems quite quickly. These diets are definitely unadvisable for growing children.

Choosing a balanced diet

Lacto- and ovo-vegetarians may not have nutritional difficulties as long as they eat a variety of foods and include foods from all the four main food groups. Vegans, however, have to be much more careful. They have to include a wide variety of foods, such as cereals, pulses, leafy vegetables, nuts and fruits, because restricting to one or two kinds of food may lead to nutritional difficulties.

The iron in vegetable foods is not as well absorbed as the iron in meat. Some vegetarians therefore run the risk of become anaemic. However, a well balanced vegetarian or vegan diet can provide plenty of iron.

Summary

- It is possible to eat a balanced diet containing little or no animal foods.
- Careful food choice is necessary to ensure all the nutrients are present.
- Vitamin supplements may be necessary for some types of vegetarians.

Questions

1. Explain how vegetarian and vegan diets differ.
2. Why do vegetarian diets need careful planning?
3. Which nutrients are most likely to be in short supply in a vegetarian diet?
4. Plan a day's diet suitable for a 16-year-old vegetarian which would supply the RDAs for all nutrients.

SECTION 4 The nutrients in our food

4.1 | Dietary energy

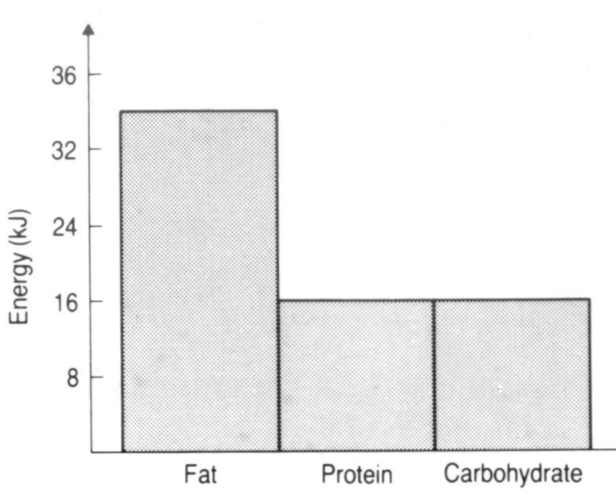

Fig. 1 Bar chart to show the energy provided per gram of fat, protein and carbohydrate

A jacket potato
Weight = 200 g
Energy = 728 kJ

A boiled egg
Weight = 50 g
Energy = 306 kJ

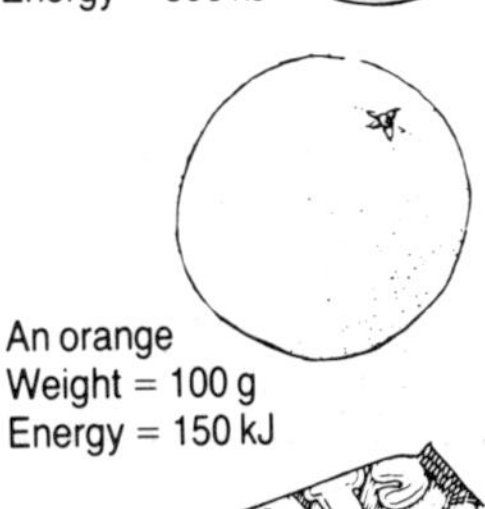

An orange
Weight = 100 g
Energy = 150 kJ

A Mars bar
Weight = 68 g
Energy 1,260 kJ

Fig. 2 The energy provided by different foods

In order for our bodies to work we must have a source of **energy**. In the same way as a car requires petrol to provide the energy it needs to move, and a fridge and cooker need gas or electricity to make them work, so the human body needs **fuel**. We need energy to fuel all the chemical reactions in our bodies, to allow our muscles to contract and to keep our body temperature even. This energy comes from our food. The food you eat is broken down by your body and is eventually used as fuel to be 'burnt up' in your muscles. The energy is stored in the chemical bonds of the fat, carbohydrate and protein molecules (Fig. 1). In order for the energy to be released, **oxygen** must be present. This comes from the air we breathe in.

Different types of food give us different amounts of dietary energy (Fig. 2).

The rate at which our bodies use up energy is called our **metabolic rate**. Even when we are fast asleep, our bodies still use up energy. Our hearts, lungs, brains, digestive systems and many other bodily activities are working and using energy. The rate at which energy is used to keep all this happening is called the **basal metabolic rate** (BMR).

In working out our BMR we need to know what our body mass is as well as the total surface area of our body. The BMR is about 160 kJ per square metre of body surface per hour for men and about 150 kJ for women. This is approximately 4.7 kJ per kg per hour for both.

Everybody is different but there are some general recommendations about how much dietary energy we are likely to need to get from our diets. These are called **Recommended Daily Amounts** (see p. 12).

People can check their right weight for their height by looking at standard height/weight tables. These are designed for people who are 18 years and over and have stopped growing. Special height/weight charts exist for children and teenagers. On these you have to take into account age and sex as well as height and weight. They are called **growth charts** (Fig. 3).

Keeping your weight right for your height is called being in **energy balance**, i.e. your diet is providing the same amount of energy as you are using. If you are getting thinner you are using up more energy than your diet is providing and you are said to be in **negative energy balance**. If you are getting fatter you are said to be in **positive energy balance**, because your diet is providing more energy than you are using and your body is storing the extra as fat.

Groups of people have different energy needs depending on their size, sex and the amount of physical activity they do. For example, the dietary energy recommendations for an 18- to 34-year-old man are as follows:

Sedentary e.g. office job with little other exercise – 10.5 MJ per day;

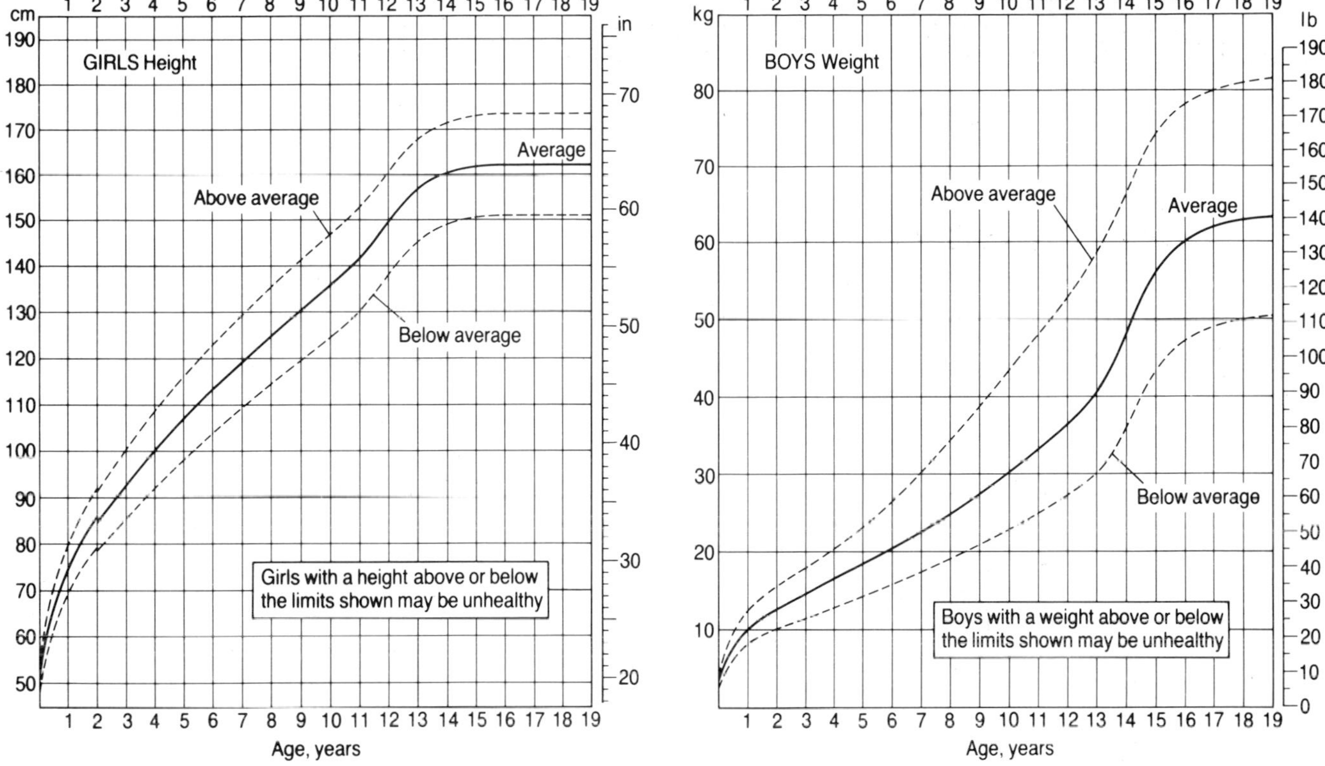

Fig. 3 Growth charts

Moderately active e.g. office job but taking some exercise – 12.0 MJ per day;
Very active e.g. work involves heavy manual labour, such as manually digging coal from the coal face – 14.0 MJ per day.

Some examples of the amount of dietary energy required for different activities are:

Activities	*kJ per hour* (approx.)
Sleeping	150
Sitting quietly	190
Playing football	1200
Riding a bicycle	1030
Swimming	1470
Walking up stairs	2570

The requirement for **salt** also depends on the amount of physical activity involved in the work. The more activity, the greater the need. This is related to the amount of sweat produced. Salt is lost from the body in sweat. If too much is lost, muscle cramps will result.

Summary

- A healthy balanced diet keeps a person in energy balance at their optimum weight.
- Requirements for dietary energy depend on age, sex, physiological state and activity levels.
- Salt requirements vary with activity and the amount of sweat produced.

Questions

1. How much dietary energy is contained in (a) 5 g fat, (b) 5 g carbohydrate?
2. Explain what is meant by Basal Metabolic Rate (BMR).
3. How would you know if your body was in (a) positive energy balance, (b) energy balance?
4. How much energy is used for each of the following activities: (a) sleeping, (b) riding a bicycle, (c) swimming?

4.2 Carbohydrates

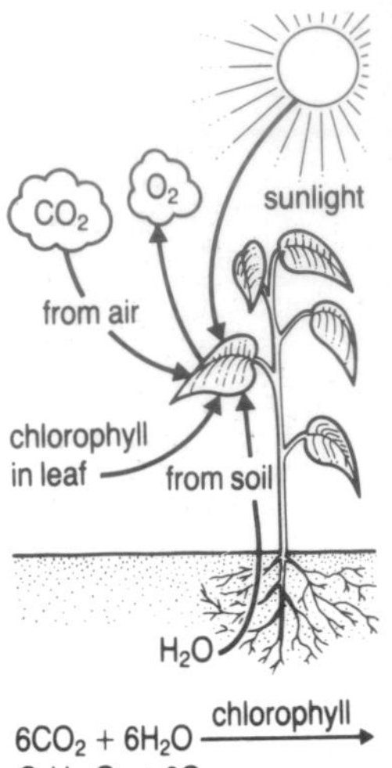

$6CO_2 + 6H_2O \xrightarrow{\text{chlorophyll}} C_6H_{12}O_6 + 6O_2$

Fig. 1 Photosynthesis

All carbohydrates have the same basic chemical structure. They consist of **carbon**, **hydrogen** and **oxygen**, containing twice as much hydrogen as oxygen. They are produced in green plants by the action of sunlight on the green pigment in the plant called **chlorophyll**. This process is called **photosynthesis** (Fig. 1). The energy from the sun's rays is used by the plants chemically to convert water, from the plant, and carbon dioxide, from the air, into glucose (a carbohydrate) and oxygen. The oxygen is then released back into the air and the glucose is converted, by the plant, into other types of carbohydrate.

$6CO_2$ (six molecules of carbon dioxide) + $6H_2O$ (six molecules of water) $\xrightarrow{\text{photo-synthesis}}$ $C_6H_{12}O_6$ (one molecule of glucose) + $6O_2$ (six molecules of oxygen)

Carbohydrates are one of the main sources of dietary energy. They are also known as **saccharides** and are classified according to the number of saccharide units they contain. They have different functions in the body (Fig. 2). The three main types of carbohydrate in the diet are **sugars**, **starches** and **dietary fibre**.

Sugars

The most simple carbohydrates are **monosaccharides** (i.e. they are made up of single saccharide units). They are also known as 'simple sugars'. **Glucose** is found in small quantities in fruit and vegetables, **fructose** in fruit and **galactose** in milk.

The most common saccharide we know is a **disaccharide**, **sucrose**. This is what we call **sugar**. It occurs naturally in sugar cane and sugar beet (Fig. 3) and is extracted, refined and used very widely in food processing and as a sweetener. Sucrose is also found naturally in some fruits. The other commonly found disaccharide is **lactose**, which is found in milk. **Maltose**, the third disaccharide, does not occur naturally in many foods.

All these disaccharides are made of pairs of monosaccharides joined together in a simple chemical reaction.

monosaccharide	**+ monosaccharide**	**= disaccharide**
glucose	+ fructose	= sucrose
glucose	+ glucose	= maltose
glucose	+ galactose	= lactose

The names of all these sugars end in the letters OSE. Any nutrient or substance added to food during processing ending with the letters OSE is a type of sugar or carbohydrate.

Starch

Starch is a **polysaccharide** and is made up of a complicated chain of glucose units. It is contained in cereals and starchy vegetables in the form of granules (Fig. 4). The size and shape of the granule varies according to the source of the starch. Each granule consists of many millions of starch molecules. There are two kinds of starch molecule. One is a straight chain and is called **amylose**, the other is a branched chain and is called **amylopectin**.

Starch in foods is usually found in combination with dietary fibre. Food processing and refining can alter this natural balance.

Fig. 2 Classification of carbohydrates

MONOSACCHARIDES (1 saccharide unit)
- PENTOSE (5 carbon atoms) → Component of dietary fibre
- HEXOSE (6 carbon atoms) → Glucose (fruit, vegetables), Fructose (fruit), Galactose (milk)

DISACCHARIDES (2 saccharide units)
- SUCROSE (Glucose + Fructose) Extracted from sugar cane, and beet. Found in fruit and vegetables
- MALTOSE (Glucose + Glucose) Breakdown of starch, e.g. in malting of barley.
- LACTOSE (Glucose + Galactose) Milk.

POLYSACCHARIDES (Many saccharide units)
- STARCH (manufactured by plants)
  DEXTRINS (breakdown of starch)
  GLYCOGEN (annimal equivalent of starch)
- DIETARY FIBRES:
  Cellulose (plant cells)
  Hemicellulose (plant cells)
  Lignin (woody tissue)
  Pectin (soft tissues of fruit and vegetables)
  Gum (plant tissues)

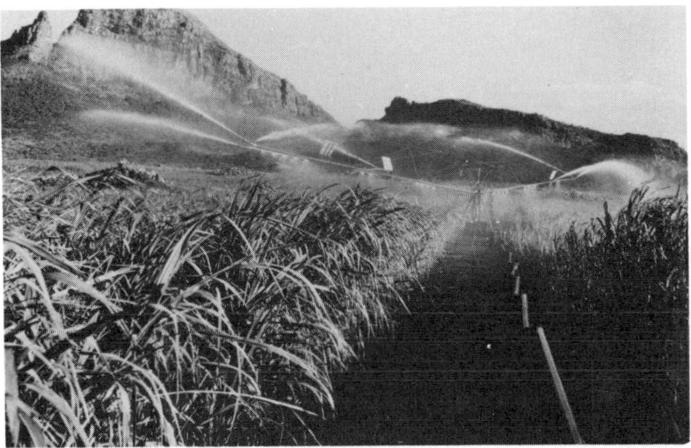

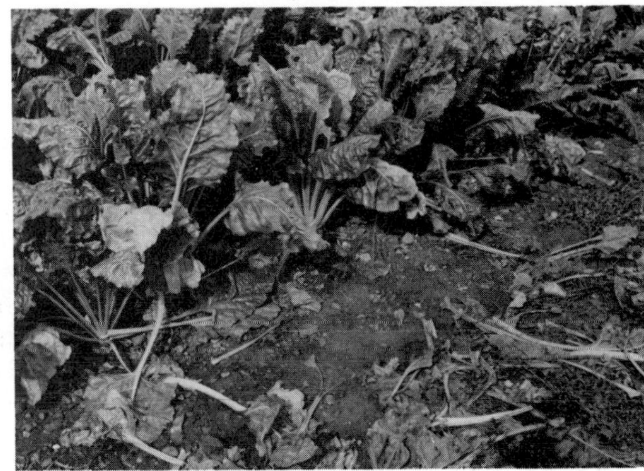

Fig. 3 (a) Sugar cane, (b) sugar beet

Glycogen

Glycogen is also a polysaccharide. Apart from glucose, it is the only carbohydrate found in the bodies of animals, including humans. It is a carbohydrate store in the liver and muscles which can be turned rapidly into glucose for use by the body.

Dietary fibre

The most complicated carbohydrates are known collectively as dietary fibre. Dietary fibre is a mixture of substances. There is cellulose and hemicellulose (the cell wall of plants), lignin (the woody part of plants), pectin (the soft tissue from fruit and vegetables) and gum (also from plants). Pentoses are also a useful form of dietary fibre. Unlike most other foods dietary fibre is not digested in the **small intestine**. It passes, relatively unchanged, into the **colon**, where evidence suggests it is partially broken down by the gut flora and fauna. Dietary fibre helps to keep the gut healthy.

cellulose cell wall

starch granules

Fig. 4 Starch granules in raw potato

Specific RDAs do not exist for carbohydrates, but current nutrition guidelines recommend average intakes of dietary fibre and sugar (sucrose) for the whole population. Within these averages there will be wide variations between individuals and groups of people. NACNE recommend that over the next 15 years people should try to achieve an average sugar intake of not more than 20 kg per head per year. This is approximately half the estimated current intake. The recommended intake of dietary fibre for the whole population is approximately 30 g. Current intakes are estimated at around 20 g.

Summary

- Carbohydrates are made by plants during photosynthesis.
- Carbohydrates are a major energy source.
- The body uses different types of carbohydrate in different ways. Some types may be harmful, others beneficial.

Questions

1. Explain how sugar is made by green plants.
2. Copy and complete this chart

Monosaccharide + Monosaccharide		=	....
Glucose	+	=	Sucrose
....	+ Galactose	=	....

3. In what form is sugar stored in the liver?
4. What is dietary fibre?
5. Describe a starch granule.

4.3 Fats

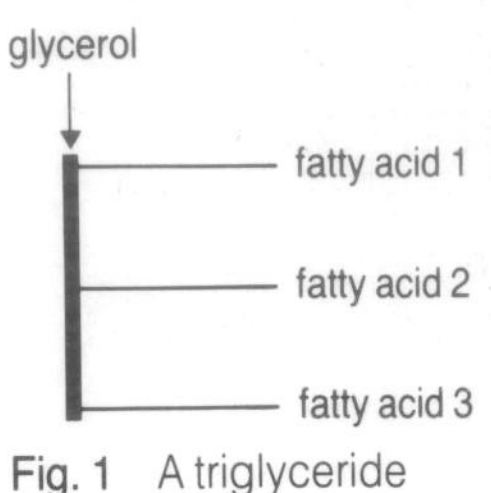

Fig. 1 A triglyceride

Fats are the other main energy source in the diet. They also carry with them some important vitamins. Like carbohydrates, fats contain carbon, hydrogen and oxygen, but in different proportions. Fats are made up of units called **triglycerides**. A triglyceride consists of a molecule of an alcohol called **glycerol**, which is attached to three molecules of **fatty acids** (Fig. 1).

The actual fatty acids present have an important effect on the way the fat behaves both before and after it is eaten. Fatty acids contain long chains of carbon (and hydrogen) atoms. They have an acid group at one end. The length of the carbon chain determines the type of fat, and it can vary from 4 to 24 carbon atoms long. Each fat is given a shorthand name based on the number of carbon atoms it contains. For example butyric acid, which is a 'short chain fatty acid', contains only 4 carbon atoms and is known as C4:O (the O refers to the number of double bonds – see below). Stearic acid (C18:O) contains 18 carbon atoms and is a 'long chain fatty acid'.

```
  H H H ¦  O  ¦
  | | | ¦ //  ¦
H-C-C-C-C     ├── Acid group
  | | | ¦ \   ¦
  H H H ¦  O-H¦
```

Butyric acid (found in butter) (C4:O)

```
  H H H H H H H H H H H H H H H H H   O
  | | | | | | | | | | | | | | | | |  //
H-C-C-C-C-C-C-C-C-C-C-C-C-C-C-C-C-C-C
  | | | | | | | | | | | | | | | | |  \
  H H H H H H H H H H H H H H H H H   O-H
```

Stearic acid (C18:O)

Fatty acids are divided into three main types.

Saturated fatty acids have each of the carbon atoms (except the end two) attached to two hydrogen atoms, e.g. stearic acid (C18:O) above. They are the most **stable** types of fatty acids and are solid at room temperature. A diet high in saturated fatty acids seems to increase the risk of developing **heart disease**. The mechanism for this is not fully understood but is discussed later in the book (see page 121).

Monounsaturated fatty acids have two hydrogen atoms missing. The spare bond this causes is attached to the next carbon atom. This creates what is known as a 'double bond'. Double bonds are not very stable.

```
  H H H H H H H H H H H H H H H H H   O
  | | | | | | | | | | | | | | | | |  //
H-C-C-C-C-C-C-C-C-C=C-C-C-C-C-C-C-C-C
  | | | | | | | |     | | | | | | | \
  H H H H H H H H     H H H H H H H H O-H
```

Oleic acid (C18:1) double bond

Polyunsaturated fatty acids contain more than one double bond. They are quite **unstable** and tend to be liquid at room temperature. They can easily become saturated by repeated heating, e.g. when using the same oil for cooking chips. In this process, the double bonds are broken and hydrogen atoms join onto the 'open' bonds so that the fatty acids become saturated.

```
  H H H H H H H H H H H H H H H H H   O
  | | | | | | | | | | | | | | | | |  //
H-C-C-C-C-C-C-C-C-C=C-C-C-C=C-C-C-C-C
  | | | | | | | |     | |     | | | \
  H H H H H H H H     H H     H H H   O-H
```

Linoleic acid (C18:2)

Most fatty acids needed in the body can be made from others. However, there are a few which cannot. These are called **essential fatty acids** and must be present in the diet. These may be important in protecting the body against heart disease. The proportion of each type of fatty acid in different fats varies (Fig. 2).

Cholesterol is a substance in the same chemical group as fat. It is found in all animal tissues and is present in small amounts in all foods of animal origin. It is necessary for the body and if it does not exist in the diet the body will make its own. The only foods containing significant amounts are egg yolk, shellfish and offal like kidney and liver. Some people believe that eating too much cholesterol is also connected with the high incidence of **heart disease** in this country although this is not generally agreed.

There are no specific RDAs for fat in the UK as there are none for carbohydrates. However, both the NACNE and COMA reports made recommendations about fat. NACNE proposed that over the next 15 years the average fat intake for the whole of the population should drop by about one fifth. At the same time the intake of saturated fatty acids should drop by approximately 45%. COMA recommended that anyone over 5 with a fat intake which provided more than 35% of their dietary energy, or a saturated fat intake providing more than 15% of their dietary energy, should attempt to reduce it to these levels (Fig. 3).

Fig. 2 Foods containing more than 40% of their fat in specific fatty acids

Type of fatty acid	*Dietary fat*	*Foods in which it is found*
Saturated	Animal fats	Meat, meat products, suet, dripping, milk, butter, cheese, cream, some margarine
	Vegetable fats	Coconut, palm oil, some rapeseed
Monounsaturated	Fish	Sardines in oil, tuna in oil
	Animal fats	Dripping, lard, some margarine, meat, meat products, eggs
	Vegetable fats	Some margarine, olive oil, palm oil, peanut oil, avocado pears, olives, most nuts
Polyunsaturated	Cereal fats (only small quantities)	Barley, wheat, oats, rye
	Vegetable fats	Polyunsaturated margarines, cottonseed oil, corn oil, safflower seed oil, sunflower oil, soya oil, walnuts, some rapeseed
	Meat fats	Grouse
	Fish	Herring

Rancidity

When fats or oils 'go rancid' they develop an unpleasant taste and smell. This can occur in two ways.

(a) By **hydrolysis** (addition of water). The fatty acids break away from the glycerol. These free fatty acids are unpleasant tasting and smelly, e.g. butyric acid in rancid butter.

(b) By **oxidation**. Oxygen reacts at the point of the double bond 'using up' these extra bonds. This can happen only in unsaturated fatty acids. Antioxidants are used as preservatives in foods containing fats. They prevent this kind of rancidity.

Summary

- Fats are a major source of dietary energy.
- The way a fat affects the body depends on the type of fatty acids it contains.
- Current dietary guidelines for protection against heart disease recommend cutting down fat intakes.

Questions

1. What is a triglyceride?
2. Describe three differences between fats and oils.
3. Name the three types of fatty acids and suggest two sources of each.
4. Apart from the spreading and cooking fats/oils, where does the fat in your diet come from?

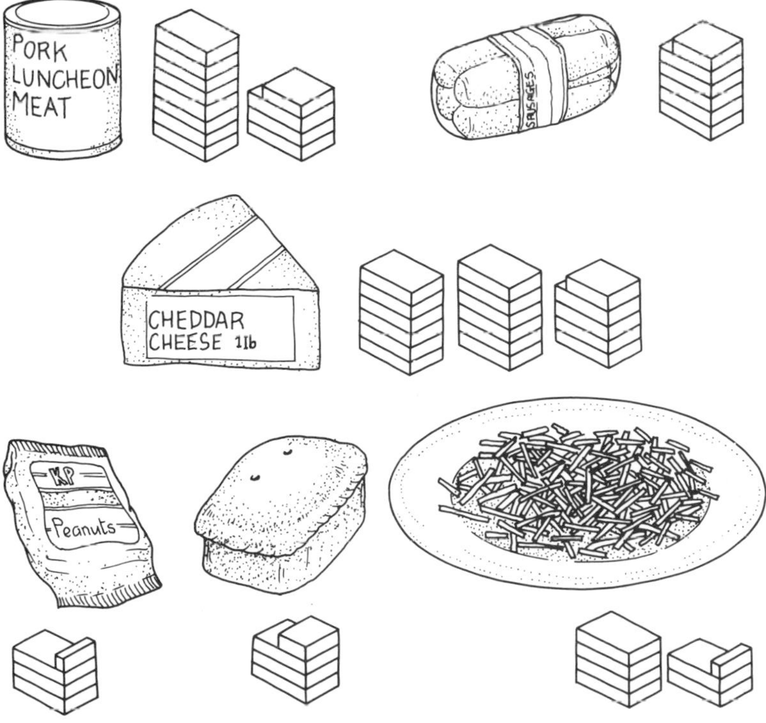

Fig. 3 The amounts of fat contained in some popular foods are shown here by small wedges, each representing 8 grams of fat.

4.4 Protein

Protein is one of the nutrients essential for the **formation, growth** and **repair** of all the muscles and other tissues in the body. It also forms part of the **blood** and the many chemicals which keep our bodies working properly. Every cell in the body contains protein.

Protein needs differ with individuals, but relatively more is needed for growing children and teenagers and for women who are pregnant or breastfeeding. RDAs exist for protein as well as for dietary energy.

The role of protein in the diet

We need protein to build up new tissues and to replace damaged and worn out tissues. It is important in the production of body fluids such as blood, enzymes and hormones, and it is needed to make **antibodies**. Antibodies protect us against infection. Protein is also an energy source.

The structure of protein

Proteins are made up of individual units called **amino acids** (Fig. 1). All amino acids contain hydrogen, carbon, oxygen and nitrogen. Some contain sulphur and/or phosphorus as well. There are thousands of proteins, but there are only 20 commonly found amino acids. These are combined in different ways to make the different proteins. Most of the amino acids can be made in the body from others. Eight cannot. They are called **essential amino acids** and must be present in the diet.

During digestion, the proteins in foods are broken down to their individual amino acids. These are then absorbed into the blood and rebuilt to form different proteins in the body.

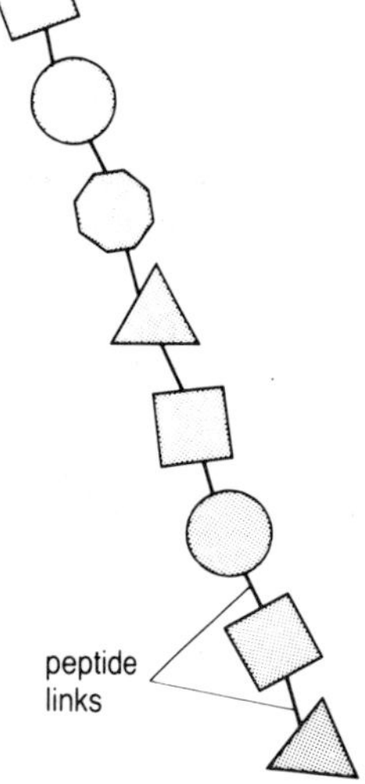

Fig. 1 A chain of amino acids making up part of a protein molecule. The different shapes represent different amino acids

Different types of protein

The actual combination of amino acids in a protein affects the way in which the body will use it. Proteins which are well used by the body are said to have a **high biological value**. Proteins with a biological value of 100 have their amino acids in a combination similar to that found in the proteins in the human body. If the protein in a food is low in one of the essential amino acids, it is said to have a **low biological value** and the one which it lacks is said to be the limiting amino acid. Only a relatively small amount of that protein is used by the body. The rest is wasted. Foods which contain protein with a high biological value are meat, fish, eggs, milk, cheese and soya beans. With the exception of soya beans, the protein in pulses and cereals is of a low biological value. The protein in cereals is low on the amino acid lycine. The protein in pulses is low in sulphur amino acid. However, when cereals and pulses are eaten together the amino acids in the one complement the other. One food makes up what is lacking in the other. The protein in this combination of foods is then of high biological value and just as useful as any protein from animal sources. The cereals and pulses must be eaten at the same meal in order to have this complementary effect. Many traditional and commonly eaten dishes fulfil this need for complementation: for example corn and beans, rice and dahl, wheat and beans, rice and peas, beans and rice, tortilla and beans, and baked beans on toast (Fig. 2).

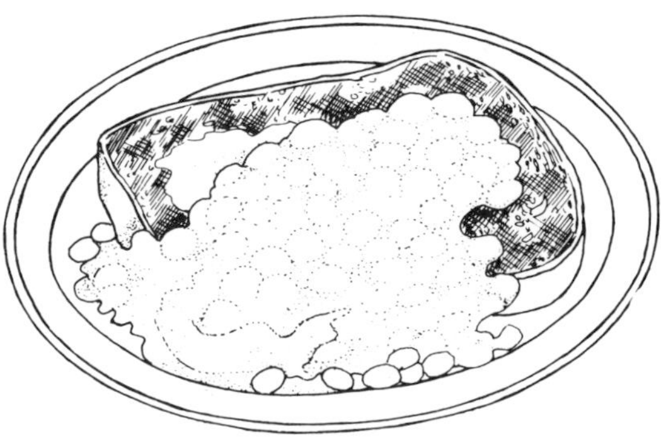

Fig. 2 The proteins in baked beans on toast are complementary

The protein in cereals is also complemented by the protein in milk and milk products in the same way. The biological value of bread and cheese is therefore much higher than the biological value of the protein in a piece of bread.

Nuts and pulses also complement each other.

Fig. 3 This child in Ethiopia is suffering from protein energy malnutrition

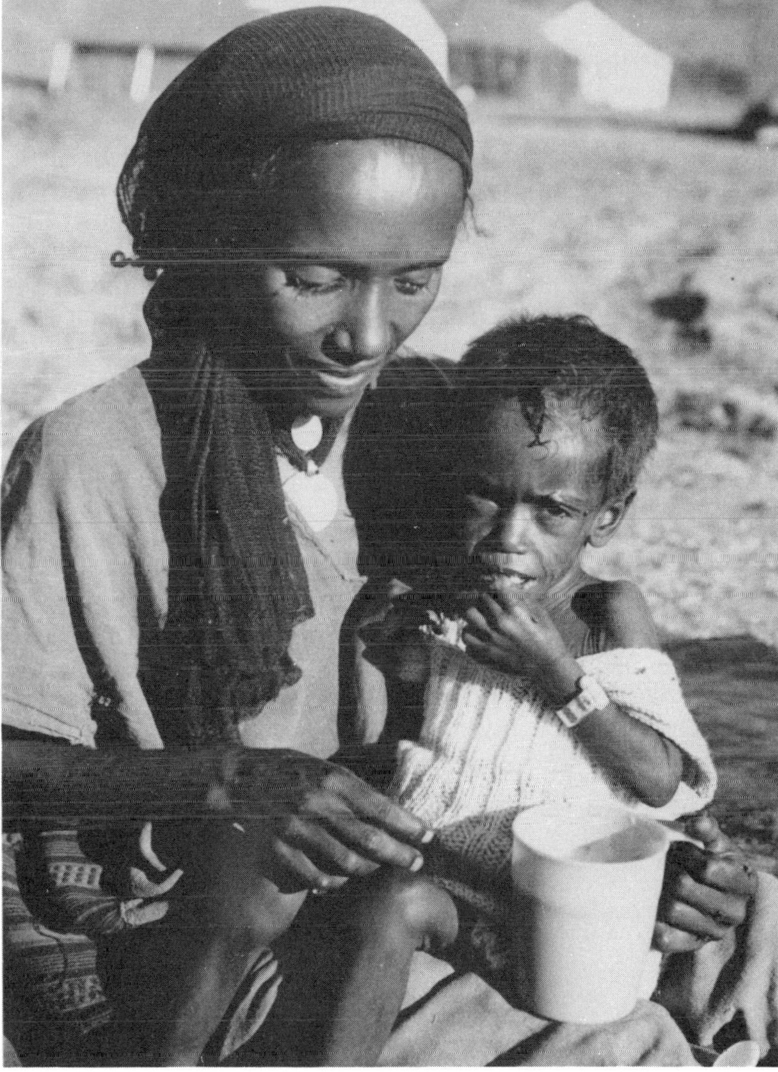

Protein deficiency

Protein deficiency is not found in the UK. It is found in poor parts of the world. This is usually a result of insufficient food rather than insufficient protein. During its **metabolism**, protein gives off energy. So if there is insufficient dietary energy from fat and carbohydrates, protein will be used to provide energy in preference to its use for the growth, maintenance and repair of tissues. This eventually results in **protein energy malnutrition** (PEM) which is an important consideration when famine affects children.

PEM is found mostly in growing children between the ages of two and three years. Growth is retarded, the stomach swells and diarrhoea and infections are common. The skin and hair also become in very poor condition. This is called **kwashiorkor**. Another type of protein energy malnutrition is called **marasmus**. This is most common in infants in their first year in countries where there is famine. It results in wasting of muscles, no body fat, pot bellies and a very thin, sick appearance. Infections and diarrhoea are very common in malnourished children. These conditions can be cured if sufficient food is made available (Fig. 3).

Summary

- Protein is necessary for growth, repair and the maintenance of tissues.
- Protein from vegetable foods needs to be eaten in specific combinations to get the best value from it.
- Protein deficiency is not found in the UK.

Questions

1. What is your own RDA for protein?
2. Which groups have a particular need for extra protein?
3. What is meant by the term 'essential amino acids'?
4. What is meant by 'complementary proteins'? In what ways do traditional meals provide complementary proteins?
5. Describe how protein is used in the body if the food intake is low. What disease results from this poor diet?

4.5 Protein-calorie deficiency

A diet containing adequate quantities of protein and calories is essential for normal mental and physical development of children. If children under five suffer from a lack of either protein or calories, they are frequently stunted for life.

Children in poorer countries are particularly vulnerable to malnutrition and are likely to slip into **cyclic malnutrition**. This cycle must be broken by intervention strategies (Fig. 1). If not, the child may die. Malnutrition is the root cause of poor social and economic conditions. Hungry children cannot concentrate at school and will underachieve. Hungry adults will not be efficient workers.

If a varied diet supplies enough calories, it is likely to supply adequate protein. When poverty reduces the variety in the diet, problems arise.

- Protein sources, both animal and plant, are more expensive than carbohydrate and are likely to be reduced. (For example, in West Africa cassava is the staple. It has almost no protein value and would normally be eaten with a pulse. But if people are too poor to buy pulses, then cassava is eaten on its own.)
- Some staples like rice are not calorie dense, so that it is not possible for a small child to eat enough bulk to supply enough calories.
- When insufficient calories are eaten, what little protein is present is used by the body as an energy source.

The most vulnerable age for a child is from **weaning** to five years old. Human milk is **energy dense** and contains a good supply of protein (Fig. 2). Breastfeeding is very important for children of the poor, for not only is it a good food, but it is also clean and does not need a hygienic water supply. Formula milks which were promoted by companies wanting markets in the developing world are expensive and unsuitable in poor rural conditions.

Fig. 1 Cyclic malnutrition

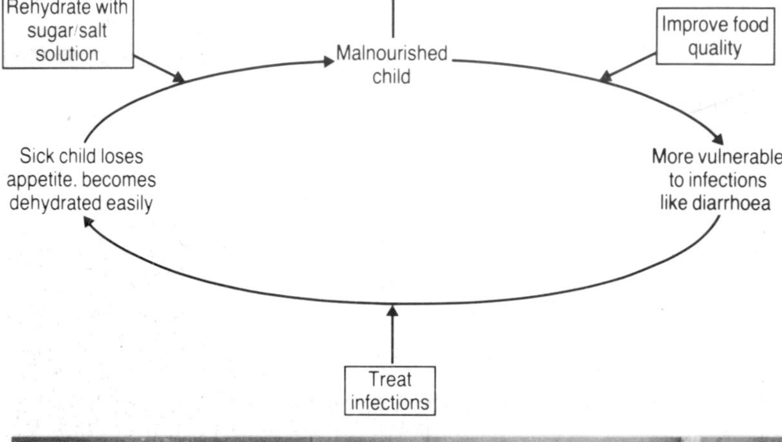

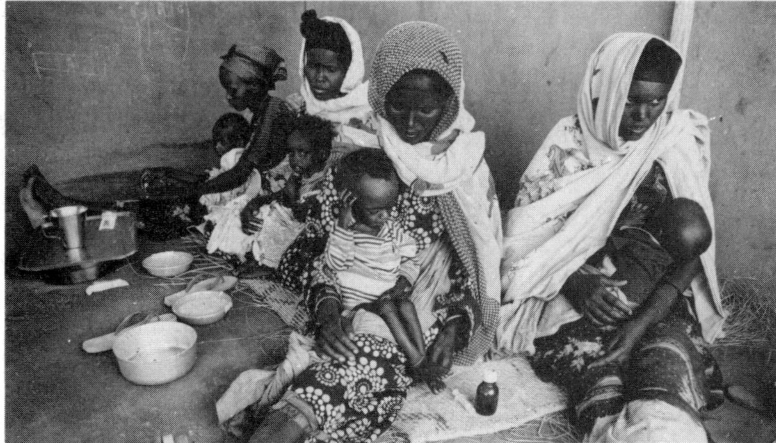

Fig. 2 A child is more likely to suffer from malnutrition after breastfeeding has finished

Summary

- Children are particularly vulnerable to malnutrition.
- Poverty is the root cause of malnutrition. Malnutrition is a cause of poverty.

Questions

1. Why are children most vulnerable to malnutrition?
2. What is the root cause of malnutrition?
3. Why are energy dense foods important for young children?
4. Explain why breastfeeding is to be encouraged in third world countries.

4.6 *Vitamins and minerals*

Vitamins

Vitamins are substances which are required by the body in very small amounts to grow, reproduce and remain healthy. Vitamins can be divided into two groups – those which are soluble in water and those which are soluble in fat. The types of food which contain vitamins depend on these properties. There are at least 13 vitamins which are known and whose function is understood to a certain extent (Fig. 1). These are discussed in more detail later on in the book.

Minerals

About 15 minerals are known to be essential to human life and must be produced by the diet. The most important of these are calcium, iron, phosphorus, magnesium, potassium, sodium and chlorine. Most is known about these. Some minerals are only required in minute amounts. These are known as **trace elements** and are also known to be important, although their exact role in the diet is not well understood. They have only recently been found to be essential and dietary deficiencies have still not been recognized. These trace elements include cobalt, copper, chromium, fluorine, iodine, manganese, zinc and selenium.

Summary

- There are at least 13 known vitamins needed for the body to grow, reproduce and remain healthy.
- The body also requires a number of minerals.

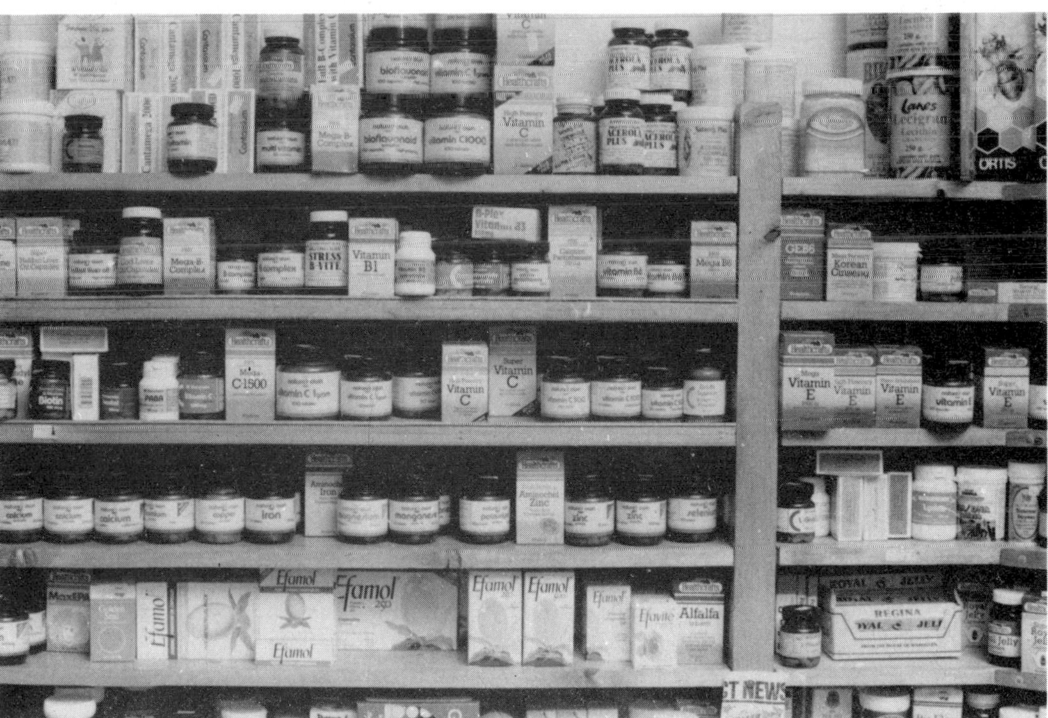

Fig. 1 Vitamins for sale

Questions

1. Write a sentence to describe vitamins.
2. What are 'trace elements'?
3. Name any six minerals which are essential to human life.

4.7 *The nutritional role of cereal foods and starchy vegetables*

A Dietary energy, starch and protein

Dietary energy

In a balanced diet which does not contain too much fat and sugar, these foods are the most important single source of **dietary energy**. Currently, sugar and fat supply much of our dietary energy. If we are to eat less of these, the dietary energy that they supply has to be replaced by cereal foods and starchy vegetables. According to current dietary guidelines (NACNE), cereal foods and starchy vegetables should provide over 40% of our daily dietary energy needs.

In 1983 cereal foods and starchy vegetables supplied about 27% of the UK dietary energy intake. Over the next 15 years, i.e. by the end of this century, the average consumption of cereal foods and starchy vegetables in the UK needs to go up by about 50% (Fig. 1).

Dietary energy is supplied by all foods in the form of carbohydrates (starch and sugars), protein and fats. Cereal foods provide energy mainly from their starch and protein content. Starchy vegetables provide energy mainly from their starch content. In the past starchy foods have been regarded as fattening foods. In fact, because they are not energy dense foods, this is quite untrue.

Starch

Cereal food and starchy vegetables are the main sources of starch in the diet. Starch is important nutritionally for a variety of reasons. First, it is an important source of dietary energy. In plants it is the chief food store. It is converted, as needed, into sugars. It can be stored in the stem or root of a plant, e.g. in the sago palm or cassava respectively. It is also found in edible unripe fruits, such as green bananas. Mainly, however, it is found in tubers and seeds of cereals and pulses. One gram of starch provides approximately 16 kJ of dietary energy. It has a lower energy density than fat (see page 120).

Starch is broken down during digestion into individual **glucose** molecules. These are absorbed into the blood and carried round the body to be used for the production of energy. As starch in food is normally combined with some dietary fibre, vitamins, minerals and often protein, it is a preferable source of dietary energy to sugar (sucrose) (see page 116).

Starch in the diet is also important because the foods in which it occurs tend to be high in **dietary fibre**. The presence of this dietary fibre slows down the rate

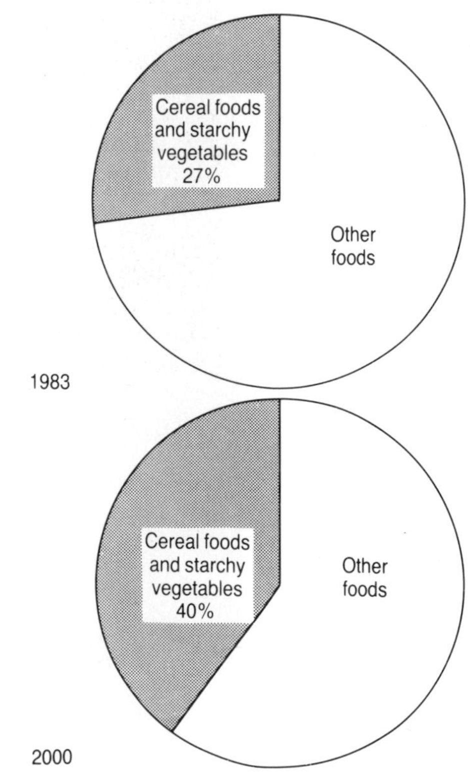

Fig. 1 Proportions of dietary energy intake supplied by cereal foods and starchy vegetables

at which glucose from starch is absorbed into the blood stream. This helps keep blood glucose levels steady by avoiding rapid surges of glucose from the intestine into the gut.

Cereal foods and starchy vegetables can, however, be **refined**. This process removes the starch, which is then used in food processing. It is often used as a thickening agent in canned and dried foods, for example in soups (Fig. 2). When it is cooked with water the starch grains swell up and burst, thickening the mixture. When refined in this way the starch loses its dietary fibre and all the other nutrients it is usually associated with. It is no longer such a nutritionally useful food.

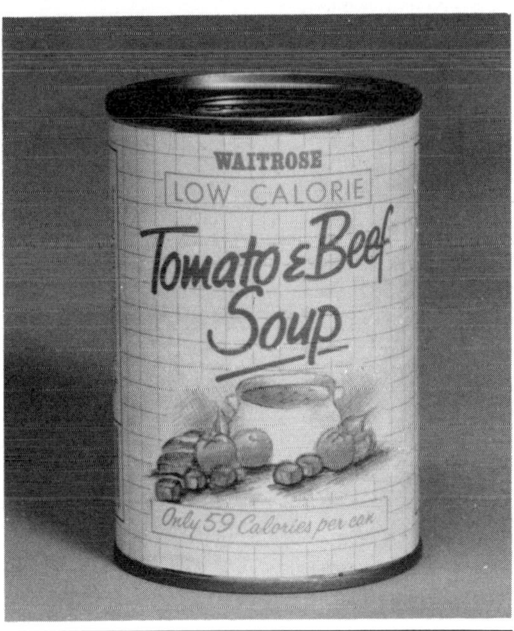

Ingredients: Beef Stock, Beef, Tomatoes, Tomato Purée, Wheatflour, Food Starch, Salt, Hydrolised Vegetable Protein, Flavour Enhancer – Monosodium Glutamate, Onion Extract, Spices, Garlic Powder

Fig. 2 Tinned soup

Protein

For most people in the UK cereal foods currently contribute about 20% of their daily protein intake. Cereal foods are, therefore, a very important source of protein. Current nutritional recommendations are that intakes of protein from vegetable sources, such as cereal foods, should be increased while those from animal sources should be reduced. This is because protein in animal foods is often associated with relatively large amounts of **saturated fats**. These are the kind of fats we should cut down on.

Cereal foods are one of the main sources of protein for people who eat little or no meat, fish, milk, eggs or cheese. They rely on plant foods to get most of their protein and need to make sure that they are eating the right combinations (see pages 72–3). Relying on protein from cereal foods alone is not enough. They need to eat a mixture of cereal foods and pulses, and cereal foods with milk and milk products. The amino acids in the proteins from cereal foods are not in the best proportions for human use. If they are eaten with other proteins from pulses or milk products, the amino acids in those products complement those from the cereal foods, making the whole protein more useful to the body.

Summary

- Cereal foods and starchy vegetables are important sources of dietary energy.
- These foods are the main source of starch in the diet.
- These foods contain protein, which is particularly important in vegetarian diets and diets which are low in animal fats.

Questions

1. Approximately how much of our dietary energy is supplied by cereal and starchy food?
2. What are the recommendations for intake of cereal and starchy foods for the future?
3. What makes starch a healthier source of energy than sugar?
4. What is the importance of group one foods in the diet of vegetarians?

B Dietary fibre

Cereal foods and starchy vegetables are one of the most important sources of dietary fibre. It is found in the outer wall of all plant cells, mostly in the part of plants which form the outer covering (skin or peel), which is usually removed and thrown away. Cereal foods are the most important source, although starchy vegetables are also very valuable (Fig. 1).

Dietary fibre is the part of plant food which is not absorbed during its passage through the small intestine. It reaches the large intestine more or less intact. This is because we are unable to digest **cellulose**, which is one of the main constituents of dietary fibre. We do not produce the enzymes necessary to do so.

Dietary fibre is a mixture of different complex carbohydrates. It is important to eat the different types. The fibre from cereal foods (**bran**) is different from that in starchy vegetables and other vegetables and fruit.

Dietary fibre and health

Many people in the UK suffer from problems with their intestines. These include constipation, diverticular disease, appendicitis, cancer of the colon and haemorrhoids (piles). These problems are all thought to be connected with the small amounts of dietary fibre we eat. At the same time, we suffer from many other health problems not found in countries where large amounts of dietary fibre are eaten. These include diabetes melitus, obesity, tooth decay, hiatus hernia and varicose veins. All these have also been associated with low fibre intakes. The evidence for this is not conclusive.

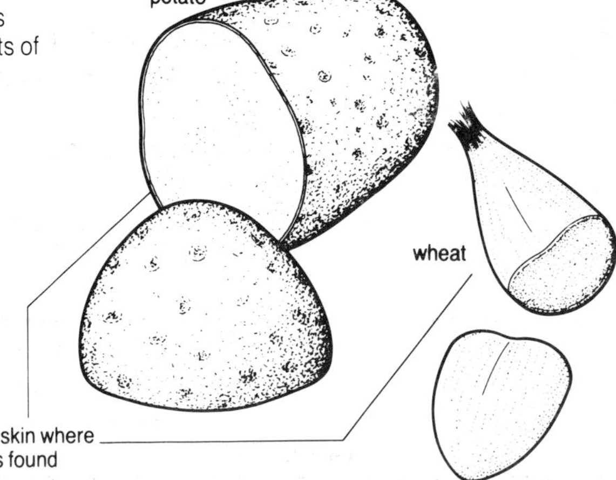

Fig. 1 Dietary fibre is often found in the parts of food which may be thrown away

The properties of dietary fibre

Dietary fibre absorbs water in the gut. The bulk and softness of the stool is affected by this absorption of water. If there is no fibre and no water is absorbed into the stool, the stool becomes hard, small and difficult to pass. If, however, there is plenty of dietary fibre and the stool absorbs water, it becomes bulkier, softer and much easier to pass. If stools are small, hard and difficult to pass, **constipation** can occur. Dietary fibre therefore has a laxative effect. This laxative effect is related to the type of dietary fibre eaten. The fibre from cereal foods is the most effective.

Dietary fibre may also be protective against **gall stones**. The dietary fibre in the gut seems to bind some of the cholesterol and bile acids in the gut. This prevents their reabsorption into the blood and reduces their concentration in the body.

Stools rich in dietary fibre pass quickly and easily through the gut. This may well be partly responsible for the protective effect of dietary fibre against **cancer** of the colon.

Fibre in cereal foods

A cereal grain is made up of three components. The outer layer which protects the grain is called the **bran**. This contains the dietary fibre and some vitamins and minerals. The **germ** is the embryo plant. This is a very tiny proportion of the grain and provides the vitamins and minerals. It also contains a small amount of fat, which is rich in essential fatty acids. The endosperm or the bulk of the grain is the growing seed's food store. This contains some protein but is mainly starch. There are also small amounts of some vitamins and minerals.

Dietary fibre is present in all cereal foods when they are first harvested. Food processing and refining of cereals,

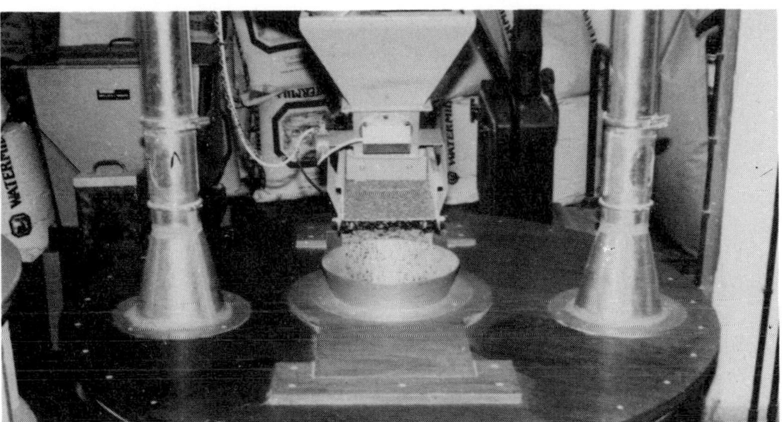

Fig. 2 This wheat is being stoneground

however, often removes it. During refining the bran and wheatgerm are removed from the grain leaving only the endosperm. This is then milled and turned into white flour. White flour is used for making bread and the many other cereal foods which are available to us. Rice is also refined in the same way and can be milled into flour, a common practice in cultures where rice is the staple food. In the UK rice is usually eaten whole.

Types of flour and bread

Wholemeal bread is made from flour which contains the whole of the wheat grain. It may be stoneground, i.e. the grains are crushed between two stones and the resulting flour is collected and used for baking (Fig. 2). Wholemeal flour which is not stoneground has been refined and divided up into its three component parts. These are then mixed together again to make the bread.

Brown bread is made from white flour with the addition of varying amounts of bran, wheatgerm and brown colouring (Fig. 3).

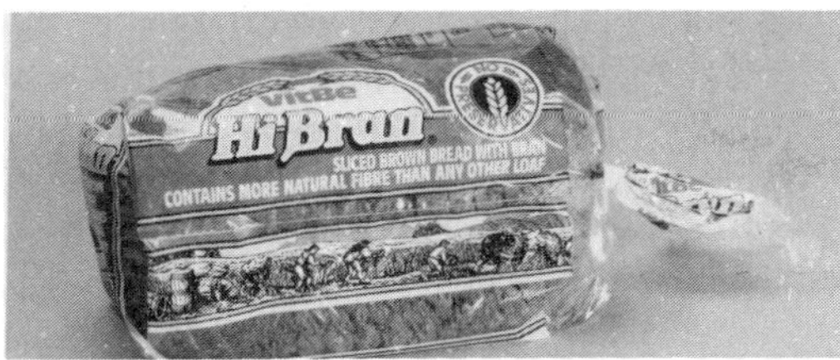

Fig. 3 Brown bread

White bread is made from refined white flour which has had all the wheatgerm and bran removed.

Intakes of dietary fibre

The NACNE report recommended that by the year 2000 the average fibre intake of the UK population should be about 30 g per person per day. The current intake is approximately 20 g. There will, of course, be very wide individual differences in intake. The amount of fibre we can get is related to the amount of cereal foods or starchy vegetables that we eat. This amount depends on our own individual energy needs.

Bran is often sold as a source of fibre in the diet. It is also used in the manufacture of a number of breakfast cereals and high fibre biscuits. 'Neat' bran should only be taken as a medicine when prescribed by a doctor or dietitian. By eating a wide variety of whole grain cereal foods and plenty of fruit and vegetables it is not too difficult to get sufficient dietary fibre.

Methods of measuring dietary fibre in foods are currently under review. It is possible that new and different information on fibre intakes and the fibre content of different foods will be available in the future.

Summary

- Cereal foods and starchy vegetables all provide dietary fibre, which is the structural part of plants.
- Dietary fibre is important to keep the gut healthy.
- Dietary fibre is often removed in the refining of food.
- Bran is a medicine, not a food.

Questions

1. What parts of the cereal grain contain (a) bran, (b) oil, (c) starch, (d) protein?
2. Explain the differences between white, wholemeal and stoneground flour.
3. What are the approximate current and recommended intakes of dietary fibre? What health problems are associated with fibre intakes?

C Iron, zinc and calcium

Cereal foods and starchy vegetables are important sources of a number of minerals. Two of the most important of these are iron and zinc.

Iron

The average dietary intake of iron in the UK is approximately 11 mg per person per day. About 40% of this comes from cereal foods and starchy vegetables, cereal foods being the most important source. The iron comes mostly from bread and breakfast cereals (Fig. 1). Wholemeal bread is naturally high in iron. White bread and many breakfast cereals have iron added during their manufacture although how much of this is actually absorbed is unclear.

The role of iron in the body

Iron is present in blood and in muscles. Some of it is stored in the liver. This store is important for young babies because breast milk contains very little iron. So babies need to rely on the store of iron in their liver.

The iron in blood is in the pigment **haemoglobin** found in the red blood cells. Haemoglobin carries oxygen from the lungs all around the body. If there is not enough iron, the blood cannot carry enough oxygen. When this happens **iron deficiency anaemia** results.

There are three main causes of anaemia. These are loss of blood because of internal or external bleeding, more rapid than normal destruction of the oxygen carrying cells in the blood, and a slowing down in the production of those cells. In the case of nutritional anaemia the last of the three is the main cause, although this may be made worse by bleeding. Anaemia caused by not having enough iron is most common in women because of the regular loss of blood during menstruation. Anaemia creeps up very slowly and most people do not know they have it. Very gradually they come to feel generally tired, irritable, breathless on exertion, and become pale or pasty to look at. People who are anaemic tend to get run down very easily, and feel tired, lazy and not able to do anything. They are lacking in enthusiasm and pick up infections easily.

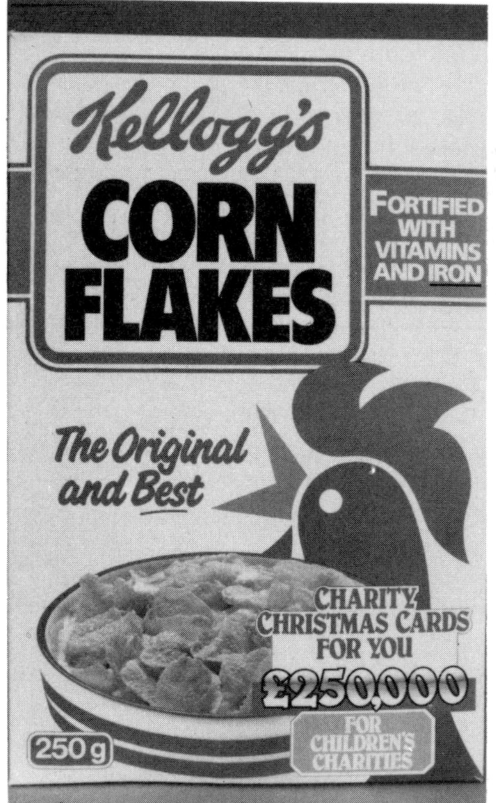

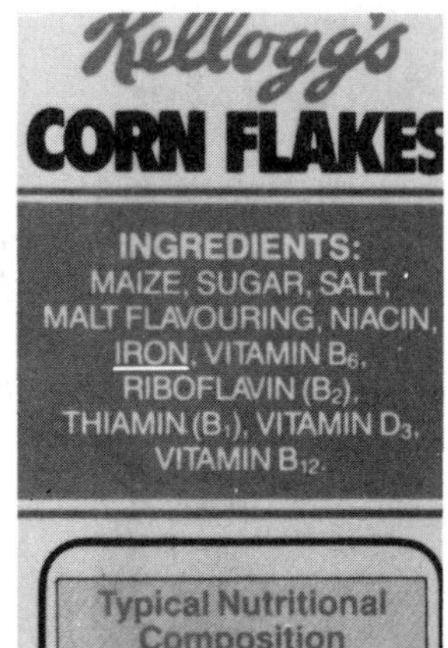

Fig. 1 Breakfast cereals may be an important source of iron

Iron in food

The amount of iron in the body is mainly controlled by the amount of iron absorbed. However, losses do occur, for example when people cut themselves or when women menstruate. The absorption of iron from food is generally low, but it is increased when the body stores are depleted. Needs for iron are greatest in growing children, menstruating women and pregnant women. Elderly people also may be short of iron because of their reduced food intakes and less efficient absorption.

There are two types of iron found in food, **haem** iron and **non-haem** iron. Haem iron is derived from the blood in animal foods and non-haem iron is found in vegetable foods.

Haem iron is more readily absorbed than non-haem iron. Up to 25% of the iron in meat and offal can be absorbed. Only about 5% of the iron from cereal foods is absorbed. The exact amount depends on other factors. For example, vitamin C from fruit and vegetables can help increase the absorption of iron. The fruit and vegetables need to be eaten at the same time as the food containing iron. There are chemicals in eggs and tea which can reduce the absorption of iron if these foods are eaten at the same time. The phytates in whole grain cereal foods also can reduce the absorption of iron. However, during the leavening of bread, enzymes split up the phytic acid so it no longer binds the minerals. This action of the phytates is probably only important in diets where cereals are eaten in the form of unleavened wholewheat bread, for example chapattis (Fig. 2), or where large amounts of pure bran are included.

Fig. 2 The phytates in the unleavened chapattis may reduce the absorption of iron from the other foods here

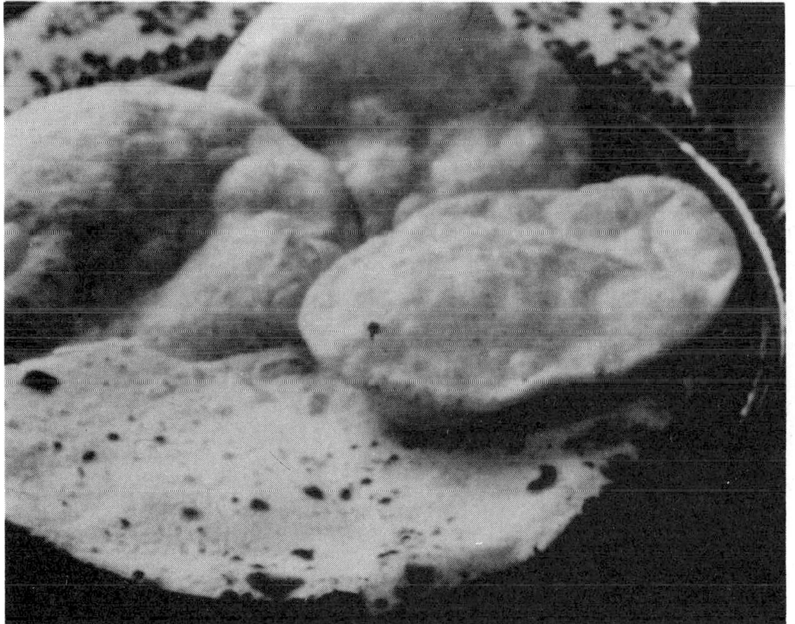

Zinc

Cereal foods and starchy vegetables are important sources of zinc in the diet. It is often associated with protein in those foods. Like iron, zinc also can be bound by phytic acid in the bran of cereals. Zinc is associated with a large number of reactions that go on in the body. Its function is not clearly understood but more is becoming known about it.

Calcium

Cereal foods, in particular white bread, are important sources of calcium. The calcium is added to white flour used for bread making, by law.

Other minerals

Cereal foods and starchy vegetables are also important sources of the minerals **potassium** and **phosphorus**. Small amounts of other minerals and **trace elements** are also present in cereal foods and starchy vegetables. These amounts often depend on the type of soil in which the plants were grown.

Summary

- Cereal foods are one of the most important sources of iron in the diet.
- The iron from vegetable foods is less well absorbed than the iron from animal foods.
- Some groups of people need more iron than others.
- These foods also contribute significantly to zinc and calcium intakes.

Questions

1. Why is iron needed by the body?
2. Why is the RDA for iron for teenage girls higher than that for boys?
3. What are the main causes of anaemia?
4. What are haem and non-haem iron? Which is more easily absorbed?
5. If you had wholemeal toast, orange juice, a boiled egg and a cup of tea for breakfast, how would the foods interact to affect iron absorption from your meal?

D Vitamins

Cereal foods and starchy vegetables are very important sources of vitamins B_1 (thiamin) and vitamin E. Some breakfast cereals are **fortified** with a variety of vitamins, for example B vitamins and vitamin D. They can be valuable sources of these nutrients (Fig. 1).

Thiamin (vitamin B_1)

Thiamin is needed in the body to allow release of energy from carbohydrates. Thiamin requirements are therefore related to the amount of carbohydrate and dietary energy in the diet. In unrefined foods, thiamin is usually found alongside carbohydrates. Cereal foods and starchy vegetables are major sources of carbohydrates (starch). They are therefore usually rich in thiamin too. However, when cereals are refined, the thiamin in the bran is removed. In the UK, white bread must be fortified with thiamin by law.

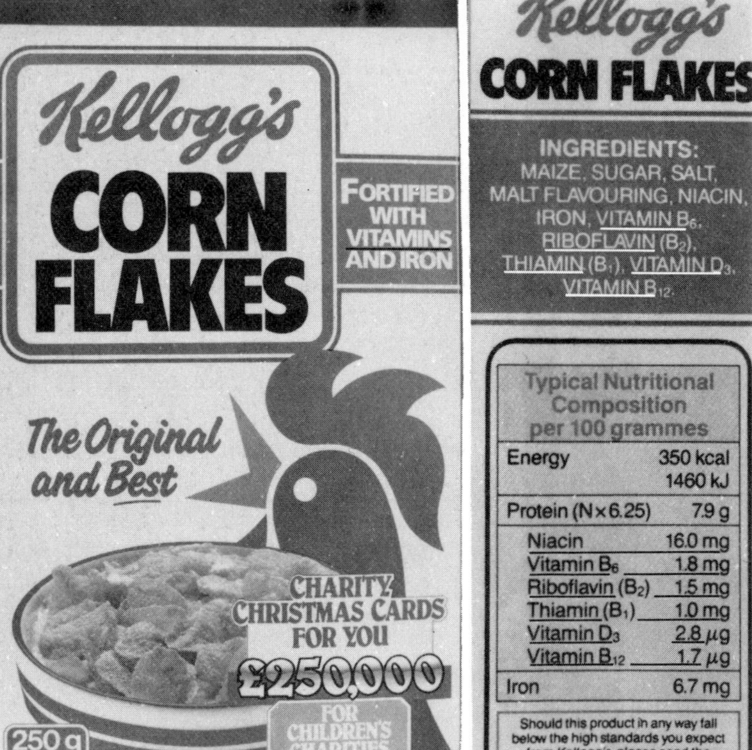

Fig. 1 Breakfast cereals may also be an important source of the B vitamins and vitamin D

People who do not have enough thiamin eventually get the disease **beri-beri**. This is not common in the UK, but it is sometimes found in people who drink a lot of alcohol and do not eat much. The alcohol increases the need for thiamin but their diet contains very little.

Thiamin easily dissolves in water and so can be lost when vegetables and cereals are cooked in too much water which is later thrown away (Fig. 2). It is relatively stable at temperatures up to boiling point, provided the cooking medium is slightly acid. It is sensitive to heat in neutral or alkaline conditions. If baking powder or an alkaline solution is used in the cooking much of the thiamin is destroyed. Freezing and canning results in the loss of only small amounts of thiamin.

Vitamin E (tocopherols)

Not much is known about the role of vitamin E in the diet. Nevertheless it is known to be an important nutrient (Fig. 3). It is found in all cell membranes and may be important in preventing the breakdown of cell tissues. Most foods contain some vitamin E but only in very small amounts. The best sources are polyunsaturated vegetable oils and whole grain cereal products. In cereal foods the vitamin E is in the germ of the cereal, so little is present in refined cereal foods. Animal fats and meat and fruit and vegetables contain very little vitamin E. It is also used in some processed foods as an antioxidant and is found in some 'fatty' fish .

Vitamin C

Starchy vegetables provide about 20% of the vitamin C in many people's diets. If fruit or vegetables are disliked, then potatoes and other starchy vegetables become very important as a source of vitamin C.

Other vitamins

Cereal foods and starchy vegetables provide important amounts of other B vitamins, including vitamin B_2

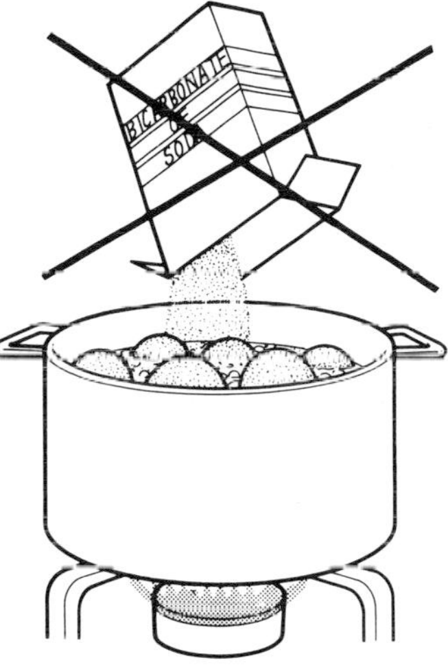

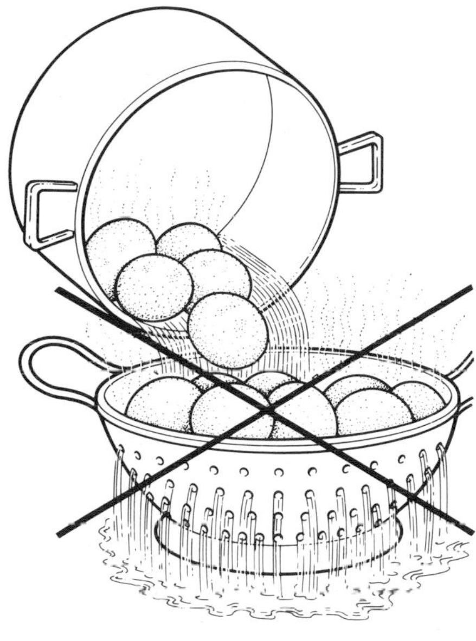

Fig. 2 Thiamin can be lost from vegetables if they are not cooked carefully

(riboflavin), vitamin B_3 (nicotinic acid), vitamin B_6 (pyridoxine), folic acid and pantothenic acid. For all these B vitamins whole grain unrefined cereal foods are better than refined cereal foods There are also small amounts of vitamin D in cereal foods which contain margarine or which have been fortified with vitamin D during processing. Breakfast cereals are sometimes fortified with vitamin D.

Summary

- Cereal foods and starchy vegetables are important sources of thiamin and vitamin E.
- Refined cereal foods contain fewer nutrients than unrefined cereal foods.
- These foods are also important sources of a number of B vitamins.
- Potatoes and other starchy vegetables make an important contribution to vitamin C in the diet.

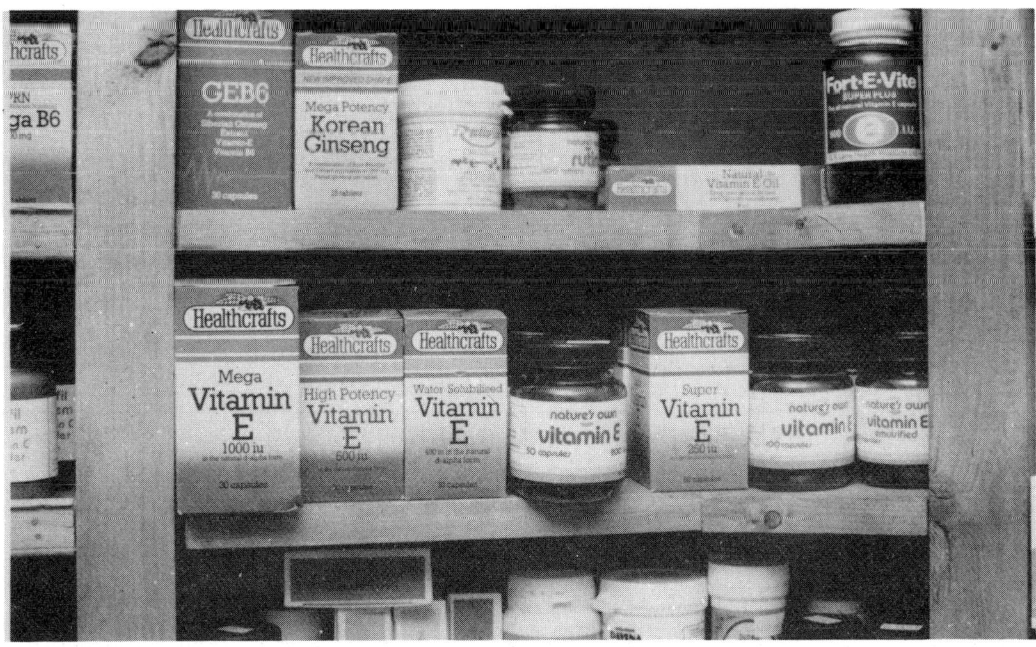

Fig. 3 Vitamin E for sale

Questions

1. Why does the body need thiamin (B_1)?
2. Where does most thiamin come from?
3. What are the best sources of vitamin E?
4. Write a few sentences about the importance of potatoes in providing vitamin C.

E Effects of cooking and processing

The foods in this group are usually referred to as **staples**. Each culture has its own range of staples depending on availability. Because the main nutrient contained in the staples is starch, which is difficult to digest in its raw state, they are normally eaten cooked. There are traditional methods of preparing, cooking and serving them, but in most cultures they are eaten with some meat or pulses and vegetables. Because they are rather dry, do not have a strong taste and are white when cooked, they are made more appetizing by the addition of sauces which make them tastier, more attractive and easier to eat.

Potatoes and other starchy vegetables

Apart from starch and protein, potatoes contain ascorbic acid (vitamin C). The amounts present vary. Freshly dug new potatoes contain about 30 mg per 100 g, whereas 'old' potatoes stored for nine months contain about 8 mg per 100 g. The cooking and preparation also affect the vitamin C content. Peeled potatoes lose some of the vitamin C, since about 15% of the total is contained just beneath the skin. The cooking method also affects the energy value of starchy vegetables (Fig. 1).

Cassava must be processed before being eaten as it contains a substance from which hydrogen cyanide is released. It is grated, then dried in the sun. Cassava pulp is made into tapioca which is eaten as a milk pudding in the UK. Sago, a similar product, is made from the sago palm.

Rice

Parboiling is a traditional way of processing rice. This involves soaking it with its husk, from which the B vitamins are taken into the grain, then steaming or boiling it before husking. This is very important since thiamin losses are minimized and beri beri, a vitamin deficiency disease, is prevented.

Milling, polishing, washing and cooking rice all result in vitamin losses. B group vitamins are all soluble and present in the highest concentration in the outer layers, which may be discarded during milling and polishing, and the loss of thiamin and nicotinic acid is heavy. This is important in the diets of rice eaters who eat a low proportion of other foods.

Malting

The process of malting involves moistening cereal grains and allowing them to sprout in a warm atmosphere.

Fig. 1 The effects of cooking and preparation on vitamin content and energy value

Vegetable	*Cooking method*	*Vitamin C lost*	*Energy value*
Potato	Boiled (peeled)	30–50%	343 kJ/100 g
	Mashed	30–50%	343 kJ/100 g
	Baked in skin	20–40%	365 kJ/100 g
	Roast	20–40%	662 kJ/100 g
	Steamed	20–40%	343 kJ/100 g
	Chips (fried in deep fat)	25–35%	1065 kJ/100 g
Plantain	Boiled	85%	518 kJ/100 g
	Fried	40%	1126 kg/100 g

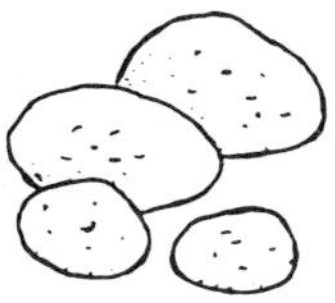

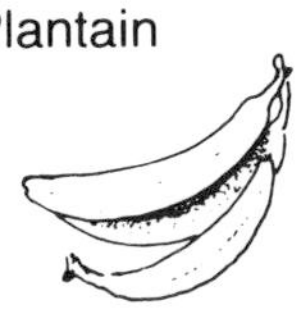

(a)

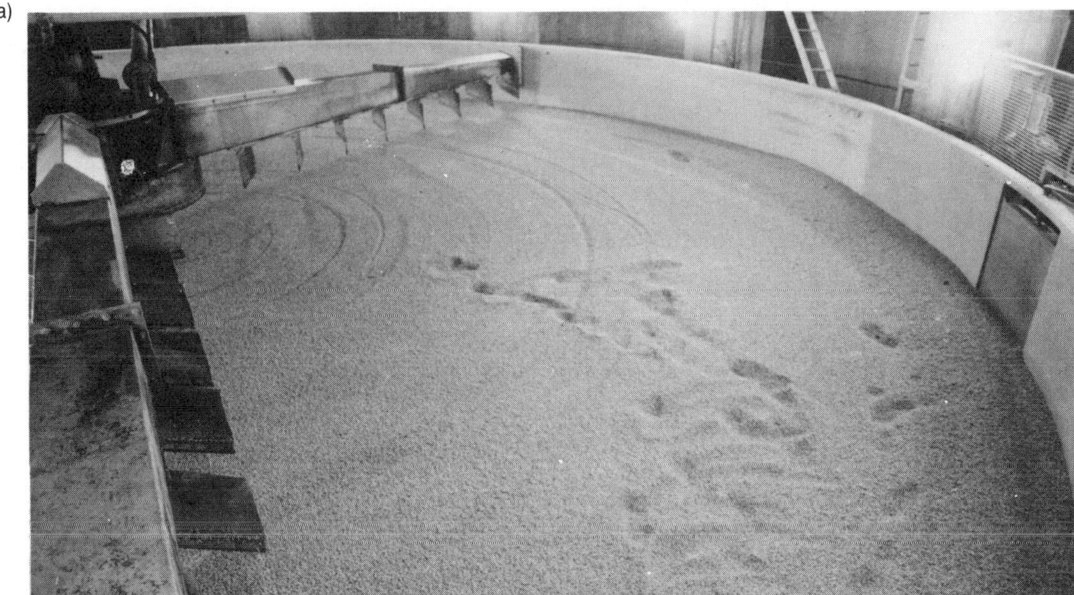

Fig. 2 (a) Barley is used at a brewery for malting into beer
(b) Drinks produced by malting various grains

(b)

Grain	Drink
Barley	Beer, Ale, Stout, Whisky
Maize/Wheat, barley	Bourbon
Rye	Rye Whisky, Vodka

The enzyme diastase is activated and this changes the starch into dextrins and maltose, some of which is changed into glucose by maltose. Heat then inactivates the enzyme. Yeast ferments the sugars into alcohol (Fig. 2).

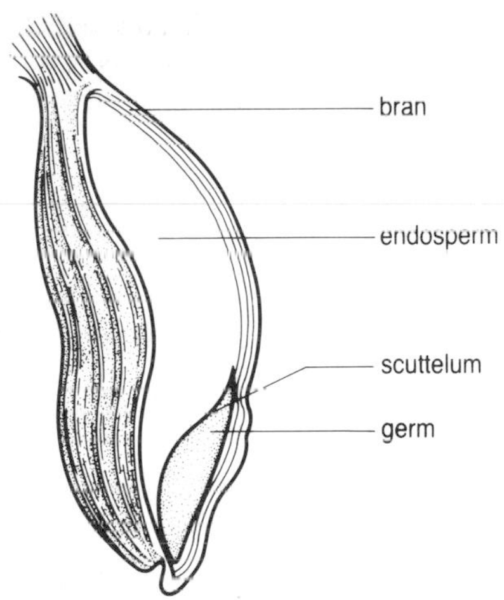

Fig. 3 Wheat grain

Wheat

Wheat is an important staple in many parts of the world, including the UK. There are a number of varieties. **Winter wheat** like that grown in the UK contains less than 10% protein and is called 'soft' and gives a weak dough. **Spring wheat** like that grown in Canada is rich in protein and is called 'hard' – it gives a strong dough. Durum wheat is particularly hard and used for making pasta. The nutrients in wheat grains are not distributed evenly (Fig. 3). The germ and scuttelum are relatively rich in protein, fat and vitamins. The scuttelum contains 50% of the thiamin. The outer endosperm contains a higher concentration of proteins, vitamins and phytic acid than the inner endosperm, which is mainly starch with some protein. The nutrient loss on milling depends on how much is removed. (Eighty-five % extraction means 15% bran is discarded.)

The minerals present in wholewheat flour are not well absorbed due to the presence of phytic acid, which binds them as insoluble phytates. Leavening (using yeast as a raising agent) prevents this binding, so that the eating of unleavened wholemeal bread as a major part of the diet may affect the absorption of minerals like calcium and zinc.

Breadmaking needs a strong flour. When flour is mixed with water to form a dough two proteins present in wheat combine with water to make **gluten**. Gluten forms an elastic like network which is the basic structure of bread (Fig. 4). When **fermentation** due to yeast acting on sugar produces carbon dioxide, the gas is trapped in pockets by the gluten. It stretches and rises and forms the shape of the dough. Baking **coagulates** the protein and a loaf is produced.

Commercial bakers use various processes to speed up fermentation (Fig. 5). The Chorleywood process requires more yeast and water than the traditional method, and the addition of fat and vitamin C. Good bread can be made with weak (English) flour and the whole process of breadmaking takes under 2 hours. The fat in bread makes it keep longer.

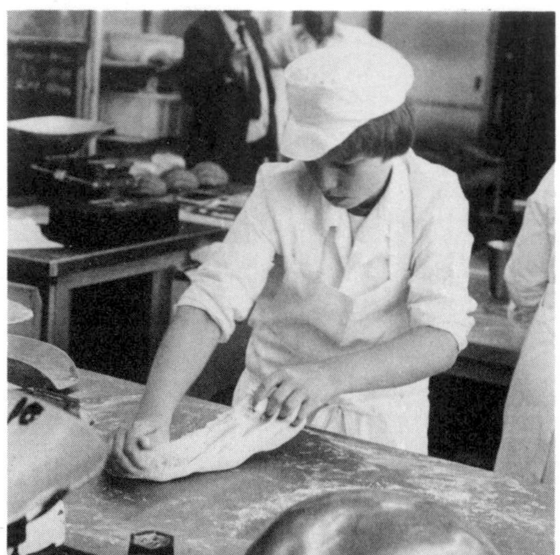

Fig. 4 Gluten in kneaded dough gives it its elasticity

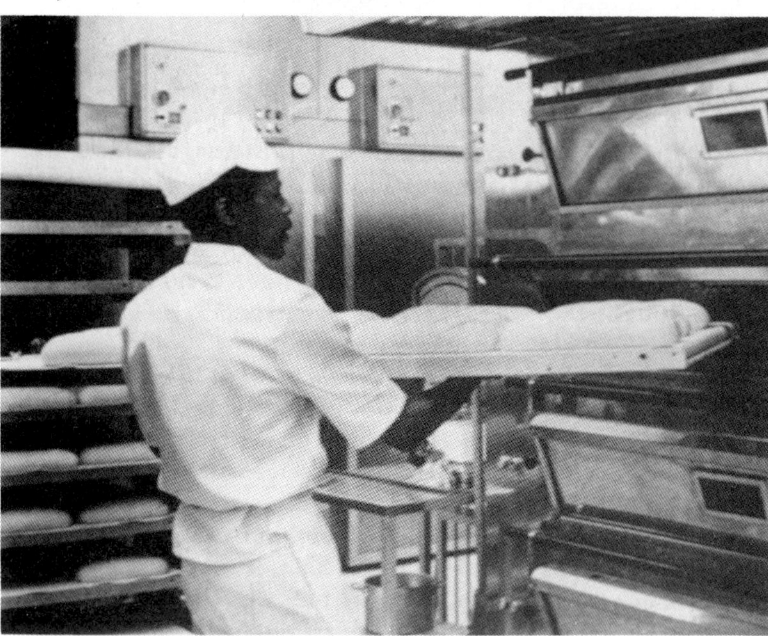

Fig. 5 A commercial bakery

Biscuits and **cakes** are made from weak flour. They can be made from wholewheat (100% extraction) or white flour. The weak flour gives the crumb required in cake making. The texture of a cake depends on the interaction of the ingredients before and during baking (Fig. 6).

The attractive brown crust on bread and cakes and toast is brought about by the **Maillard reaction**. This is a chemical reaction between protein and sugar. This reaction is sometimes called non-enzymic browning and is caused by cooking food in dry heat. It is responsible for the changes in flavour of roast meat, coffee beans, nuts, biscuits and breakfast cereals, as well as bread and toast.

Undamaged starch grains are insoluble in cold water. As the temperature rises, water is absorbed by the starch granules. They swell and amylose leaches out making a sticky paste. This is the process used in making thickened sauces, etc. If a concentrated paste is allowed to cool the bonds between amylose and amylopectin are remade and a gel is formed – as in blancmange. Sometimes the gel becomes rubbery and water leaks out. This is called retrogradation. It happens when thickened products like gravy in meat pies or sauces in fruit pies are frozen. The answer to this problem is to use a waxy starch like maize starch as a stabilizer.

Summary

- Staples are normally eaten cooked.
- Different cultures use different staple foods.
- As well as being a source of starch, most staples provide vitamins.
- Starch is a polysaccharide. As a result of digestion it provides energy.

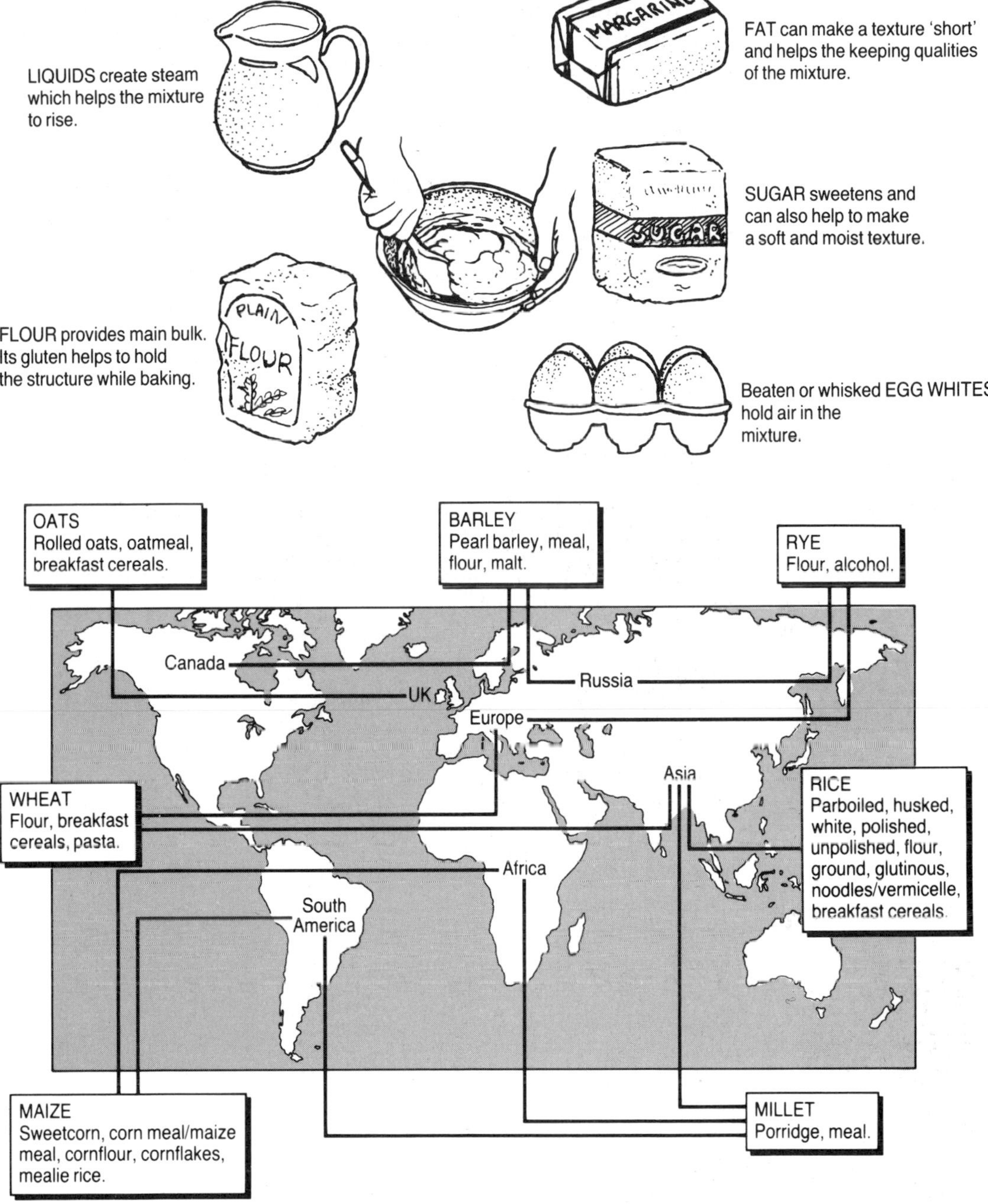

Fig. 6 Function of ingredients in baked mixtures

Fig. 7 Cereals and their products around the world

Questions

1. How does the way in which potatoes are processed affect (a) their vitamin C content, (b) their calorific value?
2. What is meant by parboiling rice? Why is it important in diets of people living mainly on rice?
3. Explain what is meant by soft and hard flour and how they are used in baking.
4. What is the Maillard reaction?
5. Explain what happens to starch grains when they are heated with water.

F Digestion

Starch

Starch is a **polysaccharide**, i.e. a polymer consisting of long chains of glucose molecules bonded together. Starch molecules are large and more or less insoluble in water. Before it can be used as a source of energy by the body, it must be broken down into glucose molecules. This process is brought about by **enzymes**. Enzymes are specialized in their functions. Each enzyme brings about one change – splitting larger molecules into smaller ones (Fig. 1).

Dietary fibre

Dietary fibre passes through the gut. It absorbs water in the colon, making the faeces larger and softer. It prevents constipation.

Polysaccharide = Starch
ENZYME AMYLASE
Disaccharide = Maltose
ENZYME MALTASE
Monosaccharide = Glucose

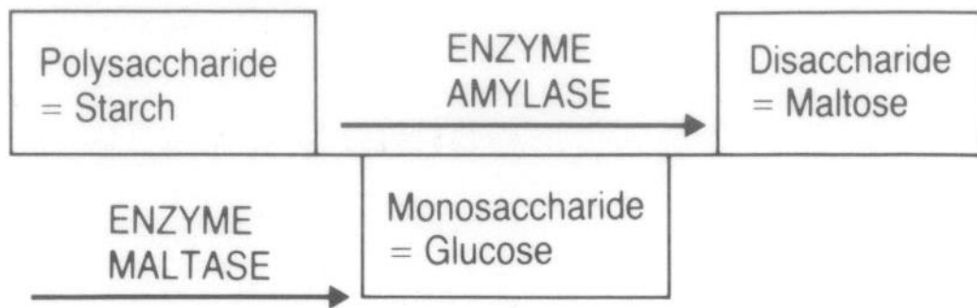

Fig. 1 The breakdown of polysaccharides

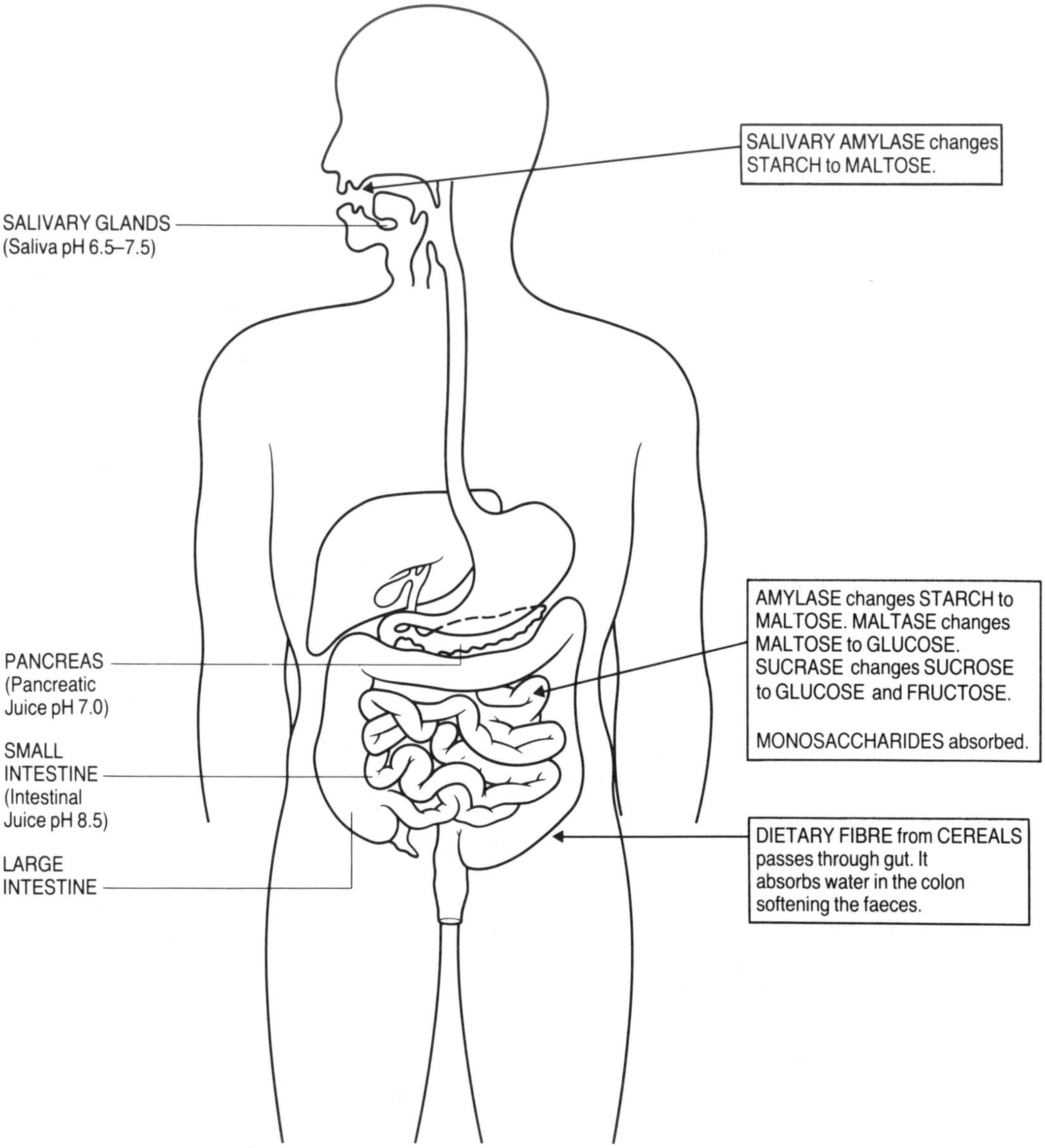

SALIVARY AMYLASE changes STARCH to MALTOSE.
SALIVARY GLANDS (Saliva pH 6.5–7.5)
AMYLASE changes STARCH to MALTOSE. MALTASE changes MALTOSE to GLUCOSE. SUCRASE changes SUCROSE to GLUCOSE and FRUCTOSE.
MONOSACCHARIDES absorbed.
PANCREAS (Pancreatic Juice pH 7.0)
SMALL INTESTINE (Intestinal Juice pH 8.5)
LARGE INTESTINE
DIETARY FIBRE from CEREALS passes through gut. It absorbs water in the colon softening the faeces.

Fig. 2 Digestion of cereal foods and starchy vegetables

4.8 The nutritional role of fruit and vegetables

A Dietary energy, dietary fibre and carbohydrate

Dietary energy

Nearly all fruit and vegetables contain more than 75% water. They contain very little fat and protein and small amounts of simple carbohydrates. They are high in dietary fibre, which is of a different type to that found in cereal foods and just as important. Vegetables and fruit therefore are **low energy dense foods** (Fig. 1).

Dietary fibre

In most UK diets approximately 60% of dietary fibre is provided by fruit and vegetables. The dietary fibre found in these foods is mainly in the form of **cellulose**, **hemicellulose** and **pectin**. Cellulose is the fibre which plants depend on for support. It is a **polymer** of glucose units. Hemicelluloses are closely associated with the cellulose in plant tissues. Pectins are found in the soft tissues of plants and vegetables. They are soluble in hot water. In the presence of sugars and a warm, slightly acid dilute solution they turn into jelly. This property is what makes jams set.

The use of dietary fibre has been discussed more fully on page 69.

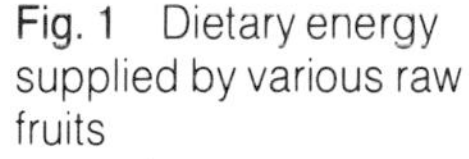

Fig. 1 Dietary energy supplied by various raw fruits

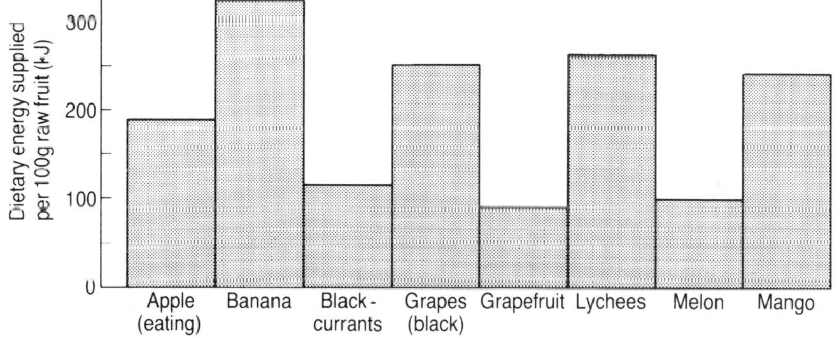

Carbohydrates

Most fruit contains between 5% and 20% carbohydrate. This is in the form of the simple sugars **fructose** and **glucose** (and **sucrose** in some fruits). There is more fructose than glucose. Bananas contain more carbohydrate than most fruit, i.e. about 20% (Fig. 2). When they are not ripe this is in the form of starch. Ripe bananas are about 2% starch and 18% fructose, sucrose and glucose. During ripening, enzymes in the raw fruit change the starch to fructose and glucose and most ripe fruit contains no starch. Unripe fruit is usually sour. This is because of organic acids in the fruit. These are broken down by reactions controlled by enzymes during ripening and the sourness disappears.

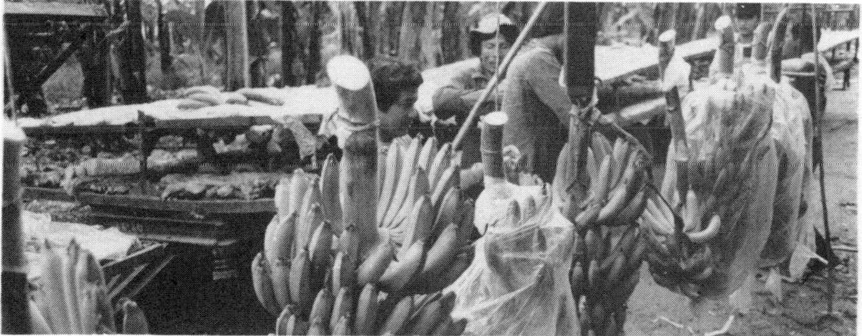

Fig. 2 Bananas contain about 20% carbohydrate. In the unripe fruit it is mainly in the form of starch

Summary

- Fruit and vegetables have a low energy density.
- Fruit and vegetables contain dietary fibre.
- Fruit and vegetables contain the simple sugar fructose and small amounts of glucose.

Questions

1. Why are fruit and vegetables useful in a calorie controlled diet?
2. Describe the dietary fibre found in these foods.
3. What happens to fruit as it ripens?
4. Which sugars are found in fruit?

B Vitamin C

Vegetables and fruit are the main sources of ascorbic acid (vitamin C) in our diet. Approximately 70% of our vitamin C comes from these foods. The rest comes mainly from starchy vegetables. Most plant foods except cereals and pulses contain some vitamin C. The amount of vitamin C in different fruits and vegetables varies widely. For example, oranges contain about 50 mg of vitamin C per 100 g. Apples contain only about 3 mg of vitamin C per 100 g. The same is true for vegetables. Cooked Brussels sprouts contain approximately 40 mg of vitamin C per 100 g. Boiled carrots only contain about 4 mg of vitamin C per 100 g (Fig. 1). (The RDA for vitamin C for an adult is 30 mg per day.)

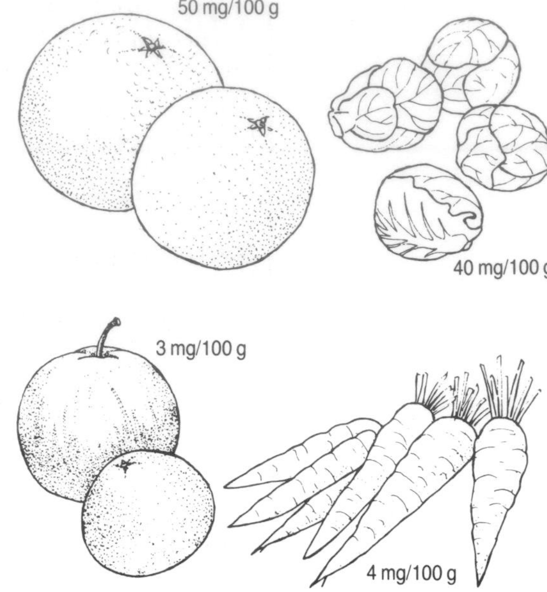

Fig. 1 The amount of vitamin C in different fruit and vegetables varies widely. Oranges and brussels sprouts, for example, contain much more than apples or carrots

The role of vitamin C

Collagen production Vitamin C is necessary to the basic structure of the healthy body. Bones, muscles and tendons all contain a protein called collagen. Collagen is an important component of the **connective tissues** in the body (Fig. 2). The function of connective tissues is to support the organs and other tissues of the body.

There are different types of connective tissues, most of which contain collagen. Connective tissues fill the spaces between **organs**. They form the **tendons** which attach muscles to bones. They are found in the **ligaments** which hold the joints together. They also form the basis of the **bones** and **cartilage**, which provide a rigid framework for the body. Bones are formed when calcium and phosphorus are deposited on the basic collagen structure. Collagen is also important for the quick healing of cuts and wounds.

Vitamin C is essential for the formation of collagen. Without it muscle tissues are unable to hold together and small blood vessels and capillaries break down. In a healthy body approximately 27% of the total protein is collagen. By maintaining collagen production vitamin C also helps the body protect itself from minor illnesses and infections.

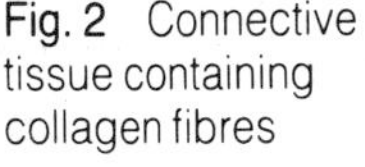
Fig. 2 Connective tissue containing collagen fibres

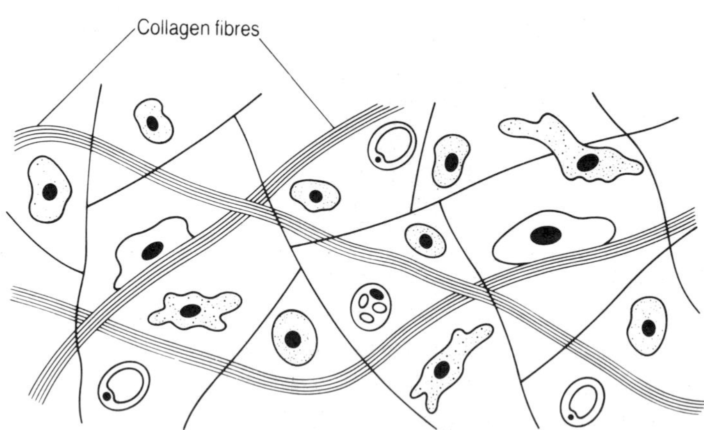

Some people believe that taking large doses of vitamin C (for example 1–5 g per day) helps protect against and cure the common cold. However, scientific evidence to support this is not clear and little is known about other effects of these very large doses.

Absorption of iron from the gut Non-haem iron found in plant foods is not as well absorbed as the haem iron found in the blood in meat. Vitamin C is a **reducing agent**. It changes the insoluble non-haem iron to the soluble form. This process happens in the stomach and is assisted by the hydrochloric acid also found in the stomach. If vitamin C containing foods are eaten at the same time as non-haem iron containing foods, more of the iron can be absorbed by the body.

Other functions Vitamin C may also be involved in other functions in the body. It is thought to be involved in the working of the brain, the breakdown of fats in the body, muscle fatigue and stamina, resistance to infections and the detoxification of potentially harmful substances such as drugs and alcohol (Fig. 3).

Fig. 3 Vitamin C may be involved in the detoxification of drugs and alcohol

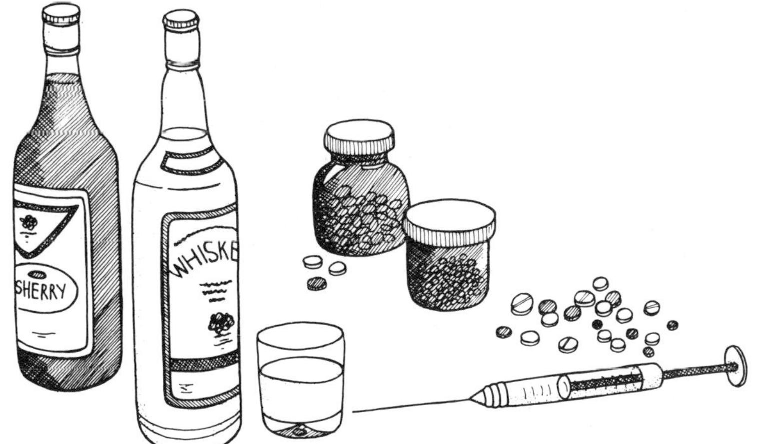

Vitamin C deficiency

If there is not enough vitamin C in the diet the collagen fibres cannot be built properly. If the diet does not contain enough vitamin C over a long period of time, **scurvy** results. The first signs are bleeding, especially from the small blood vessels under the skin, and wounds which heal very slowly. There might also be increased susceptibility of the mouth and gums to infections. As the problem becomes worse the scars of previous wounds may break down and begin to open up as sores again. At the same time the gums become soft and teeth become loose and can fall out. There is often bleeding of the gums as well. In the UK scurvy is unusual. It is sometimes found amongst elderly people, alcoholics and drug addicts who are not eating any vegetables or fruit.

Nobody knows the results of mild vitamin C deficiency. However, it is likely to show itself in tiredness, lack of resistance to infections and longer time taken for recovering from infections.

Summary

- These foods are the most important source of vitamin C.
- Vitamin C is vital for many of the body's functions.
- Vitamin C from vegetables and fruit helps the body utilize iron from other foods eaten at the same time.
- The vitamin C deficiency disease scurvy is sometimes found in the UK.

Questions

1. Where does most of the vitamin C in your diet come from?
2. What is collagen? What is its role in the body? How is it affected by vitamin C?
3. How does vitamin C affect iron absorption?
4. What other functions has vitamin C?
5. What are the results of severe vitamin C deficiency?

C Vitamins A and K

Vitamin A

Vitamin A is available to the body in two forms. The form found mostly in vegetables and fruit is **beta carotene**. (β carotene is also found in milk products.) In animal foods it is in a form called **retinol**. It is the chemical which gives some plants their bright yellow or orange colour. β carotene is widely distributed in fruit and vegetables and is often associated with chlorophyll, the green pigment. The amount of β carotene in these foods is roughly related to the depth of colour in the food. The darker the colour the more β carotene. Before it is used, β carotene is converted by the body into retinol. It takes about 6 μg of β carotene to produce 1 μg of retinol. On average, about 20% of the retinol in our diet comes from the β carotene in vegetables and fruit, milk, cheese and butter, and over 90% of this comes from the vegetables and fruit.

The best animal source of vitamin A is liver. Most people who do not eat liver probably get over half of their vitamin A from the β carotene in fruit and vegetables (Fig. 1). Whole milk is also a useful source of Vitamin A.

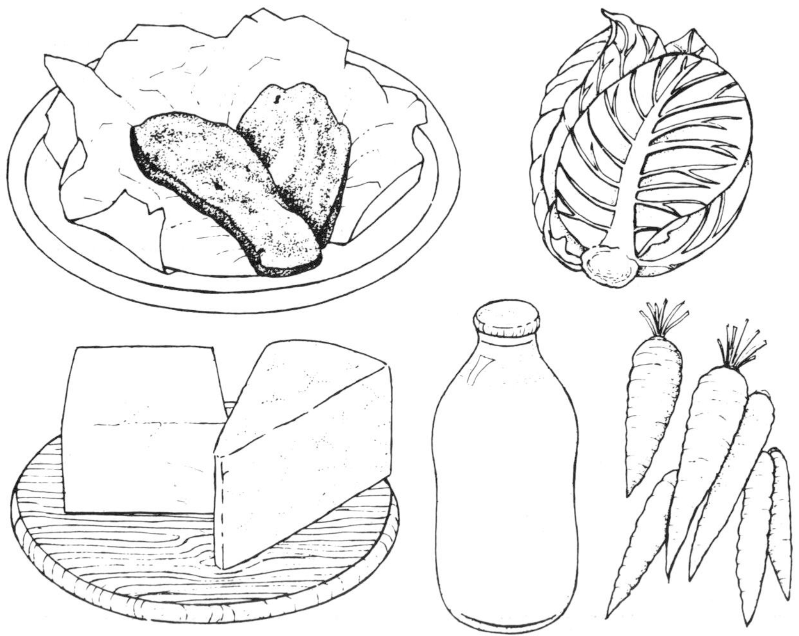

Fig. 1 These products contribute the most vitamin A

The role of vitamin A

Vitamin A has two very important functions. It is necessary for the health of our skin and other surface tissues. These other surface tissues include the lining and outer surfaces of all the body's organs. Vitamin A is also required for vision in dim light. It is an essential component of a substance called **visual purple**. Visual purple is found at the back of the eye and allows us to see in dim light (Fig. 2)

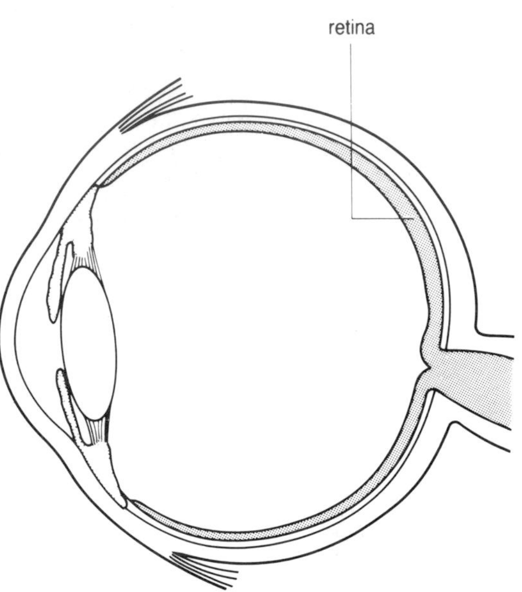

Fig. 2 Visual purple is part of the structure of the retina

Vitamin A deficiency

Vitamin A is a fat soluble vitamin and is therefore stored in the body. The main store is in the liver. Well nourished people can survive for one or two years on low intakes of vitamin A. Vitamin A deficiency is not found in the UK. In other parts of the world where poverty and malnutrition are widespread it is a problem. The first signs are night blindness and inability to see in dim light. Eventually, if no vitamin A is given, the person will go blind.

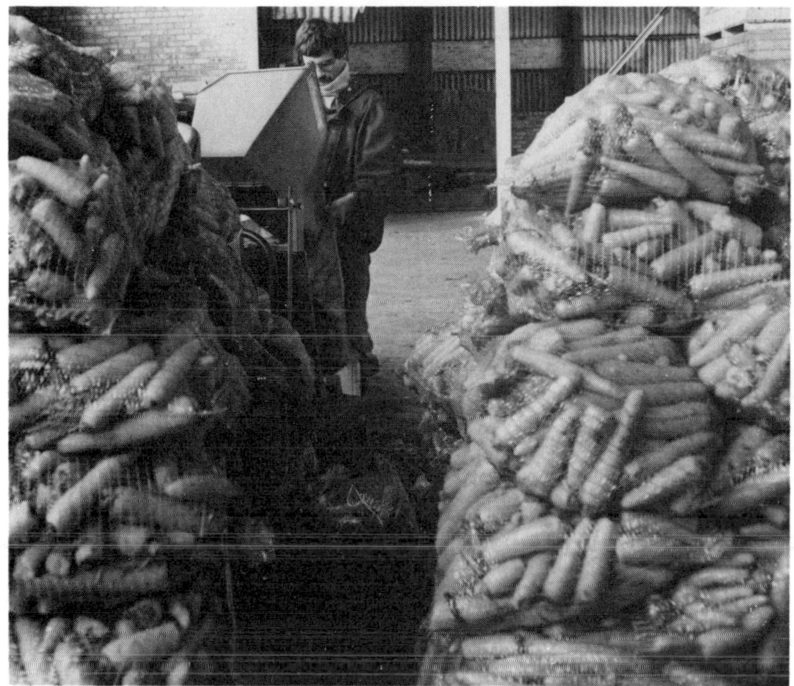

Fig. 3 Too much vitamin A is poisonous

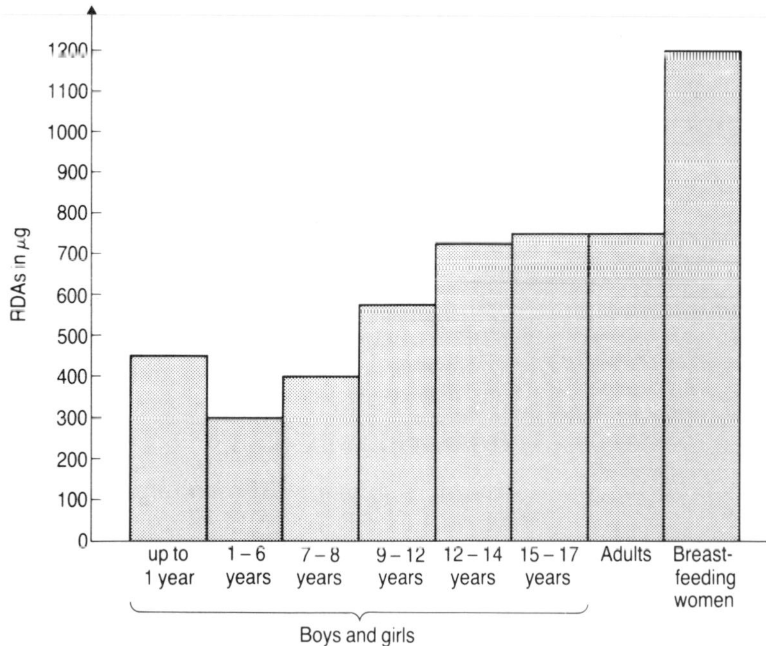

Fig. 4 RDAs for vitamin A

Too much vitamin A

Because vitamin A can be stored in the body if it is eaten in very large quantities, it can be poisonous. At least one person is known to have died in the UK from eating too many carrots (Fig. 3). He lived on virtually nothing else. Eventually his skin turned yellow and he died of vitamin A poisoning. Taking vitamin supplements can also lead to overdoses of vitamin A. If for any reason vitamin supplements are being used, great care should be taken to ensure that the recommended dose is not exceeded.

RDAs for vitamin A

RDAs for vitamin A are expressed in retinol equivalents. These include the contribution from β carotene (Fig. 4).

Vitamin K

Not much is known about vitamin K except that it is necessary for the normal **clotting** of blood. It is found in a wide variety of foods and dietary deficiency is unlikely. The best sources are green leafy vegetables and beef liver. Most other animal foods, cereals and fruit are relatively poor sources. Bacteria within our intestines can synthesize vitamin K.

Summary

- Fruit and vegetables are the main source of β carotene which becomes vitamin A in the body.
- Vitamin A is needed for seeing in dim light and for healthy skin and surface tissues.

Questions

1. Describe the different forms of vitamin A.
2. Where does most of our vitamin A come from? Why do we need it?
3. What are the effects of vitamin A deficiency?
4. Where in the body is it stored?

D B vitamins and minerals

Folic acid

Folic acid is the name given to a group of closely related chemical compounds known as **folates**. It is present in food in several different forms. The rate of absorption in the gut depends on the folate. Folates which are readily absorbed are called **free folates**. Vegetables and some fruit are important dietary sources. The best are green leafy vegetables like spinach, cabbage, broccoli and lettuce (Fig. 1). A few fruits contain useful amounts of folates. These are avocado pears, cantaloupe melons, oranges and bananas (Fig. 2). Folates are also found in offal and pulses. Other meat and dairy foods contain relatively little. Folates are destroyed very easily during cooking.

Fig. 1 Green leafy vegetables are a good source of free folates

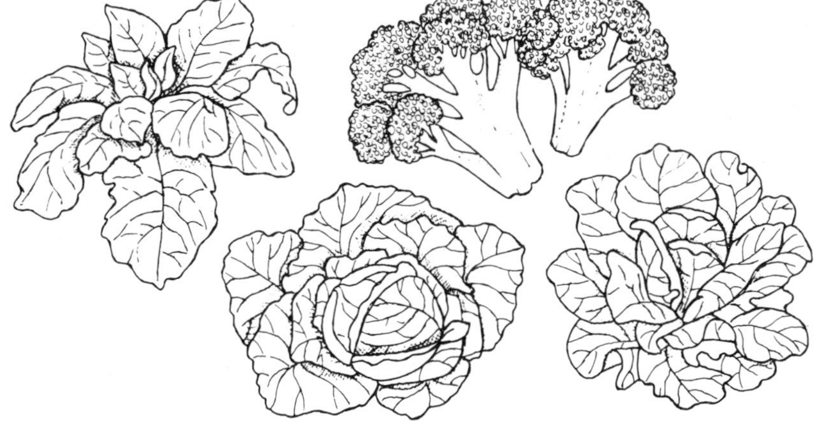

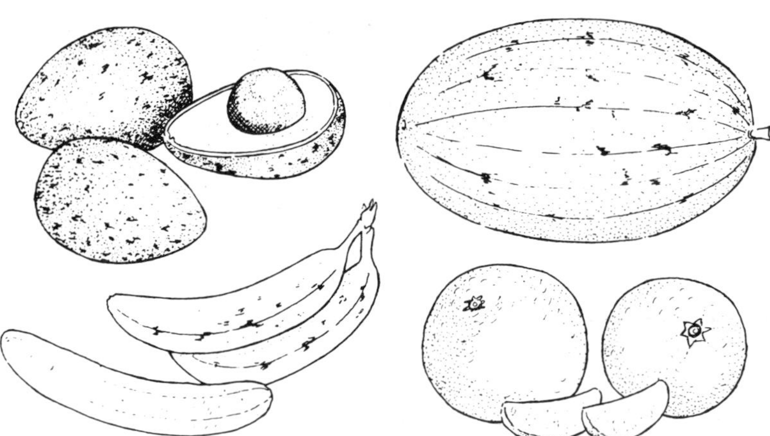

Fig. 2 A few fruits contain some folates

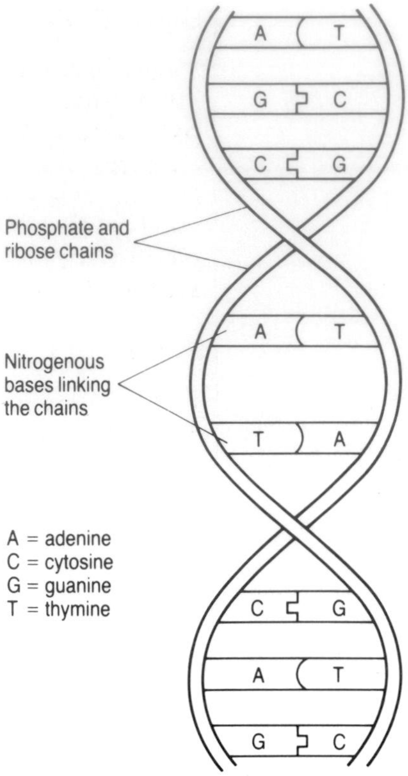

Phosphate and ribose chains

Nitrogenous bases linking the chains

A = adenine
C = cytosine
G = guanine
T = thymine

Fig. 3 Part of a molecule of DNA

The role of folic acid

Folic acid has several functions. The main function is the formation of DNA in rapidly dividing cells (Fig. 3). It is also important for the formation and maintenance of healthy blood. Folic acid is used in conjunction with vitamin B12 in these processes.

Folic acid deficiency

Requirements for folic acid are increased when the body is rapidly increasing its cell number. For example, it is needed during pregnancy when the foetus is being formed or at times of rapid growth. Elderly people who do not eat enough vegetables and fruit are also likely to suffer from folic acid deficiency. Deficiency causes a type of anaemia. Oral contraceptives and alcohol may also increase requirements for folic acid. Most pregnant women in the UK are given a folic acid supplement during their pregnancy.

Other B vitamins

Vegetables and fruit provide an important contribution to the **thiamin**, **pyridoxine** and **pantothenic acid** in a balanced diet. Pantothenic acid comes from some vegetables but is not found much in fruit. Also small amounts of **riboflavin**, **nicotinic acid** and **biotin** are found in some vegetables and fruit.

Potassium

Potassium is present in most of the fluids within the body. Its concentration is very carefully controlled. The amount in the body is related to the amount of lean tissue. It has a complementary relationship with sodium in the functioning of the cells. It is thought possible that the relationship between potassium and sodium in the diet may be connected with high blood pressure (Fig. 4). Diets which are relatively low in potassium and relatively high in sodium may contribute to high blood pressure.

Vegetables and fruit are one of the most important sources of potassium in the diet. Most of the potassium in the diet is absorbed and any extra to requirement is excreted through the kidneys.

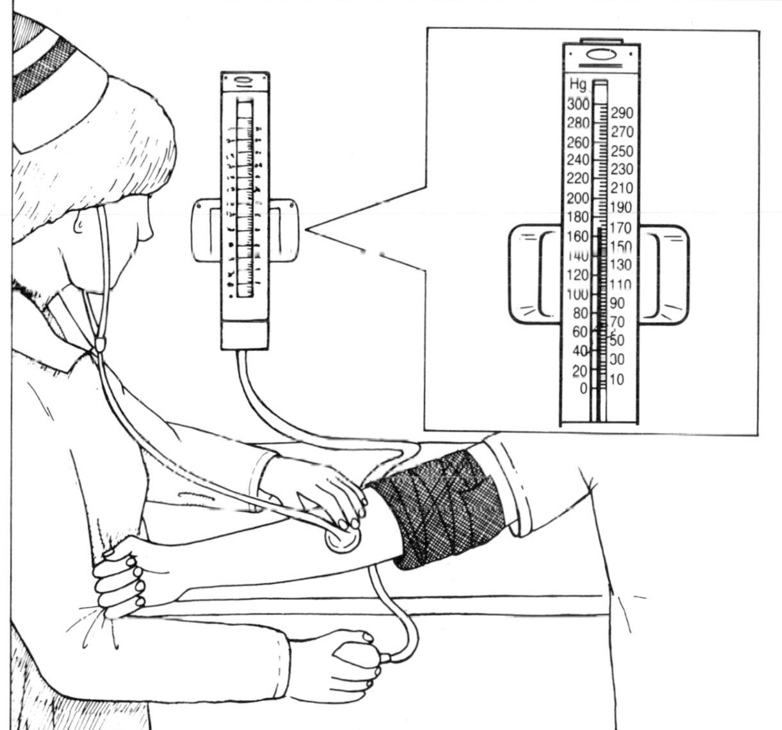

Fig. 4 High blood pressure

Other minerals

Fruit and vegetables make an important contribution to the amount of iron in the diet. On average they provide over 15%. The iron in vegetables and fruit is non-haem iron and the amount varies greatly between different types of vegetables and fruit. The vitamin C also present in these foods may help the body to absorb some of this iron. Fruit and vegetables also provide small amounts of zinc and phosphorus.

Summary

- Vegetables, especially green leafy ones, are good sources of the B vitamin called folic acid.
- Folic acid is needed for healthy blood and at times of rapid growth and cell division.
- Vegetables and fruit provide useful quantities of other B vitamins.
- These foods provide a variety of useful minerals including potassium, iron and zinc.

Questions

1. Which fruit and vegetables are good sources of folates?
2. Why do we need folates in the diet?
3. Which other B vitamins are found in fruit and vegetables?
4. Which minerals are found in fruit and vegetables in significant amounts?

E Effects of processing, storage and cooking

Cooking and processing can involve the use of heat and water. This leads to some **nutrient losses** in fruit and vegetables. The greatest losses occur with vitamin C, folic acid and thiamin.

Vitamin C

Vitamin C is very unstable. Fruit and vegetables contain enzymes which destroy vitamin C in the presence of oxygen. Destruction begins as soon as the crop is harvested. Damaging the cells by bruising, wilting and cutting of the fruit or vegetables increases the rate at which vitamin C is destroyed (Fig. 1). The broken cell membranes no longer separate the enzymes from the vitamin C. Careful storage and packing of vegetables and fruits is therefore essential to preserve as much vitamin C as possible. Preserving fruit and vegetables affects the vitamim C in different ways.

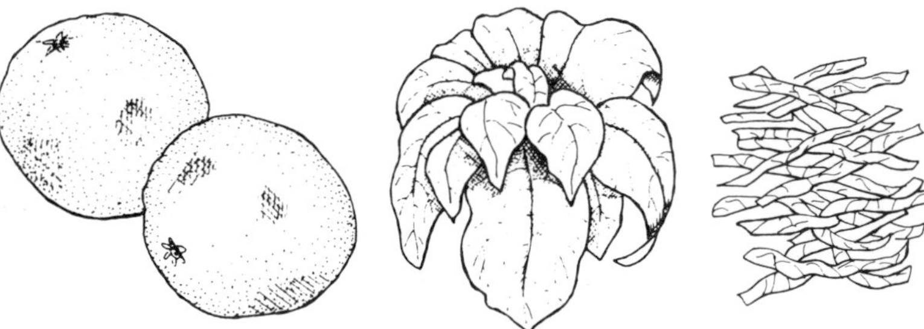

Fig. 1 More vitamin C is destroyed in bruised, wilting or cut fruit and vegetables

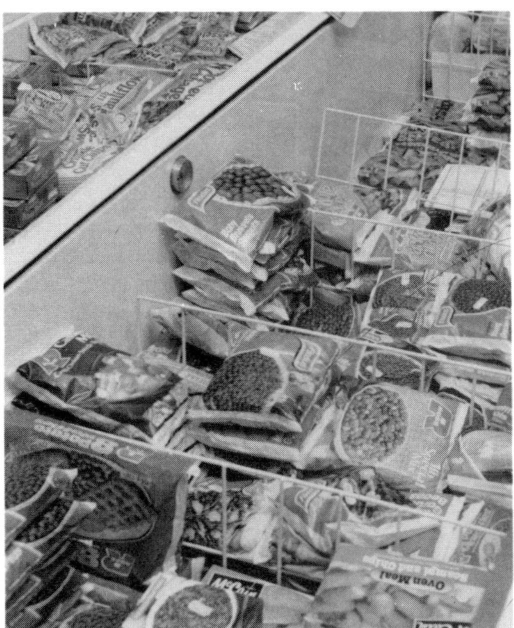

Fig. 2 Frozen fruit and vegetables

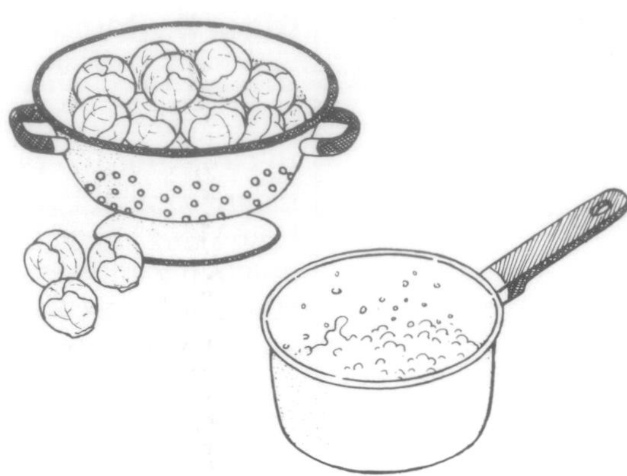

Fig. 3 Careful preparation and cooking can reduce the destruction of vitamin C

Frozen vegetables and fruit contain almost as much vitamin C as fresh ones (Fig. 2). There are greater losses during canning. After dehydration, there is very little vitamin C left at all. Vitamin C dissolves very easily in water, so if vegetables are cut up and soaked in water much of the vitamin C is removed from the vegetables. The smaller the pieces, the more vitamin C will be lost. Vitamin C is also destroyed by heat, so the cooking of vegetables over heat also adds to the loss of vitamin C. Cooking in an alkaline solution, for example in bicarbonate of soda, results in even greater losses.

If vegetables are prepared immediately before cooking and put straight into rapidly boiling water, the destruction of vitamin C is minimal (Fig. 3). Boiling the water before adding the vegetables helps reduce the vitamin C losses. Cooked vegetables should be eaten as soon as possible to preserve the maximum amount of vitamin C.

Vitamin C is often added to foods during **processing** (Fig. 4). It helps to stop changes which alter the colour of the food during storage. For example, it is used to stop preserved chips from going brown and also to speed up the proving of bread. The vitamin C used for these reasons in food processing may be destroyed during processing and is not always available to the body.

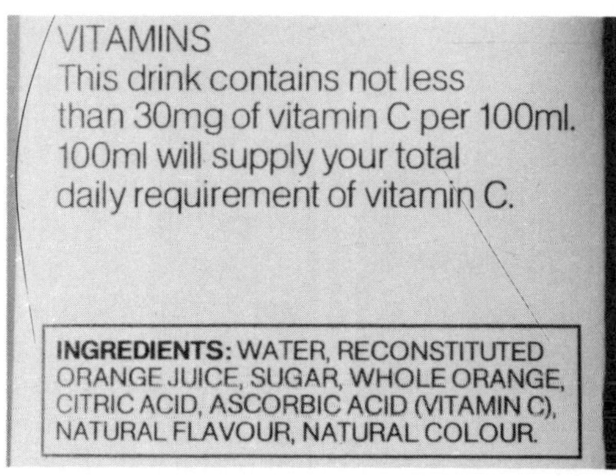
VITAMINS
This drink contains not less than 30mg of vitamin C per 100ml. 100ml will supply your total daily requirement of vitamin C.

INGREDIENTS: WATER, RECONSTITUTED ORANGE JUICE, SUGAR, WHOLE ORANGE, CITRIC ACID, ASCORBIC ACID (VITAMIN C), NATURAL FLAVOUR, NATURAL COLOUR.

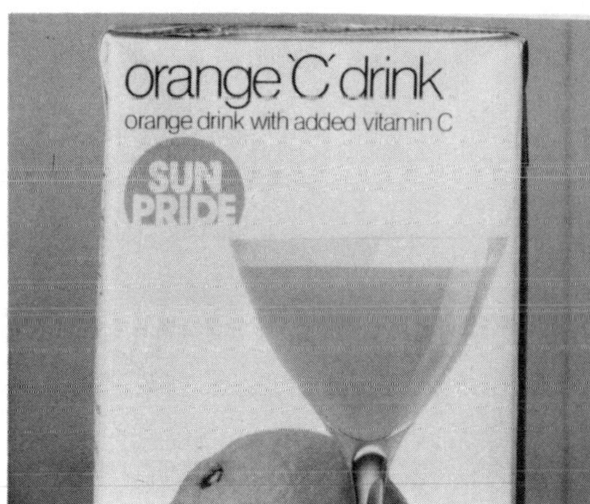

Fig. 4 Some processed foods have added vitamin C

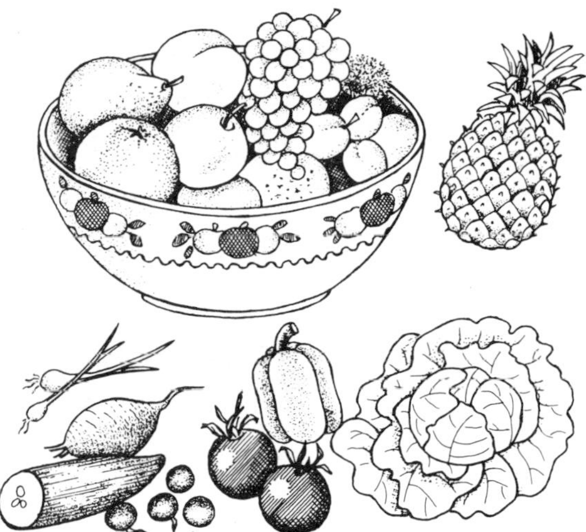

Fig. 5 Raw fruit and salad vegetables

Thiamin

All green vegetables, root vegetables and fruit contain some thiamin. None of them are rich sources but their contribution to the diet is important. Thiamin dissolves easily in water and the greatest losses occur during cooking. Adding sodium bicarbonate to water also speeds up the destruction of thiamin.

Because some of the most useful vitamins supplied by fruit and vegetables are so easily destroyed by processing, storage and cooking, it is important to eat at least one portion of raw fruit or salad vegetables each day (Fig. 5).

Folates

Cooking and preparing food can cause serious loss of folates. Folates are water soluble and **unstable**. They are easily destroyed by heating. Processes such as sterilization, pasteurization, canning, prolonged cooking or reheating can all destroy the folates. Destruction is increased in neutral or alkaline conditions, for example cooking in water or if sodium bicarbonate is added. On average, vegetables lose almost half of their total folates during processing and cooking. This can be as high as 90% to 100% if the vegetables are overcooked.

Summary

- Vitamin C, folates and thiamin are all very easily destroyed.
- Careful cooking and storage are essential to maintain the nutrients.
- At least one portion of fresh fruit or raw vegetables should be included in the diet daily.

Questions

1. Describe the ways in which the vitamin C found in fresh fruit or vegetables is reduced before we eat the food.
2. What kitchen practices will help retain the maximum amount of vitamin C in food?
3. What happens to folates when vegetables are cooked?
4. Why should sodium bicarbonate never be added to the water in which vegetables are cooked?

F Digestion

Fruit and vegetables are good sources of **dietary fibre**, consisting mainly of cellulose, hemicellulose and pectin. The dietary fibre reaches the colon undigested. It adds to the bulk of the faeces, absorbs water and encourages growth of gut flora and fauna. It is thought that some of the fibre is digested by the gut bacteria, forming simple sugars which add to the energy made available to the body.

Foods in this group contain very little fat and protein. The main contribution to the diet is **vitamin C**, which is absorbed directly, and **carbohydrates**.

The carbohydrates in fruit and vegetables are mainly in the form of sugars like fructose, glucose and sucrose. Sucrose is split in the small intestine by the enzyme **sucrase** into its monosaccharide components fructose and glucose. These simple sugars are directly absorbed into the blood stream.

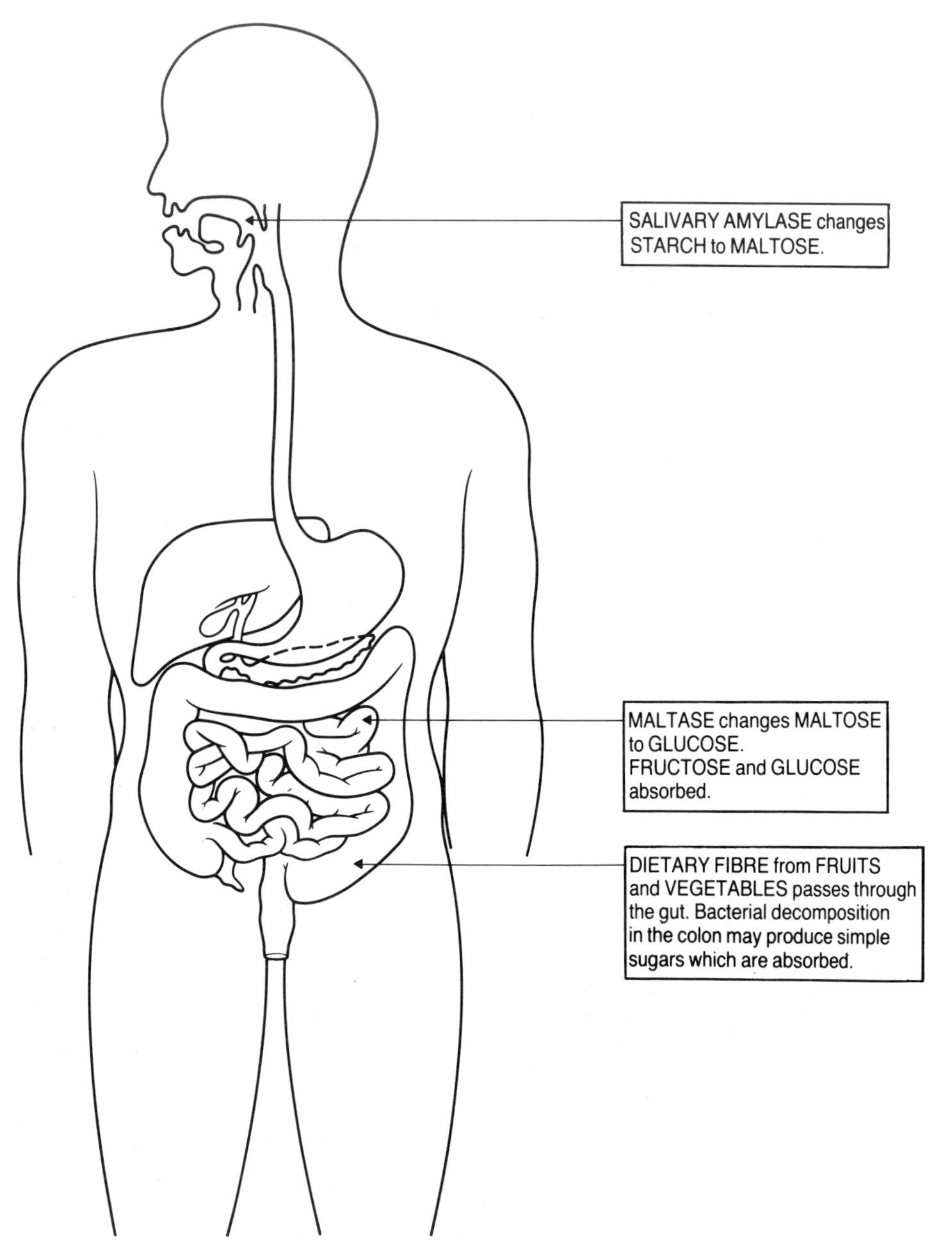

Fig. 1 Digestion of fruit and vegetables

4.9 The nutritional role of meat and its alternatives

A Dietary energy, protein, dietary fibre and fat

Dietary energy

The foods in this group provide approximately 20% of the total energy in UK diets. Most of this comes from meat, meat products, fish and eggs. Vegetarians or those whose traditional eating habits are based on pulses and nuts will get a significant proportion of their dietary energy from these foods.

The amount of dietary energy provided by these foods depends partly on their fat content and partly on the amount of water they contain. Fatty meat and meat products, for example, have a much higher energy density than lean meat (Fig. 1).

Fig. 1 Some cuts of meat have more fat than others. They provide a large amount of dietary energy

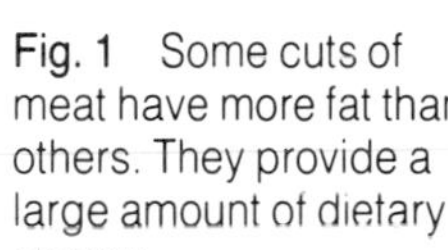

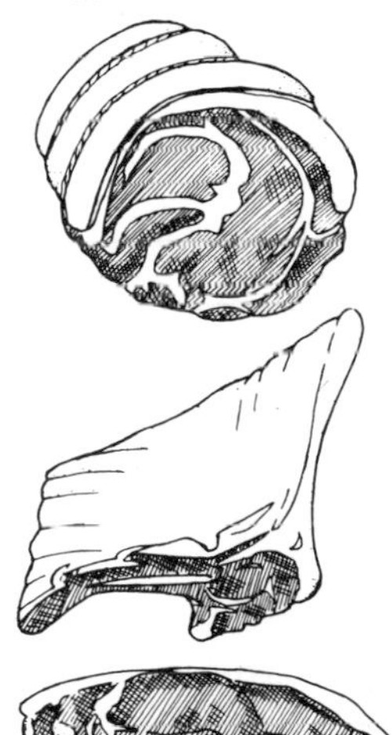

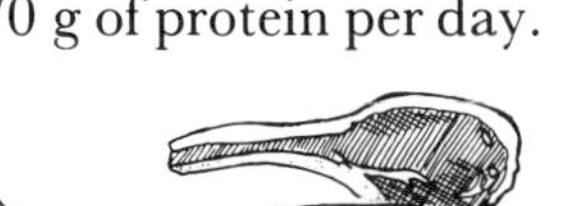

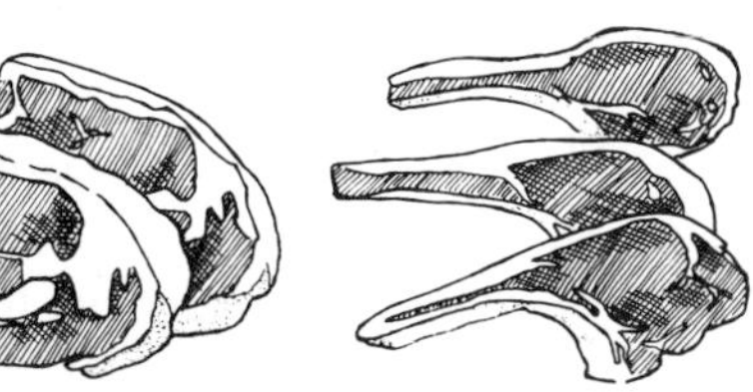

Protein

Meat and its alternatives are the most important source of protein in most people's diets. They provide approximately 40% of our dietary protein. People who do not eat animal foods get their protein from cereal foods, pulses and nuts. The amount of protein we need depends to a certain extent on our dietary energy needs. Protein should provide about 10% to 15% of the energy in our diets.

The average diet in the UK provides approximately 70 g of protein per day. The RDA for most women between 18 and 54 years is 54 g. Excess protein is converted in the body to fat where it is either stored or used for energy.

Dietary fibre

Pulses and nuts are important sources of dietary fibre. Using pulses as a meat extender or as an alternative to meat and dairy products contributes greatly towards suggested increases in dietary fibre intakes.

Fat

Food from animal sources usually contains relatively large amounts of fat. The proportion of fat in some meat and meat products can be as much as 50%. In pulses and white fish it is less than 5%. The type of fat found in most meats and meat products is high in **saturated fatty acids**, and so care should be taken over the amount eaten. The fat found in fish is less saturated and contains a higher proportion of mono- and polyunsaturated fatty acids. Poultry and white fish have relatively small amounts of fat.

The food from this group provides on average over 30% of daily fat intake. Meat and meat products provide about 25% of the saturated fat in our diets.

Summary

- Meat and its alternatives are important sources of dietary energy in our diet.
- Using pulses in place of some meat and meat products increases dietary fibre.
- Some meat and meat products are very high in saturated fat.

Questions

1. How does the amount of dietary energy provided by foods in this group differ?
2. Which foods in this group are good sources of dietary fibre?
3. What can you do to reduce the saturated fats you obtain from foods in this group?

B B group vitamins

Meat and its alternatives are the most important contributors to the B vitamins nicotinic acid (vitamin B3), pyridoxine (vitamin B6), cyanocobalamin (vitamin B12), pantothenic acid and biotin.

Fig. 1 Good sources of vitamin B3 (nicotinic acid)

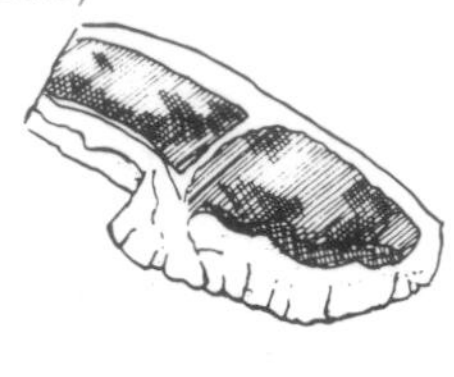

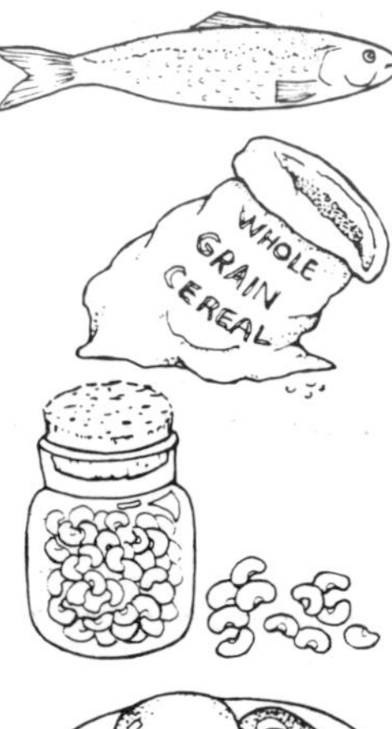

Vitamin B3 (nicotinic acid)

Nicotinic acid is found widely in plants and animal foods but only in small amounts. Meats, fish, whole grain cereal, pulses and offal foods are all useful sources (Fig. 1).

Nicotinic acid is turned in the body into **nicotinamide**. This is the form in which it is used. The amino acid tryptophan can also be converted into nicotinic acid. Sixty milligrams of tryptophan is required to make 1 mg of nicotinic acid. Nicotinic acid in the diet is measured in nicotinic acid equivalents. This includes the contribution from tryptophan.

In the UK nearly half the nicotinic acid in the diet is supplied by meat and meat products. Half of the remainder comes from cereal foods.

The role of nicotinic acid Nicotinic acid is involved in releasing energy from food. It is therefore important for growth as well as for general everyday life. It is also important for healthy skin, tongue, digestive and nervous systems.

Severe **nicotinic acid deficiency** is not found in the UK. It is usually only found in countries where maize is the staple food. Maize should be treated with an alkaline solution before use, to destroy the niacytin which prevents the nicotinic acid being absorbed. The deficiency causes sore, cracked skin, diarrhoea and nervous depression. Partial paralysis can also occur.

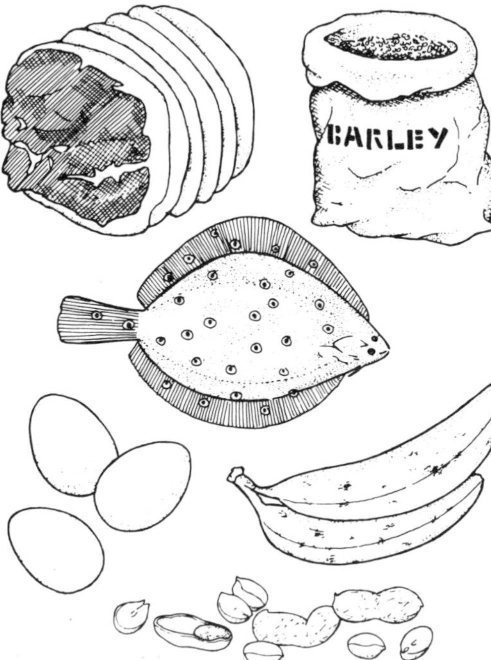

Fig. 2 Good sources of vitamin B6 (pyridoxine)

Vitamin B6 (pyridoxine)

Pyridoxine is one of the compounds which make up vitamin B6, and is found in many foods. The best sources are meat, fish, eggs, whole grain cereals, peanuts and bananas (Fig. 2). Vitamin B6 is involved in the metabolism of amino acids. It is needed for the conversion of tryptophan to nicotinic acid. Vitamin B6 requirements are therefore related to the protein content of the diet. The vitamin is also needed to make the haemoglobin in the blood.

Vitamin B6 deficiency is not thought to be a major problem in the UK. Some groups of elderly people have been found to have vitamin B6 deficiency. Women taking oral contraceptives may also need more vitamin B6 than other people.

Vitamin B12

Vitamin B12 occurs only in foods from animal sources (meat, fish, eggs, milk and milk products – Fig. 3) and in some micro-organisms which may be present in some foods as contaminants. Some B12 is found in fermented vegetable products such as tempee and meso, which are fermented soya bean products. It is required by the body in very small amounts, for the production of red blood cells and the normal functioning of the nervous system. It is also involved in the metabolism of protein, carbohydrates and fats. Together with folic acid it is needed by rapidly dividing cells such as those in the bone marrow and those which form the blood.

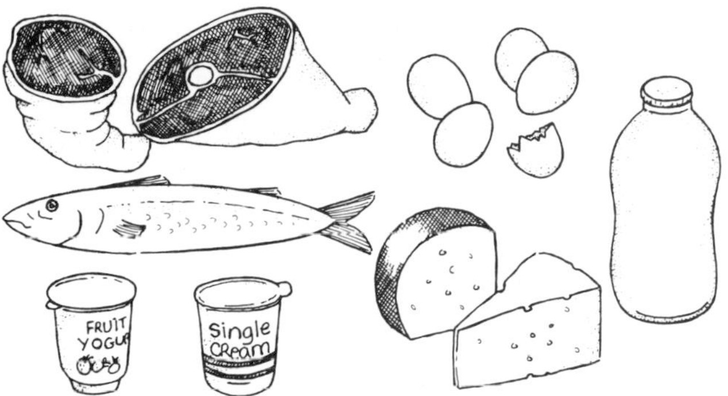

Fig. 3 Good sources of vitamin B12

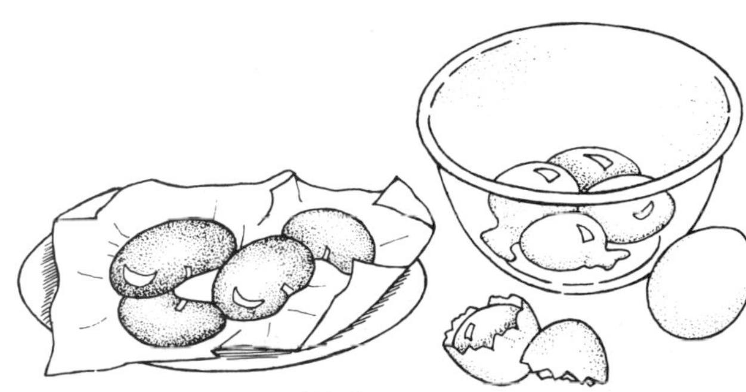

Fig. 5 Good sources of biotin

B12 deficiency is known as **pernicious anaemia**. It is more likely to result from enzyme rather than dietary deficiency. A particular enzyme is needed in the gut for the absorption of vitamin B12. If this is not present then pernicious anaemia will result. Vitamin B12 is added to some foods for vegans, such as yeast extracts and soya products.

Pantothenic acid

Pantothenic acid is found in all living tissues. The best dietary sources include liver, kidney, yeast, egg yolk, wheatgerm, peanuts and some vegetables (Fig. 4). Its main function is in the release of energy from fat and carbohydrates. Deficiency of pantothenic acid has not been found in the UK.

Fig. 4 Good sources of pantothenic acid

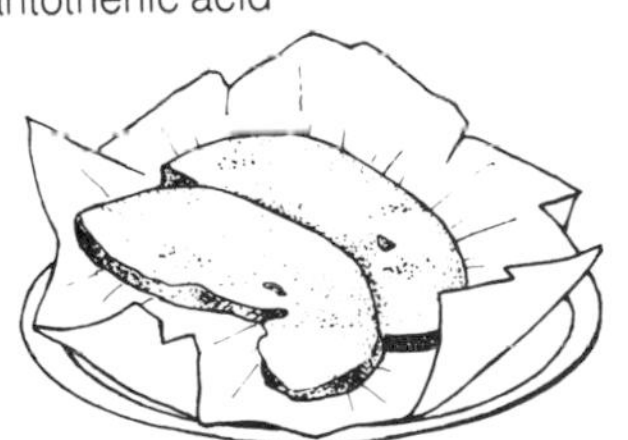

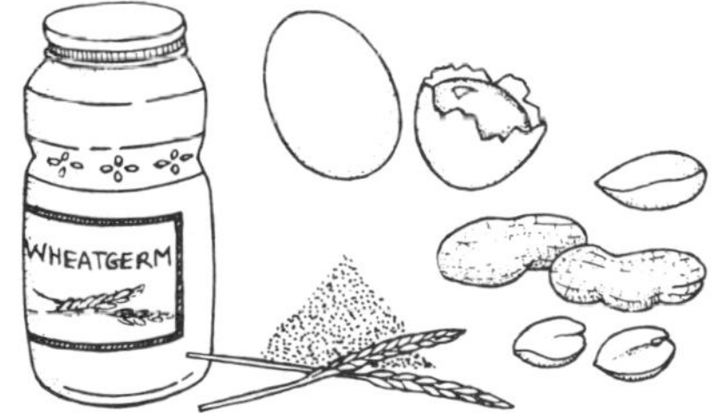

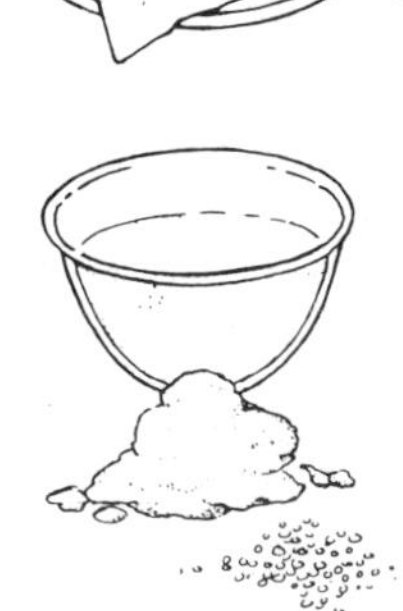

Biotin

Biotin is essential for the metabolism of fat. Rich sources of biotin include offal and egg yolk (Fig. 5). Smaller amounts are found in milk and milk products, cereals, fish and some fruit and vegetables.

Other B vitamins

Meat and its alternatives can also be important sources of **thiamin**, **riboflavin** and **folic acid**.

Summary

- These foods are the main source of nicotinic acid in the diet.
- Nicotinic acid is important for the release of energy from foods.
- The B vitamins pyridoxine, pantothenic acid and biotin are all found in useful quantities in these foods.
- The animal foods in this group are an important source of vitamin B12.
- People who do not eat animal foods need to take a vitamin B12 supplement.

Questions

1. Complete this table:

B group vitamin	Main source	Function in the body
Nicotinic acid Pyridoxine B12 Pantothenic acid Biotin		

2. Why is maize treated with limewater before being made into Mexican tortillas?
3. Why might vegans need B12 supplements?

Fig. 1 Good sources of vitamin D

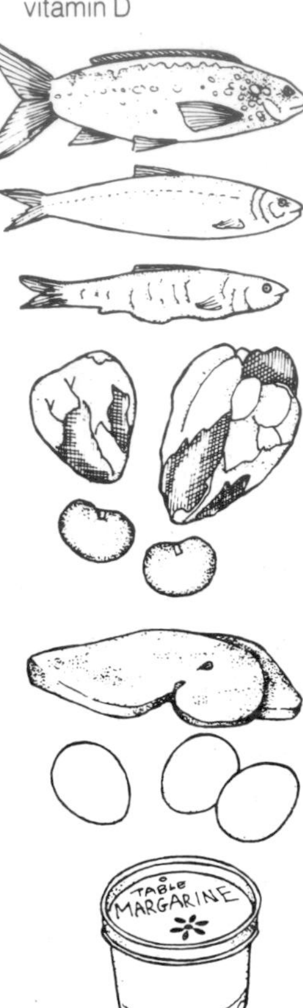

C Fat soluble vitamins

The foods in this group are important sources of fat soluble vitamins, vitamin A and vitamin D.

Vitamin D

Very few foods contain vitamin D. These include oily fish, eggs, offal and margarine (Fig. 1). Cheese, butter and milk contain only small amounts. Some breakfast cereals are fortified with vitamin D. About one third of dietary vitamin D comes from the fish, eggs and some offal in this food group.

The role of vitamin D

Vitamin D is essential for the absorption and utilization of **calcium**. It is involved in the production of a protein which binds calcium, promoting the absorption of calcium from the gut. It keeps the right amount of calcium in the bones by allowing the addition or removal of calcium as necessary. It increases the absorption of phosphate, also required for building bones, by stimulating the transport of phosphate into the blood stream.

Other sources of vitamin D

The vitamin D in our diets plays a very small role in providing the vitamin D we actually need. Mostly it is produced in the body by the action of sunlight on the skin. Even relatively small amounts of **ultraviolet rays** from the sun falling on the skin can provide useful amounts of vitamin D. Ensuring that people, especially the elderly, spend time in the summer sunshine is important for their nutritional status (Fig. 2). For most people dietary vitamin D is not essential.

RDAs for vitamin D

Dietary vitamin D is important during periods of rapid growth, during pregnancy and when women are breastfeeding. Elderly people who do not get out into the sunshine very much may also be at risk of not getting sufficient vitamin D. They too need to get plenty from their diet.

Vitamin D deficiency

In growing children vitamin D deficiency causes **rickets** (Fig. 3). Rickets occurs when the calcium cannot get to the bones to make them grow properly. Bones in the ankles and wrists become swollen and when the child begins to walk the bones bend, resulting in knock knees or bow legs. Rickets can be cured by giving large doses of vitamin D. However, if changes in the bone shape have already occurred these cannot be corrected. Vitamin D deficiency in adults is called **osteomalacia**. The bones progressively

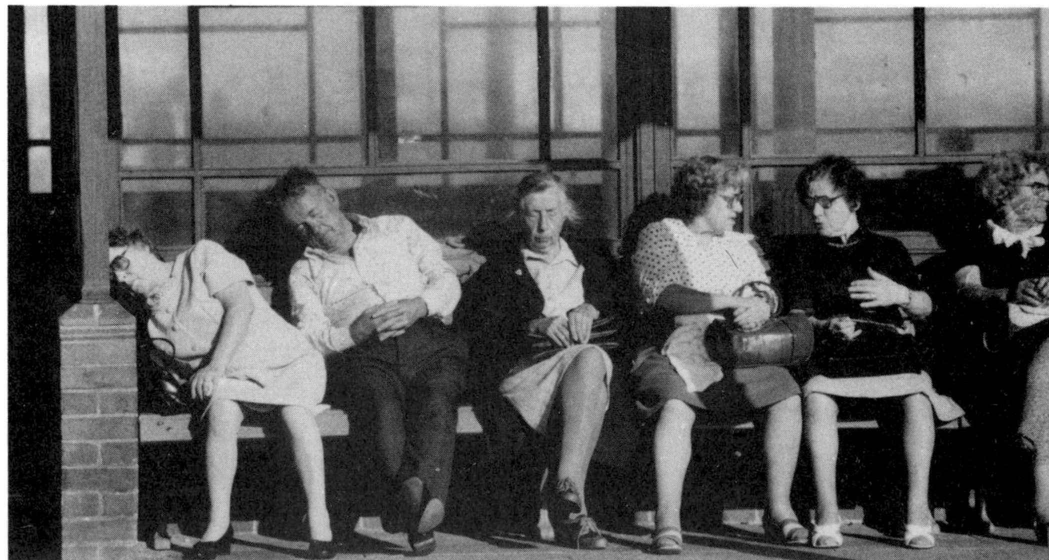

Fig. 2 Sunshine provides useful amounts of vitamin D, especially for elderly people

lose their calcium and become weak. Osteomalacia may be a problem for women who have had frequent pregnancies and for people who have had little exposure to sunlight. Tradition may dictate this. It may also be common amongst housebound elderly people in the UK and amongst those people in long stay hospitals.

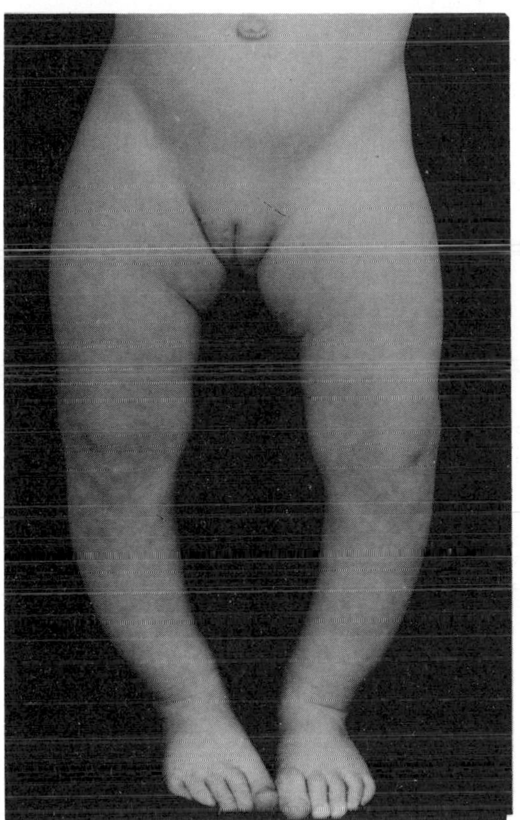

Fig. 3 A child suffering from rickets

Vitamin supplements

Vitamin D is a fat soluble vitamin and so is not excreted from the body. It is stored in the fatty tissues. Too much of it can be poisonous. As little as five times the RDA taken over prolonged periods has been shown to cause problems. If vitamin D supplements are being used care should be taken to make sure that the amount does not exceed the recommended dose. It is not possible to eat too much vitamin D in foods. Some foods such as margarine and breakfast cereals and some types of milk are fortified with vitamin D.

Vitamin A

The foods in this group can be an important source of vitamin A. Liver is the richest source there is. Eggs and oily fish are also useful sources, as are yellow or green pulses (Fig. 4). The rest of the foods in this group do not provide very much vitamin A. The vitamin A in the animal foods in this group is in the form of retinol, while in the vegetable foods it is in the form of beta carotene.

Other fat soluble vitamins

Eggs are a useful source of vitamin E, and beef liver is a useful source of vitamin K.

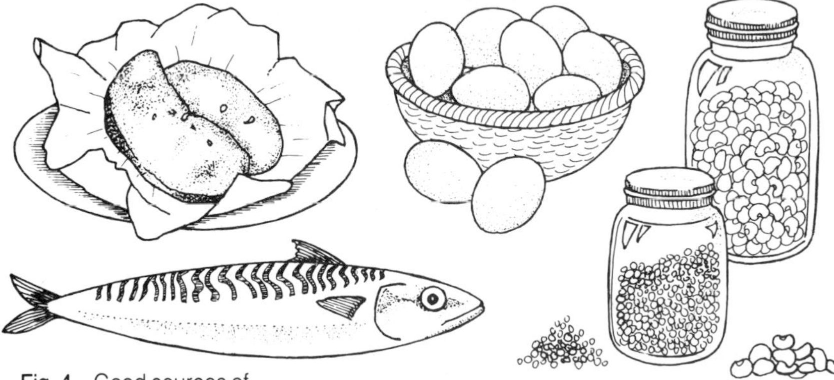

Fig. 4 Good sources of vitamin A

Summary

- Oily fish and eggs yolks are important sources of dietary vitamin D.
- We get most of our vitamin D from sunshine falling on the skin.
- Elderly people, young children and pregnant and breastfeeding women need extra vitamin D.
- The best source of vitamin A is liver.

Questions

1. Why is dietary vitamin D not essential for most people?
2. What role does vitamin D play in the body?
3. Which foods are rich sources of vitamin A, and which are rich sources of vitamin D?

D *Minerals*

The foods in this group supply a wide range of minerals and trace elements.

Iron

The iron in the animal foods in this group is in the form of **haem iron**. It is derived from the blood of the animals. As haem iron it is more easily absorbed than the non-haem iron found in the pulses in this group. The foods in this group provide nearly 30% of the dietary iron in the UK. The richest sources are liver and kidneys. The absorption of iron from egg may be reduced by **phosphor-proteins** present in the eggs. These bind the iron making it insoluble in the gut and therefore not available.

Calcium

Sardines, pilchards and other tinned fish are often eaten with their bones (Fig. 1). They are then a very important source of dietary calcium for people who do not eat or drink animal milk and its products. There are also useful amounts of calcium in the pulses in this group, but the rest of the foods contain very little.

Trace elements

Zinc, potassium and phosphorus are also present in useful quantities in the foods in this group.

Summary

- The iron in animal foods in this group is important because it is more easily absorbed than the iron in cereals, pulses and vegetables.
- Fish eaten with its bones can be a useful source of calcium.

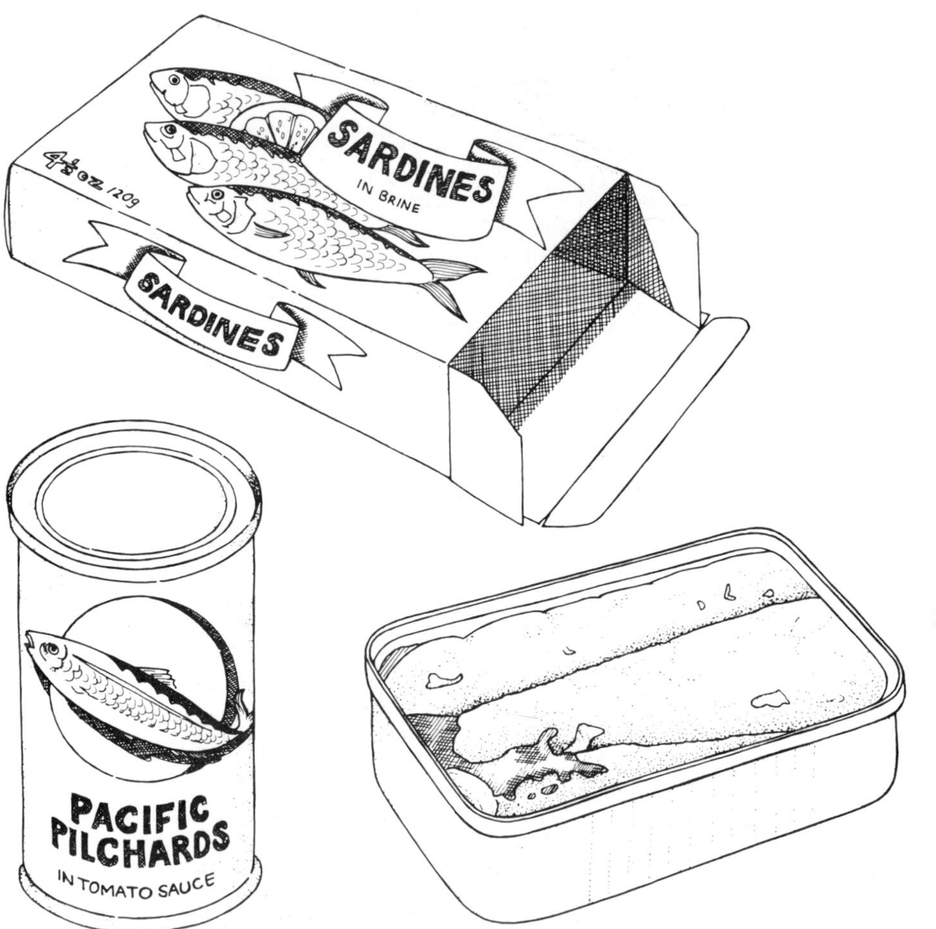

Fig. 1 Tinned fish that are eaten with their bones are a good source of calcium

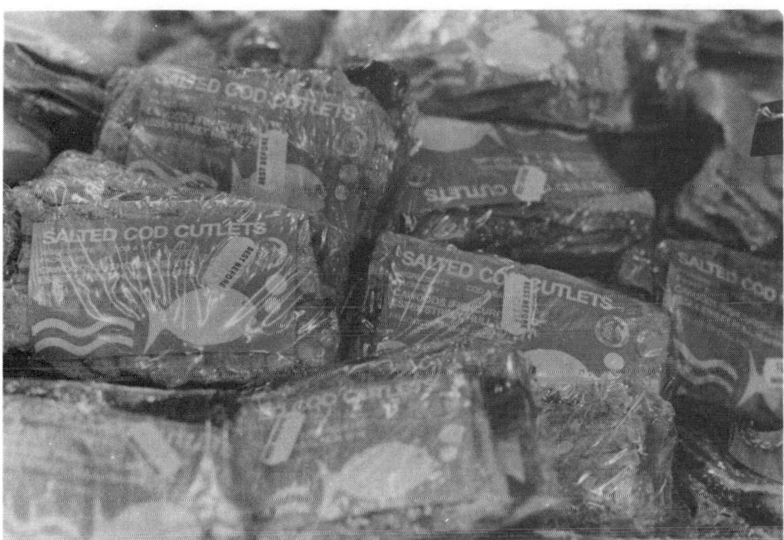

Fig. 1 Fish may be salted, canned or frozen

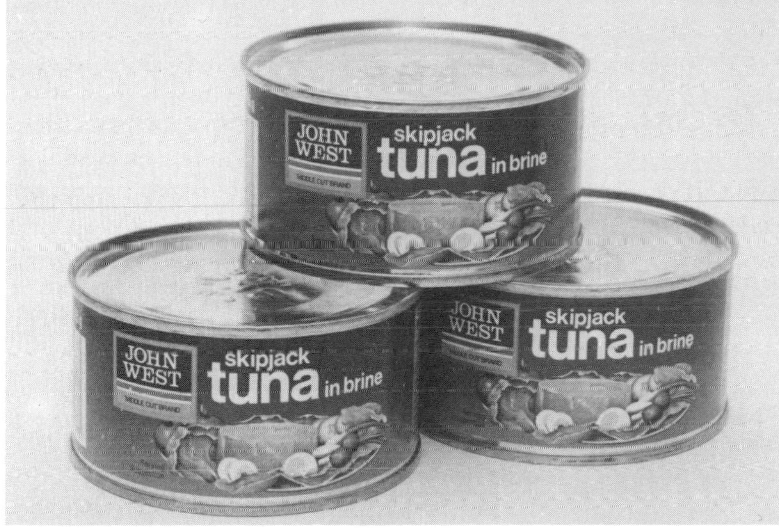

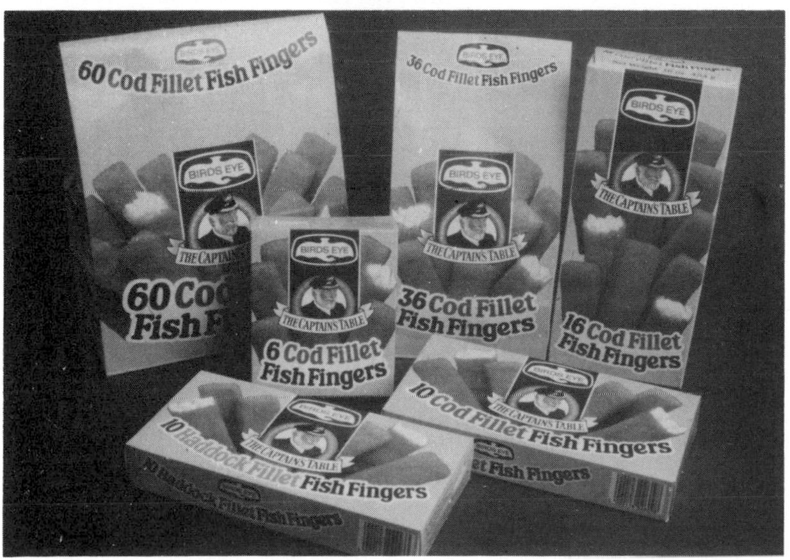

E Effects of cooking and processing

Cooking

The foods in this group are rarely eaten raw. Cooking alters the nutritional value and digestibility. Protein coagulates and becomes soluble and therefore more easily digested. The collagen in meat and fish is hydrolysed to form gelatine which is soft and easy to digest.

The B group vitamins are all sensitive to heat and, being water soluble, are lost in the fluid when frozen meat is thawed. Vitamin B12 is stable to heat but not in continued heating. Milk which has been boiled and cooled down before drinking may have lost much of its vitamin B12.

Cooking destroys poisonous micro-organisms in food. The animal foods in this group are the foods most likely to cause **food poisoning**. They are good media for the growth of micro-organisms. Careful storage and cooking is therefore essential. Most cases of food poisoning from meat, meat products and poultry result from storing them for too long at temperatures which are not low enough.

Pulses have to be cooked before they are eaten. However, mung and soya beans, for example, may be sprouted and eaten raw. Some beans, i.e. those from the kidney bean family, have to be boiled for at least 15 minutes after they have been soaked and before they are cooked slowly. These beans cannot be sprouted. If these beans are not boiled before slow cooking they are poisonous and can cause severe stomach upset.

Commercial food processing

Many of the foods in this group are changed in various ways before we eat them. They may be salted, smoked, canned, frozen, have preservatives added and be combined with other ingredients to make compound dishes such as pies, sausages, fish fingers and beefburgers (Fig. 1). This processing can alter the nutritional value of food in a number of ways.

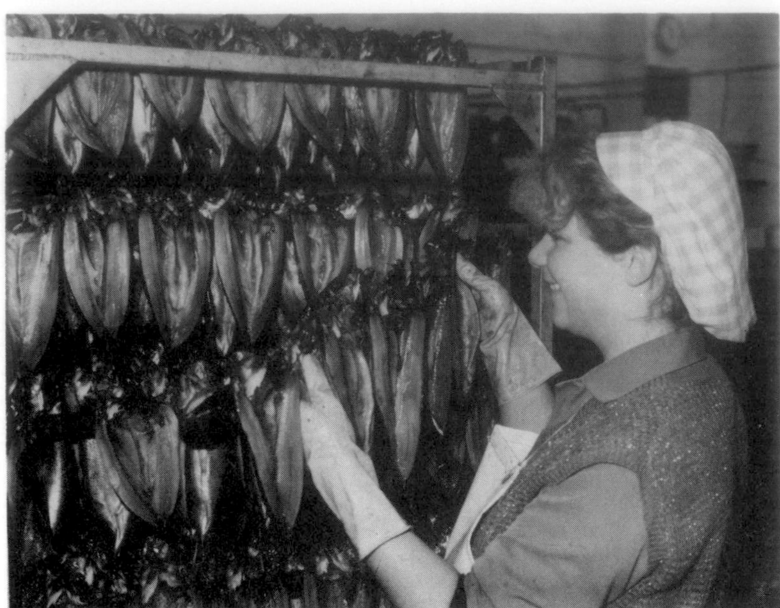

Fig. 2 Kippers being smoked

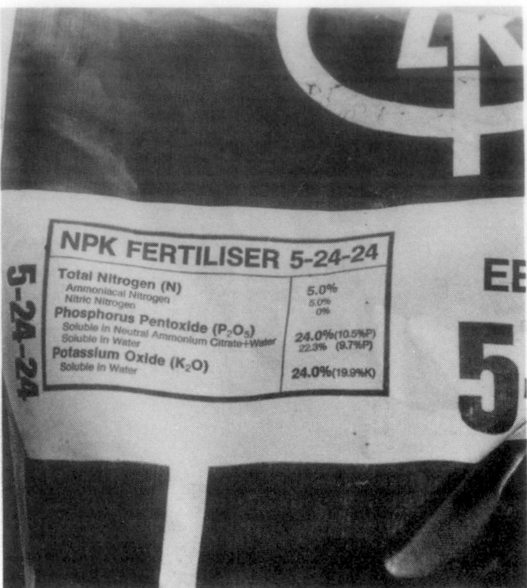

Fig. 3 Nitrates as a fertilizer

Salting Salt is added to protect meat and fish from deterioration. Examples of salted foods are ham, bacon, salt beef, salt fish, and smoked fish (Fig. 2).

Salt is also added to other processed foods in order to preserve them, add flavour and alter their texture. Most tinned foods contain relatively large amounts of salt.

Canning The foods in this group are usually cooked or processed before they are canned. They often have other ingredients such as cereals, sauces, gravy or pastry added. Many canned and processed meats have a higher fat content than their raw equivalent. Oil is often added to canned fish as well as salt. Pulses are often cooked and canned. The most popular of these is baked beans. There are also other varieties of canned beans, such as red kidney beans, butter beans and chick peas. The nutritional content of canned beans is not altered greatly from their fresh alternatives.

Freezing On the whole freezing does not result in nutritional losses. Some vitamins are, however, lost as fluid drips out of thawing meat. There is nowadays an increasing number of ready prepared frozen dishes available.

Nitrites and nitrates These are often added to foods as preservatives and to meat to enhance the red colour. Nitrites may react in the gut with other chemicals. They are widely used as fertilizers and are present in small amounts in many types of plant foods (Fig. 3). They are converted in the gut to nitrate. Although there is some evidence that nitrates can cause cancer, they are still permitted food additives in the UK.

Summary

- Cooking coagulates proteins and makes them easier to digest.
- Processing meat may result in the addition of fat and chemical additives.

Questions

1. What happens to the protein in meat when it is cooked?
2. Why is particular care needed when preparing and cooking foods from this group?
3. Why must kidney beans be well cooked?
4. Describe some ways in which foods from this group are processed.
5. Why are nitrates added to food? What are the possible dangers of this additive?

F Digestion

The main contribution to the diet made by foods in this group is **protein**. Some meats and meat products contain large amounts of fat, and the pulses contain starch and dietary fibre. The vitamins and minerals contained in these foods do not need to be digested. Protein is a large and complex molecule. Before it can be utilized by the body, the molecule must be split into smaller units called **peptides**. This can occur in the stomach as a result of the action of pepsin, but it continues in the small intestine. The other enzymes which split proteins and peptides into amino acids are erepsin from the intestinal juice and trypsin from the pancreatic juice. Some of the smaller protein or peptide units are able to pass through the gut wall. This is clear from some allergic reactions. Amino acids do not cause allergy, so an allergy to protein is a result of that protein passing through the intestinal wall.

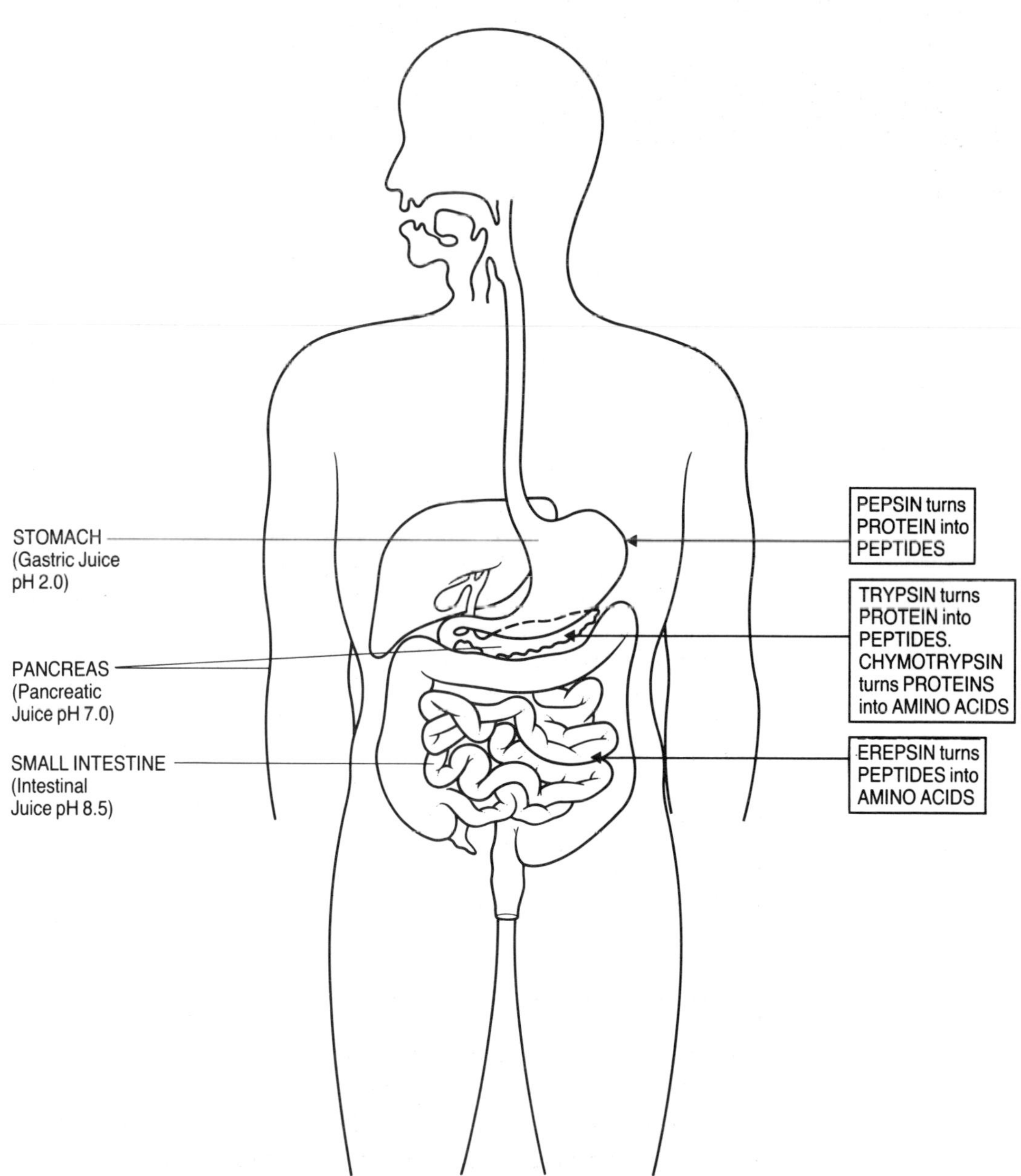

Fig. 1 Digestion of meat and alternatives

4.10 | The nutritional role of milk and milk products

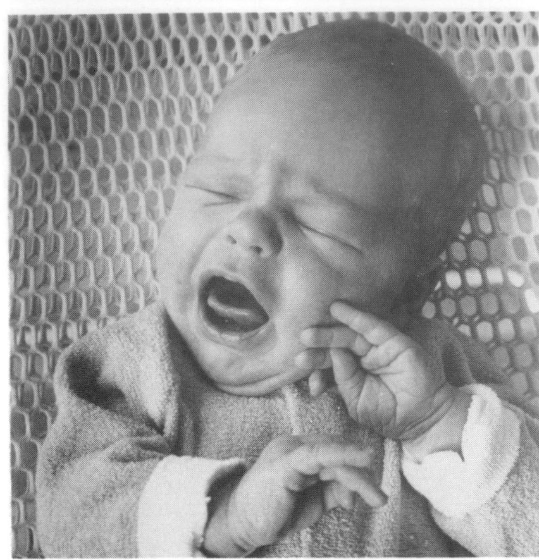

Fig. 1 A baby demanding to be fed

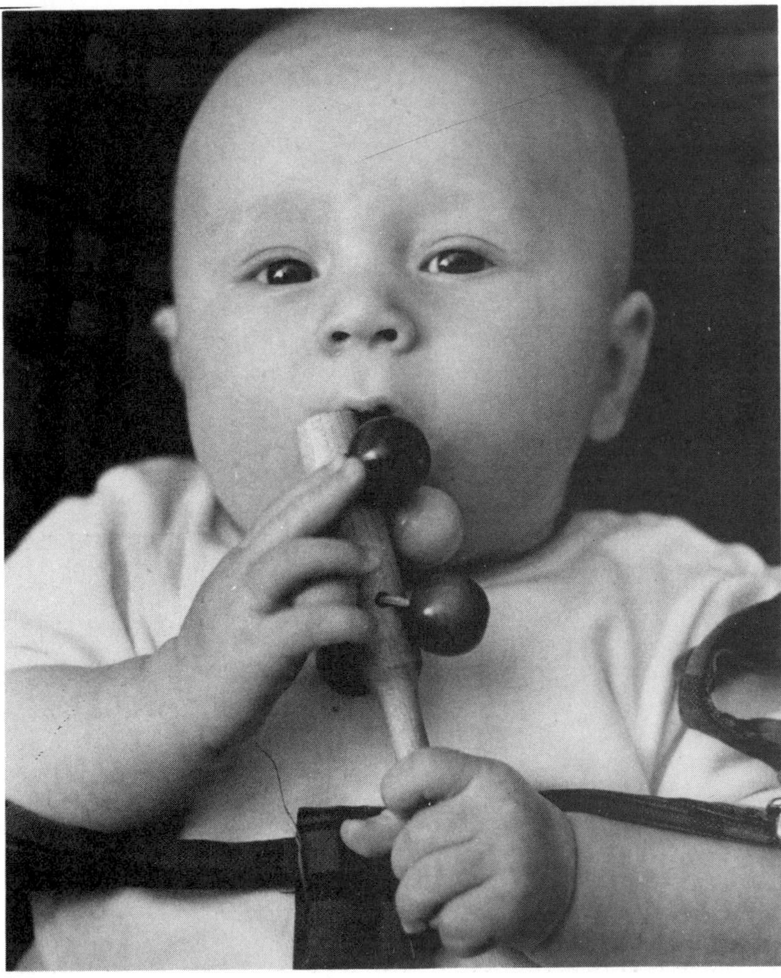

Fig. 2 An overweight breastfed baby will soon slim down

A Infant feeding

The best type of food for newborn babies is breast milk. For the first few days of life, breast milk contains only a substance called **colostrum**. Colostrum gives the baby important antibodies to protect it against infection. After two or three days, the breast milk begins to come through properly. The more the baby suckles the more breast milk there will be.

The composition of breast milk is different at the beginning and at the end of each feed. As the feed goes on the fat content of the milk increases. Eventually the baby becomes full and stops suckling. When the baby is hungry again it starts to cry and is given more breast milk (Fig. 1). This is called **demand feeding**. Feeding babies cannot be regulated by watches. They need to be fed when they are ready for it.

Breast milk is best for the baby because it contains all the nutrients, vitamins and minerals which a baby needs in the right amounts. It is different from other animal milks in the amount and type of protein and fat it contains. It contains very little iron so the baby relies on the store of iron which has been built up in its liver while it has been in the womb.

Breastfeeding is cheap, convenient, readily available and a clean way of feeding babies. It does not involve the use of feeding bottles and teats which need to be carefully sterilized to avoid infections. Breastfed babies take as much food as they need. Occasionally they eat a lot and become fat, but this overweight soon disappears when they start running around and eating a mixed diet (Fig. 2).

Occasionally women do not want to breastfeed their babies. They might find it difficult and do not want to breastfeed for social or psychological reasons. Some women return to work while their babies are still quite young. For them

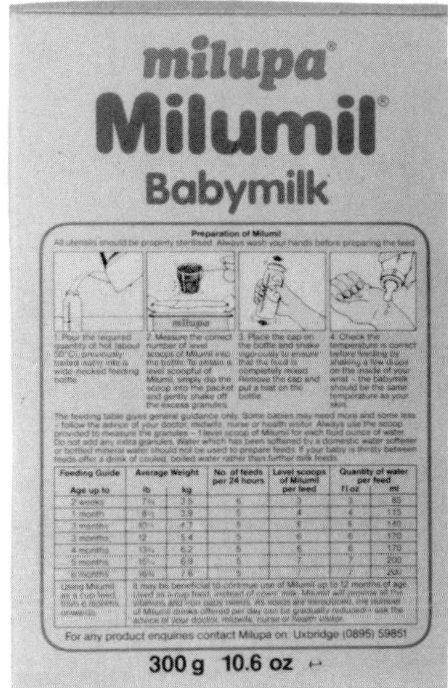

TYPICAL ANALYSIS	Per 100 g granulate	Per 100 ml prepared feed
Protein	13.3 g	1.9 g
Fat	22.0 g	3.1 g
Carbohydrate	60.0 g	8.4 g
Taurine	0.05 g	6 mg
Vitamin A (retinol equivalents)	466 µg	65 µg
Vitamin B_1	230 µg	32 µg
Vitamin B_2	350 µg	50 µg
Vitamin B_6	300 µg	42 µg
Nicotinamide	1.7 mg	0.24 mg
Folic acid	36 µg	5 µg
Vitamin B_{12}	1.5 µg	0.2 µg
Ca-D-pantothenate	1.7 mg	0.24 mg
Biotin	8.1 µg	1.1 µg
Vitamin C	54 mg	7.5 mg
Vitamin D_3 (cholecalciferol)	7.3 µg	1.0 µg
Vitamin E	5.7 mg	0.8 mg
Vitamin K_1	29 µg	4 µg
Calcium	510 mg	71 mg
Phosphorus	390 mg	55 mg
Sodium	170 mg	24 mg
Iron	3.1 mg	0.4 mg
Copper	190 µg	27 µg
Zinc	2.9 mg	0.4 mg
Iodine	15 µg	2.1 µg
Manganese	90 µg	13 µg
Energy	2060 kJ 492 kcal	288 kJ 69 kcal

Fig. 3 Specially modified infant formula

continuing breastfeeding can be very difficult. Very few work places provide facilities for women to take their young babies with them. Embarrassment also causes women to stop or give up breastfeeding. It is very difficult to breastfeed babies in public because there are not feeding facilities outside the home. Very few women are actually physically unable to breastfeed.

Women who do not want to breastfeed their babies use bottles to give them specially modified infant **formula** (Fig. 3). This is based on cows' milk. The cows' milk has been changed so that it nearly resembles human milk. Ordinary cows' milk is not suitable for young babies, nor is dried or skimmed or semi-skimmed cows' milk. If a baby is being fed then the bottles and teats must always be very carefully sterilized (Fig. 4). It is also very important to follow the instructions for making up the feed on the packet. If the feed is made up too dilute the baby will not have enough nutrients, or too strong it can give the baby digestive upsets.

A few babies are allergic to cows' milk. They need to have specially formulated plant milks. Special advice is necessary for the parents of these babies. Occasionally breastfed babies develop an allergy to milk in their mother's diet. Once again special advice is needed if a woman is to stop drinking milk while she is breastfeeding.

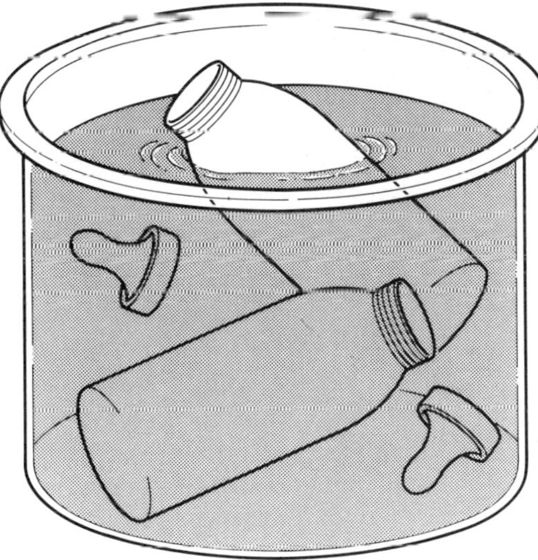

Fig. 4 Bottles and teats in sterilizing solution

Summary

- Breast feeding is best for babies.
- If a baby is not breastfed, only special infant formula should be used.
- A few babies are allergic to animal milk. Their parents need special advice.

Questions

1. What is the function of colostrum?
2. Why are mothers advised to breastfeed their babies?
3. What conditions might make this difficult?

B Dietary energy, protein, carbohydrates and fat

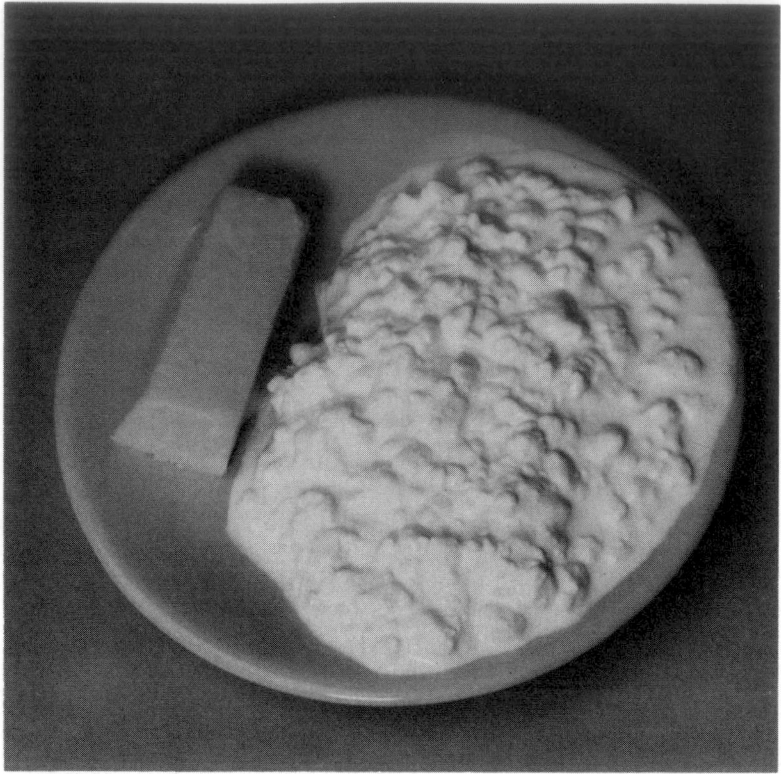

Fig. 1 Equivalent amounts of dietary energy from Cheddar cheese and cottage cheese

Fig. 2 Soya milk

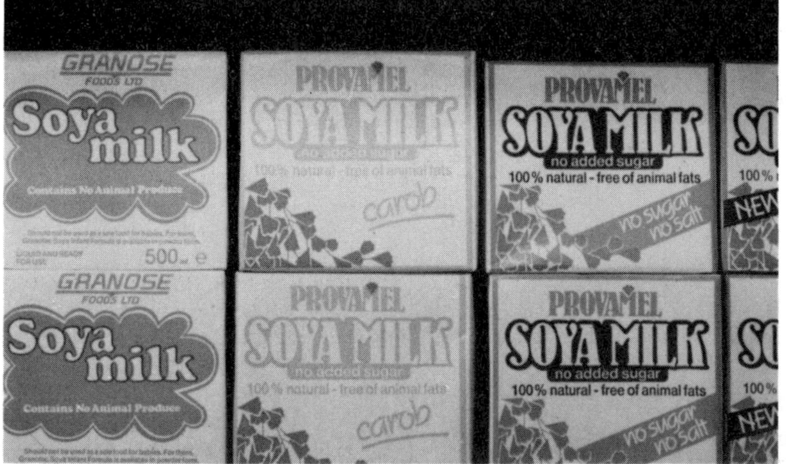

Dietary energy

Milk, cheese and yoghurt currently provide about 13% of average daily energy intakes in the UK. In young children and vegetarians this proportion is likely to be higher. The energy content of different types of milk, cheese and yoghurt varies widely. For example, whole milk provides almost twice as much energy as skimmed milk. Cheddar cheese provides over four times as much dietary energy as cottage cheese (Fig. 1). This difference is due partly to the fat content and partly to the water content. If you are trying to eat foods containing less saturated fats and are therefore cutting down on the fat from milk products, the energy contribution of these foods to your diet will be decreased.

For people who have small appetites or difficulty in swallowing food, milk can be a very useful energy source. It is often used as a basis for liquid diets.

Protein

Milk and milk products are very important sources of protein. In most diets they provide about 22% of daily protein needs. Milk itself supplies over 68% of this. In vegetarian diets this amount would be much higher. Soya milk can be an important source of protein for people who do not eat animal milks and milk products (Fig. 2).

The protein in milk and milk products is well utilized by the body, but its biological value can be increased by the addition of cereal foods. Such combinations are often eaten, for example breakfast cereal and milk, cheese on toast, rice or semolina pudding, yoghurt with rice or chapattis (Fig. 3).

Carbohydrates

Milk and yoghurt contain **lactose**. This is a disaccharide containing galactose and glucose. Human milk contains more lactose than animal milk. Most cheeses have a very low lactose content. Some adults from different parts of the world

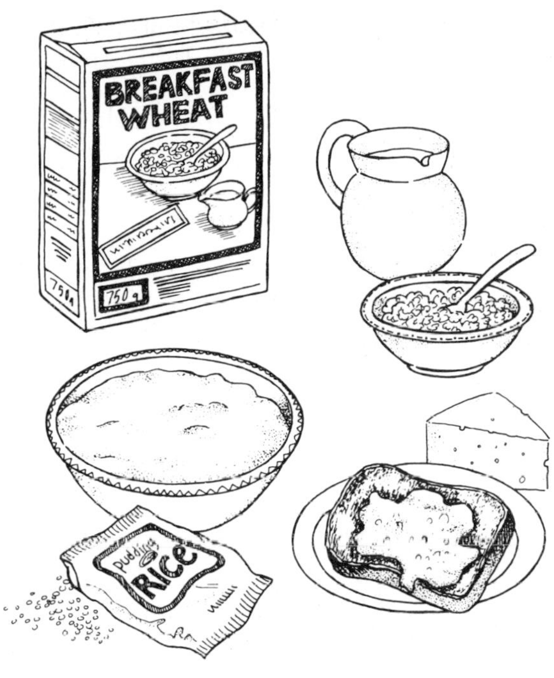

Fig. 3 Dishes that provide milk and cereal proteins

are unable to digest lactose. The enzyme they require to do so, lactase, is not present in their intestine. This is known as **lactose intolerance**. Amongst people where this is common, milk is not generally consumed by adults. They may tolerate small amounts of milk but soya milk is of major importance in their diet.

Sucrose (sugar) is added to some milks, for example in sweetened condensed milks and flavoured milks. Milk and milk products provide approximately 7% of our daily carbohydrate intake.

Fat

The fat in milk and milk products is very high in saturated fatty acids. These foods provide about 25% of the saturated fat in most UK diets. They also provide about 20% of the total fat. Reduced fat milk and milk products have become increasingly available in the UK (Fig. 4). Reducing the fat content of milk does not alter the protein, calcium or vitamin B12 content, but it does reduce the amount of the fat soluble vitamins A and D. If low fat milk and cheeses are used to replace those with a high fat content care should be taken to ensure other dietary sources of vitamins A and D are included.

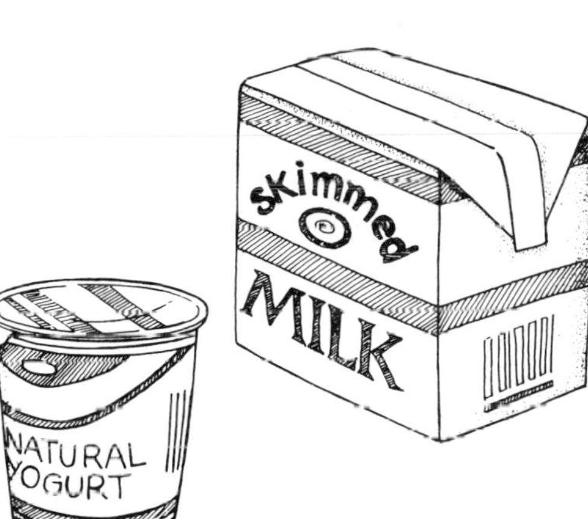

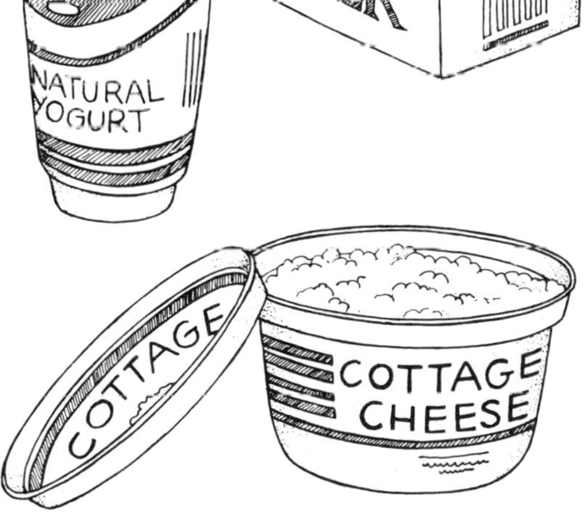

Fig. 4 Reduced fat milk and milk products

Summary

- These foods are important sources of dietary energy and protein.
- Adults from some parts of the world are intolerant to the lactose in milk.
- Whole milk and many cheeses are high in saturated fat.
- Low and medium fat milks, cheeses and yoghurt are becoming increasingly available.

Questions

1. How can the biological value of protein from foods in this group be increased?
2. What percentage of the daily protein in the average UK diet comes from milk and milk products?
3. What is meant by 'lactose intolerance'?
4. What is the effect on nutrient content of reducing the amount of fat in milk?

C *Minerals*

Milk and milk products are the most important source of calcium and phosphorus that we have.

Calcium

Nearly 60% of the calcium in our diet comes from milk, cheese and yoghurt. Soya milk is not a rich source of calcium.

Calcium is required for the formation of bones and teeth. Calcium requirements are therefore increased during periods of growth, during pregnancy and when women are breastfeeding. About 99% of the calcium in the body is actually in the skeleton (Fig. 1). The remaining 1% is in the fluid around the cells, the soft tissues and the blood. It has an important role in the nervous system and the muscles. It is essential for the clotting of blood and also for the activity of the digestive enzyme, rennin.

Only 20% to 30% of calcium is actually absorbed. **Absorption** is dependent on vitamin D (see page 102). It also needs protein and possibly lactose.

Calcium deficiency is not found in the UK. However some people feel that the disease osteoporosis suffered by elderly people may be related to low intakes of calcium when they were younger.

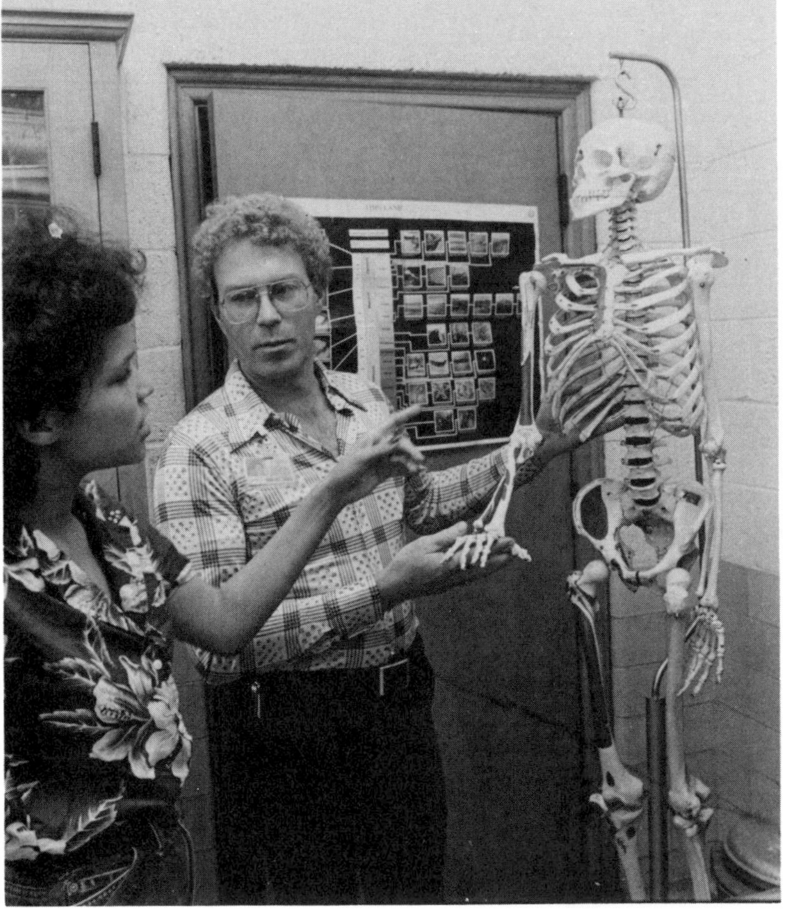

Fig. 1 The human skeleton consists of 99% of the calcium that is in the body

Phosphorus

Phosphorus is also a component of the bones and teeth. It combines with calcium to provide calcium phosphates which strengthen the skeleton. Phosphates also play an important role in releasing energy from food, and they combine with B vitamins to form the constituents of nucleic acids. Phosphorus is present in nearly all foods and so dietary deficiency is unknown in humans. Phosphates are also added to a number of processed foods.

Milk and milk products also provide a small amount of iron in the diet. These amounts are so small that they are not very important in relation to other iron sources.

Summary

- Animal milk and milk products are the main sources of calcium and phosphorus in most people's diets.
- Calcium with phosphorus is essential for the formation and maintenance of healthy bones and the formation of teeth.
- Calcium is no use without sufficient vitamin D.

Questions

1. What is the function of calcium in the body?
2. What is the role of phosphorus in the body?

D Vitamins

Riboflavin

Milk and milk products are the most important source of riboflavin in our diet. They provide nearly 40%. Riboflavin is very easily destroyed by ultraviolet light. So leaving milk on the doorstep in glass bottles results in the destruction of riboflavin (Fig. 1).

Riboflavin forms part of one of the enzymes involved in oxidation and reduction reactions, which have an important role in the release of energy in the body. Deficiency signs of riboflavin, which include sores at the corner of the mouth, are not often seen in human beings. People who eat little or no milk or milk products, however, need to make sure they get their riboflavin from other sources – yeast, liver, eggs and beef (Fig. 2).

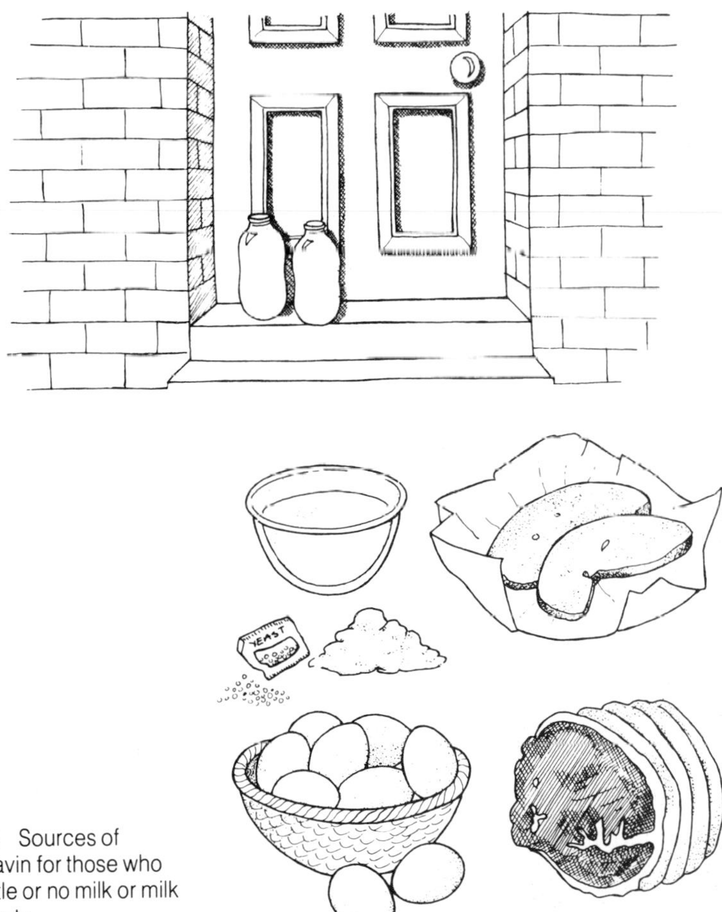

Fig. 1 Riboflavin in milk is destroyed by ultraviolet light

Fig. 2 Sources of riboflavin for those who eat little or no milk or milk products

Vitamin A

Milk and milk products are important sources of vitamin A, supplying nearly 20% of the total vitamin A in the UK diet. This vitamin A is mainly in the form of retinol, but there are also small amounts of beta carotene (see page 000). The vitamin A is a fat soluble vitamin and is therefore found in the fat component of the milk. If the fat is removed, as in the case of skimmed milk and low fat cheeses, the vitamin A is removed. This should not be a serious problem nutritionally as vitamin A intakes are generally well above the recommendations.

Vitamin D

Vitamin D is also a fat soluble vitamin and is found in the fat component of milk and milk products. There are only small amounts present and the contribution to the diet is small. However, for growing children, pregnant and breastfeeding women and elderly people who are housebound, the vitamin D in milk and milk products may be of some use nutritionally (see page 000).

Small amounts of **vitamin K** are also found in milk and milk products.

Summary

- These foods provide small but useful contributions of vitamins A and D in the diet.
- Low fat milks and cheeses contain very little vitamin A or D, unless they are fortified.

Questions

1. What is the function in the body of riboflavin?
2. How can riboflavin in milk be destroyed?
3. Why is it best not to give young children low fat milks unless the milks are fortified?

E Effects of cooking and processing

Milk has been part of people's diets since animals were first domesticated many thousands of years ago. The kind of milk which is used depends on the animals which do best in local agricultural traditions. In the UK, cows' milk is common although both sheep's and goats' milk are available and becoming more popular (Fig. 1).

Because milk does not keep for long it has always been processed to make butter, cheeses or yoghurt, which prolongs its keeping quality. The basic European process of cheese-making is to **clot** the milk – the clot is made of protein (caseinogen) and this traps the fat. Clotting is usually achieved by adding **rennet**. The curd or clot is strained and the liquid or **whey** is removed. The cheese is then salted and stored. There are 400 European varieties, whose fat content varies from 0 to 50% (Fig. 2). The variation in taste and texture is due to the maturation of fermentation processes which rely on enzyme actions.

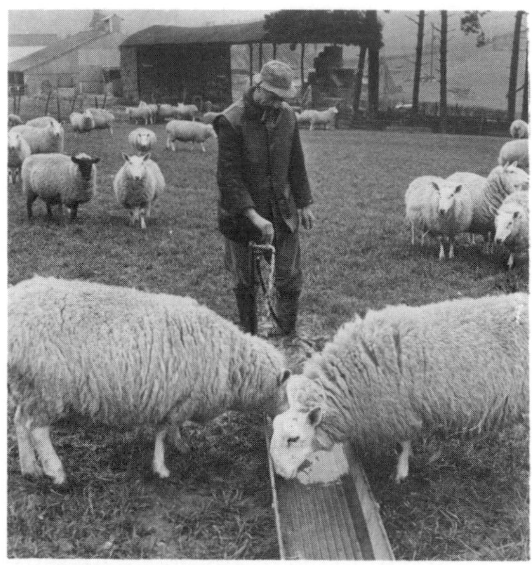

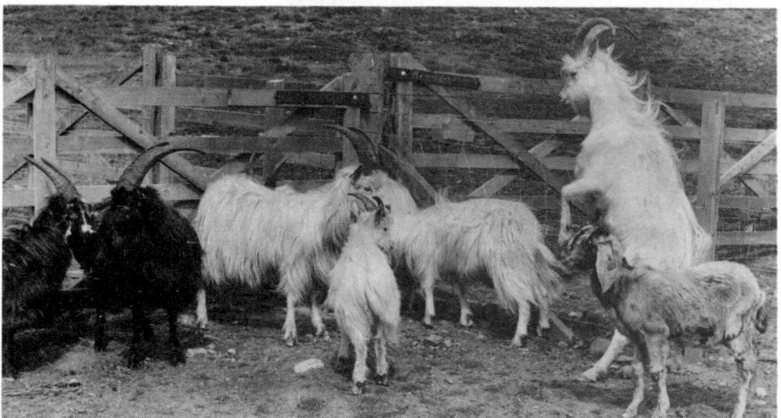

Fig. 1 Sheep and goats are widely used throughout Europe for their milk

Milk contains about 87% water, mature Cheddar cheese about 40%. Soft cheeses are not pressed to remove water and therefore contain less fat and protein than hard cheeses. The nutrient content of cheeses depends not only on the degree to which water is removed but the quality of the milk used in the cheese's manufacture. In India and other parts of the world where milk is part of the diet, a soft cheese (Khoa or Mawa) is made by boiling milk slowly to evaporate the water. When cheese is cooked, the fat in it melts and the protein coagulates and makes it soft and stringy.

Yoghurt is made when milk is first boiled, allowed to cool, then inoculated with a **bacterial culture** (usually the previous day's yoghurt) as a starter. The bacteria responsible cause the breakdown of lactose to lactic acid. Many cultures use yoghurt and it has become very popular in the UK. It contains all the fat and protein of the milk it was made from. Yoghurt will separate when used in cookery. To stabilize it, add a little waxy starch (e.g. cornflour).

Summary

- Milk has been part of people's diet for hundreds of years.
- Milk is processed to make cheeses and yoghurt which enhance its keeping qualities.

Questions

1. Describe how European cheese is made.
2. What makes cheeses taste different? How does the nutrient content of cheeses vary?
3. How is yoghurt made?

F Digestion

When milk enters the stomach it clots. This is due to **enzyme** actions. Young animals, including children, produce the enzyme **rennin** which causes milk to clot. The clotting converts **caseinogen** into **casein**, which is insoluble. This is digested by **trypsin** and other enzymes in the small intestine.

extra matured English cheddar
blue stilton
red vein cheddar
roulé
Eden Vale
Natural
Cottage Cheese
ROUNDOAK
115 g
GOATS CHEESE

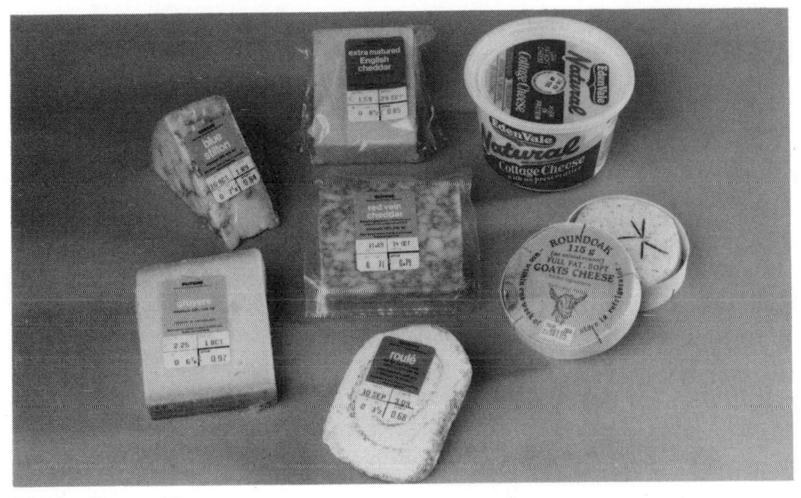

Fig. 2 Some of the many cheeses that are available

Fig. 1 Digestion of milk and milk products

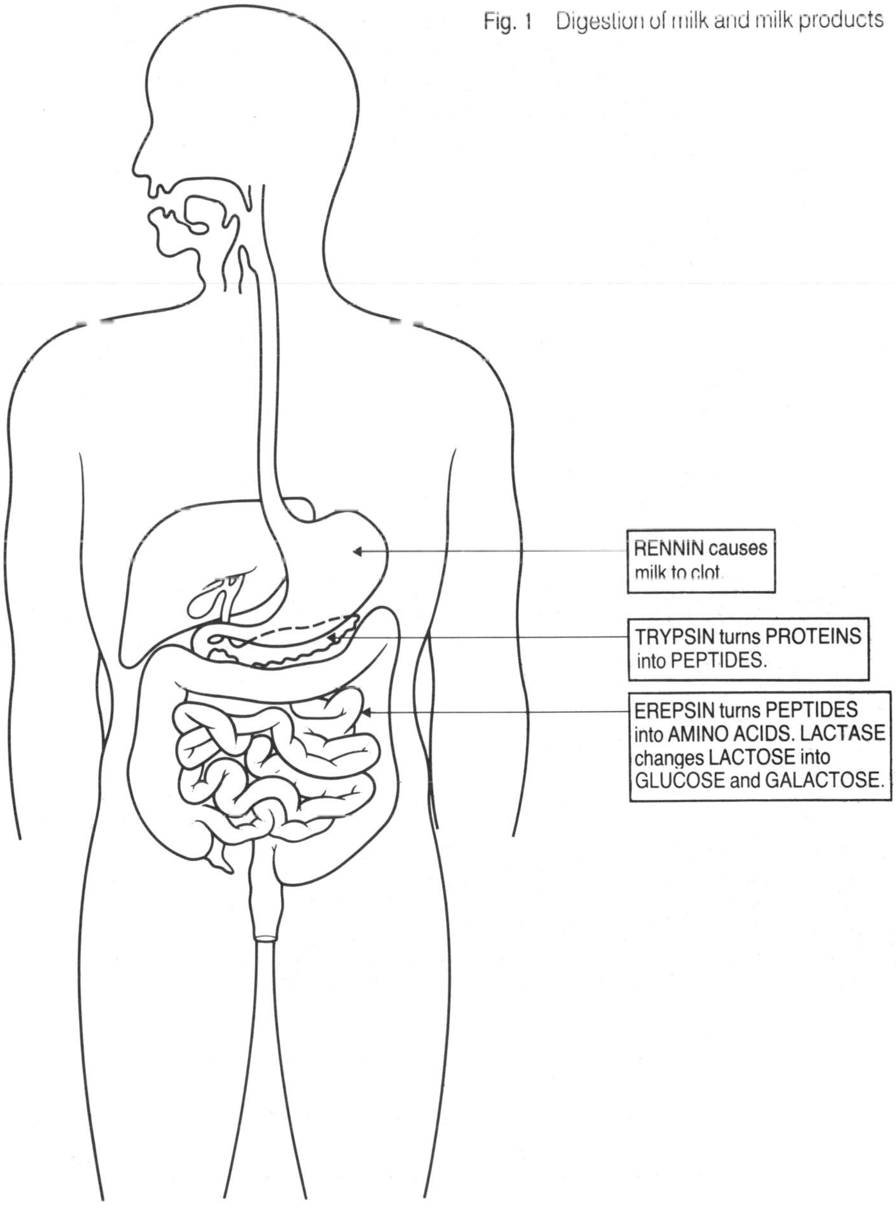
RENNIN causes milk to clot.
TRYPSIN turns PROTEINS into PEPTIDES.
EREPSIN turns PEPTIDES into AMINO ACIDS. LACTASE changes LACTOSE into GLUCOSE and GALACTOSE.

4.11 The nutritional role of sugar, sugary foods and drinks

A Dietary energy and health

All foods supply dietary energy. In most cases it is combined with other nutrients. Sugar provides only dietary energy and no other nutrients. It is rapidly digested and absorbed into the blood, and if it is not used immediately it is converted to **glycogen** or fat and stored by the body. In many foods such as confectionery, biscuits and cakes, sugar is combined with fat and refined flour (Fig. 1). Neither of these other ingredients contains many useful nutrients. These foods therefore provide many calories with very few nutrients. Refined simple sugars are often referred to as providing **empty calories**. Eating large quantities of sugar and sugary foods reduces the appetite for more nutritious foods. The more of these foods that are eaten, the less nutrient dense the diet will be.

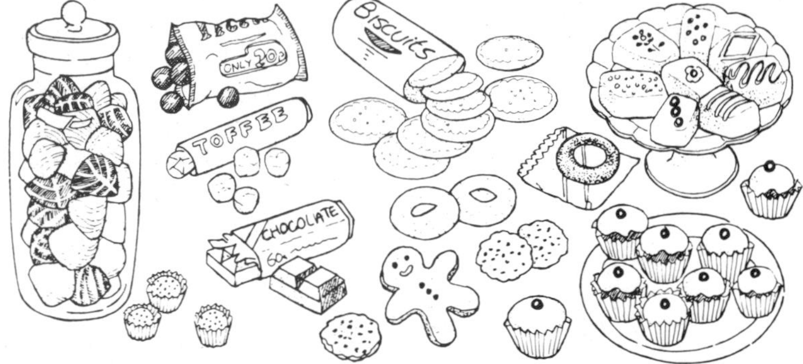

Fig. 1 These foods contain sugar combined with fat and refined flour. None of these ingredients provides significant quantities of useful nutrients

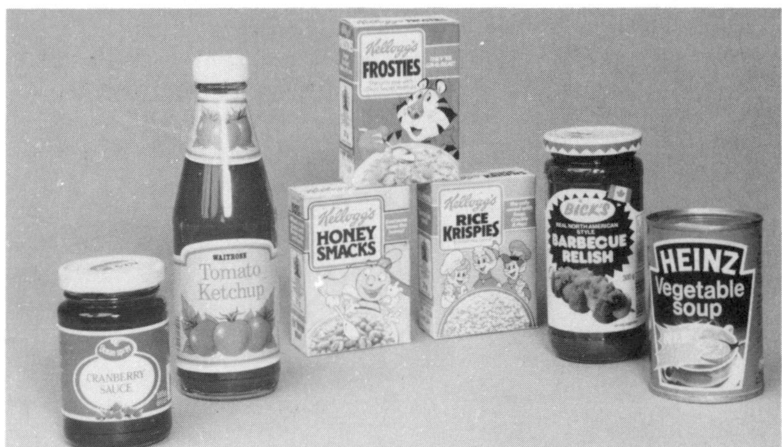

Fig. 2 It is easy to eat large amounts of sugar without realizing it

The current consumption of refined sugars in the UK is approximately 14–20% of daily energy needs. This means that on average we each eat approximately 38 kg of sugar per year, but there are very wide individual variations in intake of sugar. Much of the sugary foods and drinks consumed are taken outside the home. They are often eaten between meals and sometimes used to replace meals, curbing the appetite and leading to an unbalanced diet.

Sugar is naturally present in very small amounts in a few foods. It mainly gets into our diet during **food processing**. There are many foods which obviously contain sugar. There are others such as soups, pickles and breakfast cereals which can contain up to 35% sugar (Fig. 2). Often we are unaware of this. Most of the sugar in our diets comes from soft drinks, confectionery and packet sugar.

Many people believe that sugar is essential to provide energy. Energy is thought of as a good thing and much of the advertising of foods in this group is based on this idea. In fact, as you have already seen, all foods provide energy. Most of them provide dietary energy in much more useful forms containing other nutrients than sugar.

Tooth decay

Sugar is one of the main contributory factors in tooth decay (**dental caries**) (Fig. 3). In order for dental caries to occur there have to be three things present: the teeth, bacteria on the teeth and an acid forming substance, such as sugar, in the mouth. It is virtually impossible to remove all the **plaque** from the tooth surface, and so the only way to completely avoid caries is to cut down on the intake of sugar and other acid forming substances.

Sugar is broken down by **bacteria** in the mouth to form an **acid**. This acid then attacks the **enamel** of the tooth. If sugar is put into the mouth frequently, acid is continually produced. Within a short time of eating sugar the conditions in the mouth have become acidic. It is possible for the enamel of the tooth to recover when sugar is not present in the mouth. This is helped in alkaline conditions and especially when **fluoride** is present. Fluoride can be put on to the surface of the tooth (e.g. by using fluoride based toothpaste) or it can be consumed. If fluoride is taken when the teeth are developing it can help to strengthen the surface of the tooth and prevent decay. Saliva is normally alkaline, and increasing the flow by chewing fibrous foods helps to neutralize acids in the mouth. Foods such as milk and cheese also keep the mouth more alkaline, reducing the effects of sugar. Sugary foods and drinks taken between meals or at frequent intervals are more damaging than sugar eaten with other foods. In order to prevent tooth decay it is important to understand this and avoid eating sugary snacks between meals.

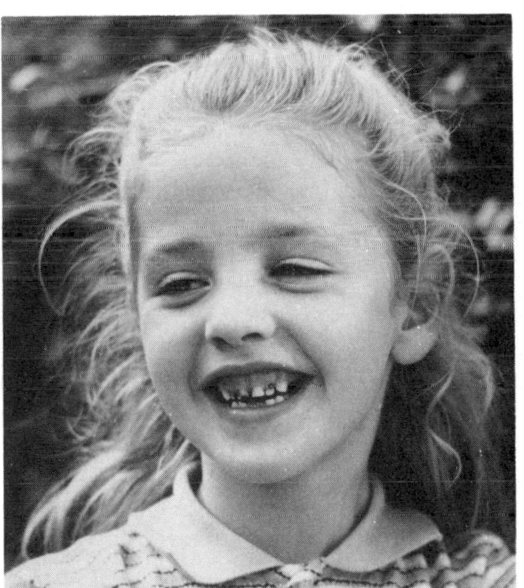

Fig. 3 Dental caries in a child's mouth

Obesity

Obesity is a major health problem today. Although eating sugar does not necessarily cause obesity, it is very easy to eat a lot of sugar. For people who are likely to put on weight easily, concentrated energy sources like sugar, sugary foods and drinks need to be avoided. Sugary foods are often high in fat and low in fibre. This, together with the fact that they are often tasty, means that they are more likely to be eaten in large amounts.

Diabetes melitus

There is no evidence to link sugar consumption with the development of diabetes, but people with diabetes need to be very careful about how and when they eat simple sugars. Obesity is a contributory factor in diabetes. People who are overweight are more likely to get diabetes when they are older. The best way to control this diabetes is by losing weight and by cutting down on the consumption of sugar and sugary foods. People with diabetes should only eat sugary foods in conjunction with foods which are high in dietary fibre. They should only eat small amounts of these sugary foods.

Summary

- Refined simple sugars provide empty calories.
- People who are overweight need to be especially careful, because it is easy to eat a lot of sugar without realizing it.
- Sugar is known to be one of the main causes of tooth decay.

Questions

1. What is the average number of 1 kg bags of sugar each person eats per year in the UK?
2. Why is refined sugar said to provide empty calories?
3. How does dental caries develop?
4. What is meant by obesity? What part in the development of obesity might be played by the foods in this group?

B Effects of cooking and processing

Sugar is used in cooking and processing for a number of reasons:
- it adds sweetness and enhances flavour
- it acts as a preservative
- it gives a texture or body to foods like tomato sauce, etc.
- it gives a good crumb texture to baked goods
- it makes baked goods keep fresher longer
- it is a relatively cheap bulk agent.

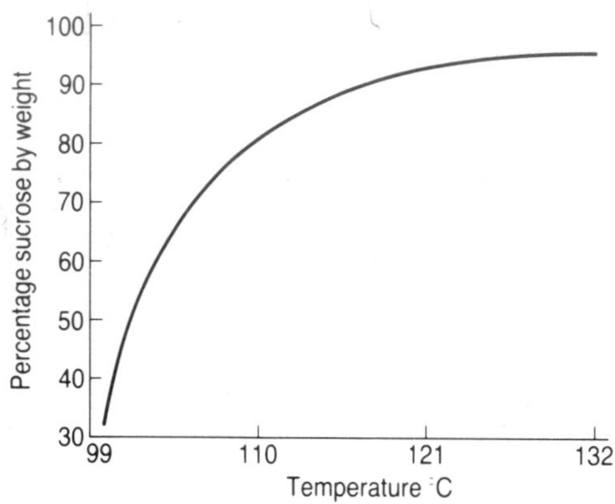

Fig. 1 The boiling points of sugar solutions

When sugar is heated in dry heat it will first go brown, becoming **caramel**. This is used to give a bitter-sweet flavour, and to give colour to foods, although much caramel used is artificial. If it is heated too much the sugar will burn leaving only **charcoal** (carbon) behind.

When heated in water sugar dissolves and forms a syrup. Its behaviour in solution varies according to the concentration or strength of the solution, and on any other substances present. When a sugar solution is heated, its boiling point depends on how much sugar is present (Fig. 1).

The higher the boiling point, the harder the cold set substance will be. To make soft toffee, the solution needs a low boiling point. Hard boiled sweets result from boiling at higher temperatures (Fig. 2). The temperatures required for confectionery are known as 'soft ball' and 'hard ball', or 'soft crack' and 'hard crack'.

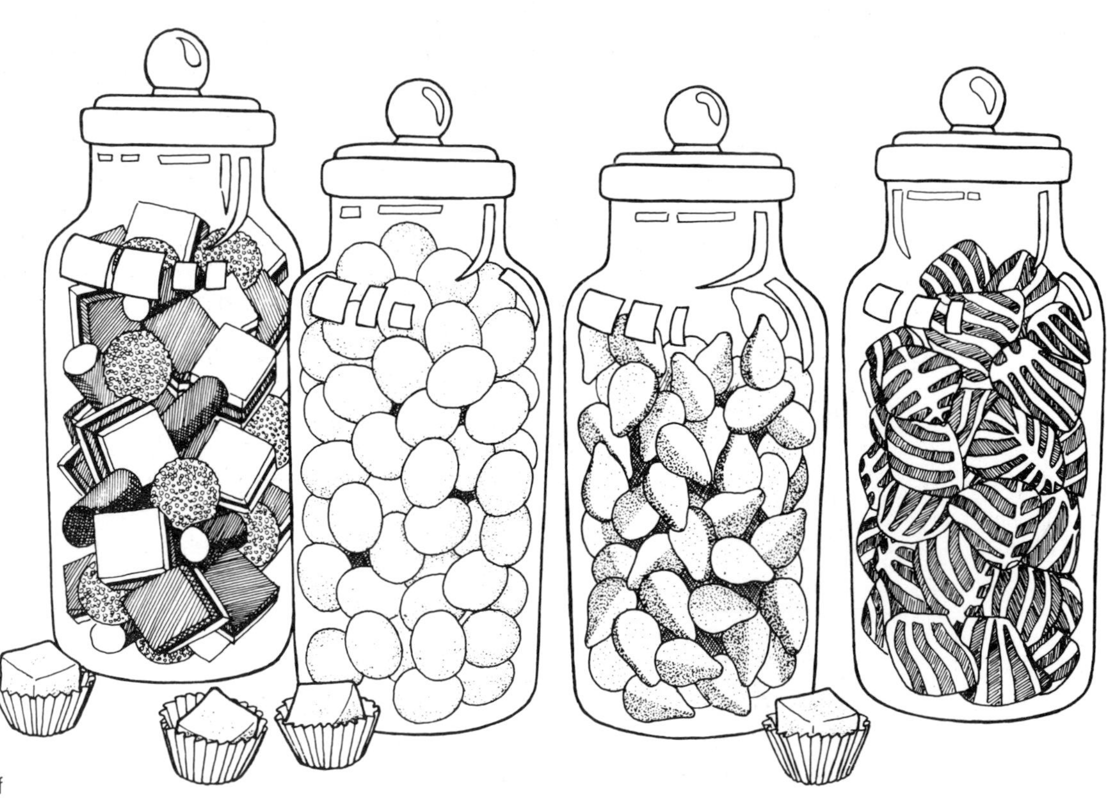

Fig. 2 These sweets are made by boiling different concentrates of sugar in solution

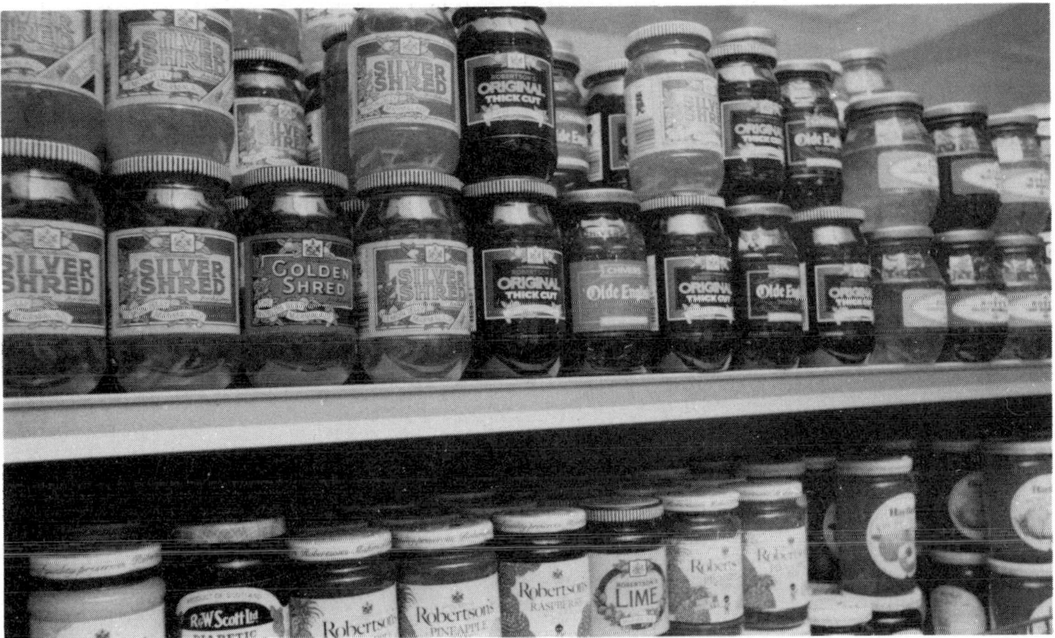

Fig. 3 Invert sugar was used to make these jams

Sucrose is very easily hydrolysed to (broken down into) its constituent monosaccharides glucose and fructose, when any acid is present. The process is called **inversion** and the product is called **invert sugar**. (It is called inversion because of the way it behaves when rays of light are passed through it.) Invert sugar, consisting of a mixture of glucose and fructose, is important in jam making as it prevents crystals of sucrose forming in the jam when it cools (Fig. 3). Honey contains a lot of invert sugar – the bee causes sucrose inversion by enzymes in its stomach where it stores nectar to make honey (Fig. 4).

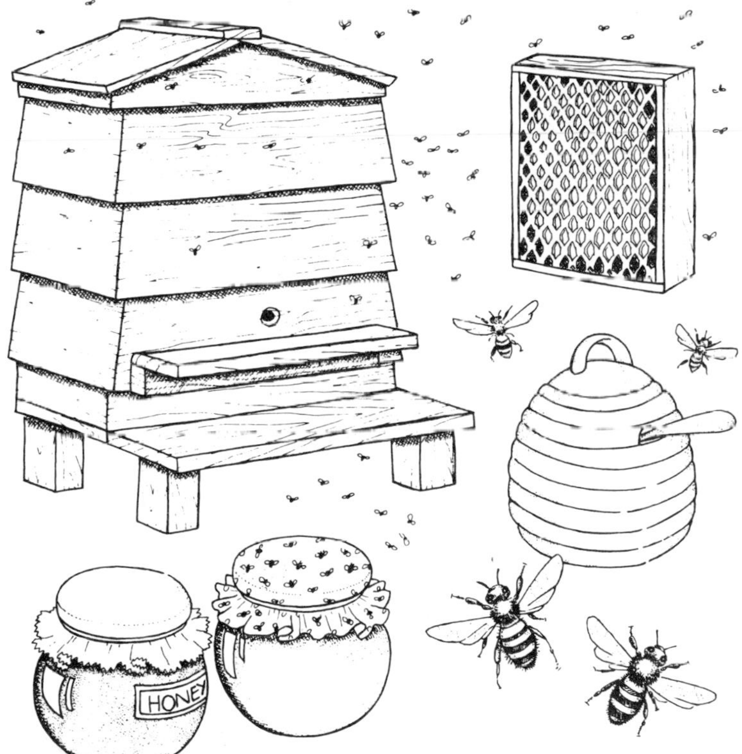

Fig. 4 The bee causes sucrose inversion in the nectar it carries

Summary

- Heating sugar in dry heat produces caramel.
- Syrup boils at different temperatures depending on concentration.
- Invert sugar is a mixture of glucose and fructose formed by the breakdown of sucrose.

Questions

1. Why is sugar used in processing and cooking?
2. What happens when sugar is heated in water?
3. Why is invert sugar important in jam making?
4. How is invert sugar made?

4.12 The nutritional role of fats and oils

A Dietary energy and fat soluble vitamins

Dietary energy

Fats and oils provide almost 16% of the dietary energy in the UK diet. They are the most **energy dense** of all foods. Fat provides more kilojoules per gram than starch, sugar, protein or alcohol. Foods in this group contain very little water. When added to foods of lower energy density they increase the amount of dietary energy supplied. Adding fats and oils to foods increases their dietary energy content but not their bulk.

Fig. 1 Butter and margarine supply vitamins A and D respectively

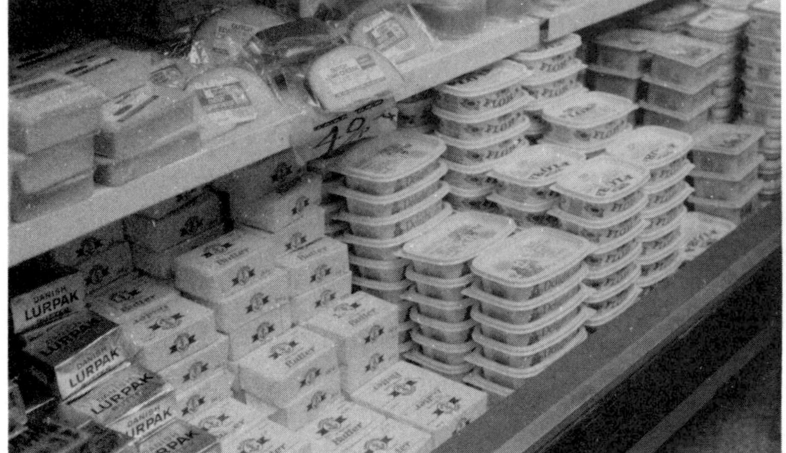

Fat soluble vitamins

Fats and oils are important sources of the vitamins A, D and E. On average, about 20% of vitamin A (in the form of retinol) and over half of the vitamin D in our diet is supplied by these foods. The vitamin A comes mainly from butter and the vitamin D mainly from margarine (Fig. 1). Margarine, by law, has to be fortified with both vitamins. Fish liver oils are also very rich sources of both but are not normally eaten. The amounts of vitamin A and D in vegetable oils are very small. Vitamin E is found only in polyunsaturated vegetable oils. Therefore vegetable margarine and cooking fats and oils are important sources in our diets.

Fat

Fats and oils supply about 36% of the **dietary fat** we consume. In plants, the fats are formed from carbohydrate. In seeds, such as sunflower, safflower, soya bean, etc., the starch in the seed decreases as the amount of fat increases. The fat from animal sources comes mainly from fat laid down around the tissues and under the skin of the animal. Butter is made by removing the fat from milk (Fig. 2).

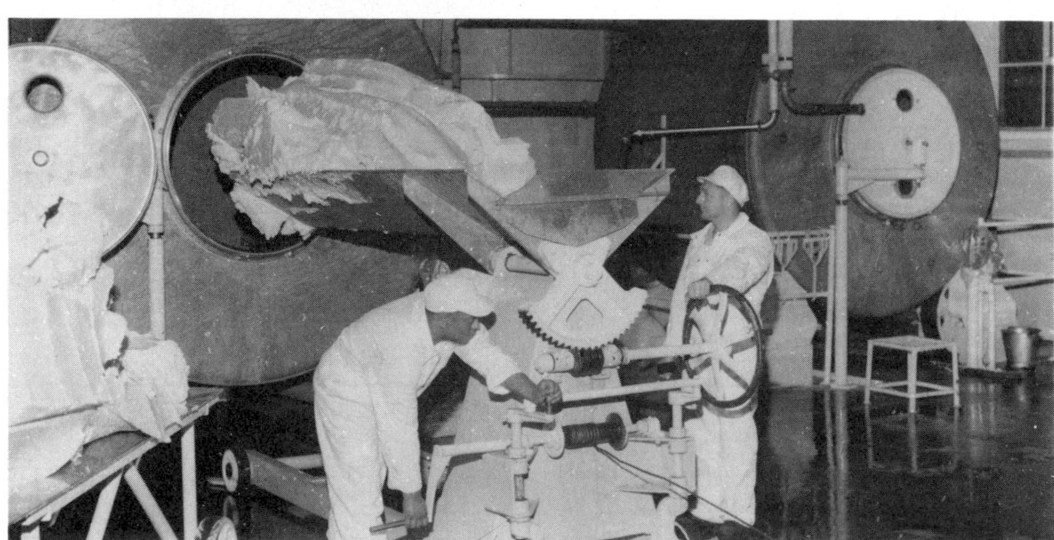

Fig. 2 Buttermaking

Different types of fat

All fats are made up of **glycerol** and **fatty acids**. There are over 40 fatty acids, and different combinations of these give fats and oils different properties. The three main types of fatty acids are polyunsaturated fatty acids, saturated fatty acids and monounsaturated fatty acids. Some of the polyunsaturated fatty acids are essential and are known as **essential fatty acids**. The main sources of polyunsaturated fatty acids are soya bean oil, corn oil, safflower seed oil, sunflower seed oil and some fish oils (Fig. 3). The fat from most animal sources, including butter, most margarines, lard, suet, dripping and other types of animal fat, are saturated. Some plant oils are also saturated. These include coconut oil and palm oil.

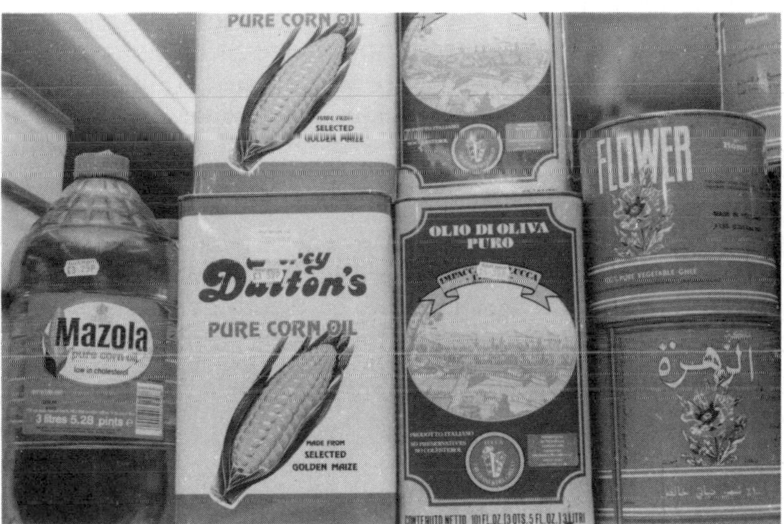

Fig. 3 Sources of polyunsaturated and monounsaturated fatty acids

Fats and health

It is generally agreed that the amount and type of fat in the diet is one of the factors affecting **heart disease**. In countries where there is a high intake of mainly saturated fats, there is a relatively high incidence of heart disease. In the UK we probably eat about 15% more fat than we need to. Most of us should try to cut down on the amount of fat we eat, particularly the saturated fats. Fat is a very energy dense food and it is possible to eat a great deal without realizing it. Obesity is common in the UK and may be a result of eating too much dietary fat. Diets containing relatively small amounts of dietary fat, with more cereal foods, starchy vegetables, fruit and other vegetables, are more bulky and less energy dense. It is harder to become overweight eating this type of diet.

The role of polyunsaturated fats and monounsaturated fats is not clear. However, it does not seem to be advisable to increase the amount of polyunsaturated fat to replace all the saturated fat from the diet. Small increases may be useful. For example, if small amounts of fat are being used in cooking it is better to use a polyunsaturated cooking oil rather than a highly saturated fat, such as lard, suet or dripping.

Summary

- Fats and oils are concentrated energy sources.
- Fats are made up of glycerol and fatty acids.
- Some fat in the diet is essential to provide the fat soluble vitamins A, D and E, and essential fatty acids.
- Eating too much fat contributes to obesity and may lead to heart problems.

Questions

1. Which vitamins are supplied by the foods in this group?
2. Approximately how much of the dietary fat we consume comes from foods in this group?
3. What are the three kinds of fatty acids? What are their differences and which fats are they found in?
4. Why do nutritionists advise a reduction in fat intake, especially saturated fat intake?

B Effects of cooking and processing

Fats and oils are used in cooking and other food processing
- for frying and roasting food (Fig. 1)
- as a shortening agent in pastry, cakes and biscuits
- to improve the texture, flavour and keeping quality of baked foods
- to provide texture in sauces and dressings.

When fat is heated for frying or baking, first it melts, then it gets hotter until it reaches smoking point, when blue smoke is produced. The temperature at which this is reached varies according to the type of oil or fat. When foods are fried the temperature should be kept below smoking point. When heated beyond this point oils and fats begin to break down into their constituent fatty acids and glycerol. This gives the oil a tainted taste and smell and changes its colour.

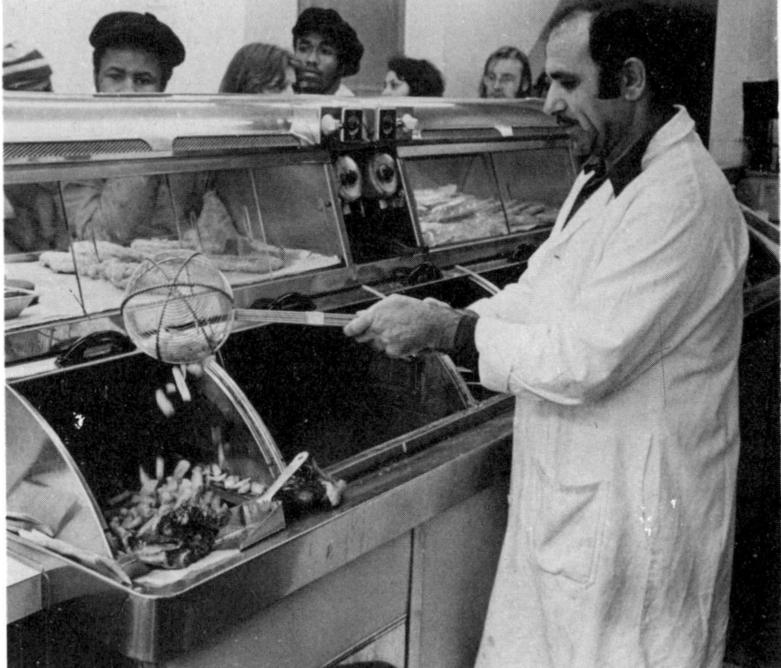

Fig. 1 A deep fryer in use in a chip shop

Repeated heating of oil, as in deep frying, can result in a build up of breakdown products, which may give the food an unpleasant flavour. The oils which are specifically made for frying have a high smoking point and can be used at temperatures below smoking point quite easily. It is important to take care when cooking with boiling oil since it boils at temperatures above that of boiling water and burns are more serious. There is also a danger of boiling oil vaporizing and the vapour bursting into flames.

Fats are used as **shortening agents** in cakes and biscuits. When fat or oil is added to a flour mixture, the fat coats the starch grains making them waterproof. This persists during cooking and gives the food a particular crumb structure and flavour. Fat is creamed with sugar in the **creaming method** of making cakes. This produces a foam whose function is to trap air and make a light risen product.

When oil and water are mixed together they produce an **emulsion**. If this is allowed to stand it will separate and the oil will float to the top. Mayonnaise is an emulsion, as are many other sauces and dressings, and mixtures which are baked. In order to prevent the emulsion separating an emulsifying agent is used. Egg yolk contains a natural emulsifying agent, lecithin. Caseinogen is another natural emulsifying agent. It is found in milk and helps milk remain as an emulsion. Starch, gums, gelatin and alginates are emulsifying agents used in processed food.

Summary

- Fats are used to fry, roast, lighten and shorten foods.
- It is dangerous to overheat fats and oils.
- Oils and water form emulsions which separate unless they contain an emulsifying agent.

Questions

1. What is meant by smoking point?
2. Why are fats used in baked goods like cakes and biscuits?
3. What happens to oils when they are heated?
4. What is an emulsion? How is it stabilized?

C Digestion

When oils and fats are eaten they pass into the warm environment of the digestive system, and the fats melt. **Bile salts**, which are manufactured by the liver and stored in the gall bladder, act as emulsifiers and break the fats and oils into small droplets. These are then acted upon by **lipases**, or fat splitting enzymes, which produce glycerol and fatty acids. These substances can then be absorbed.

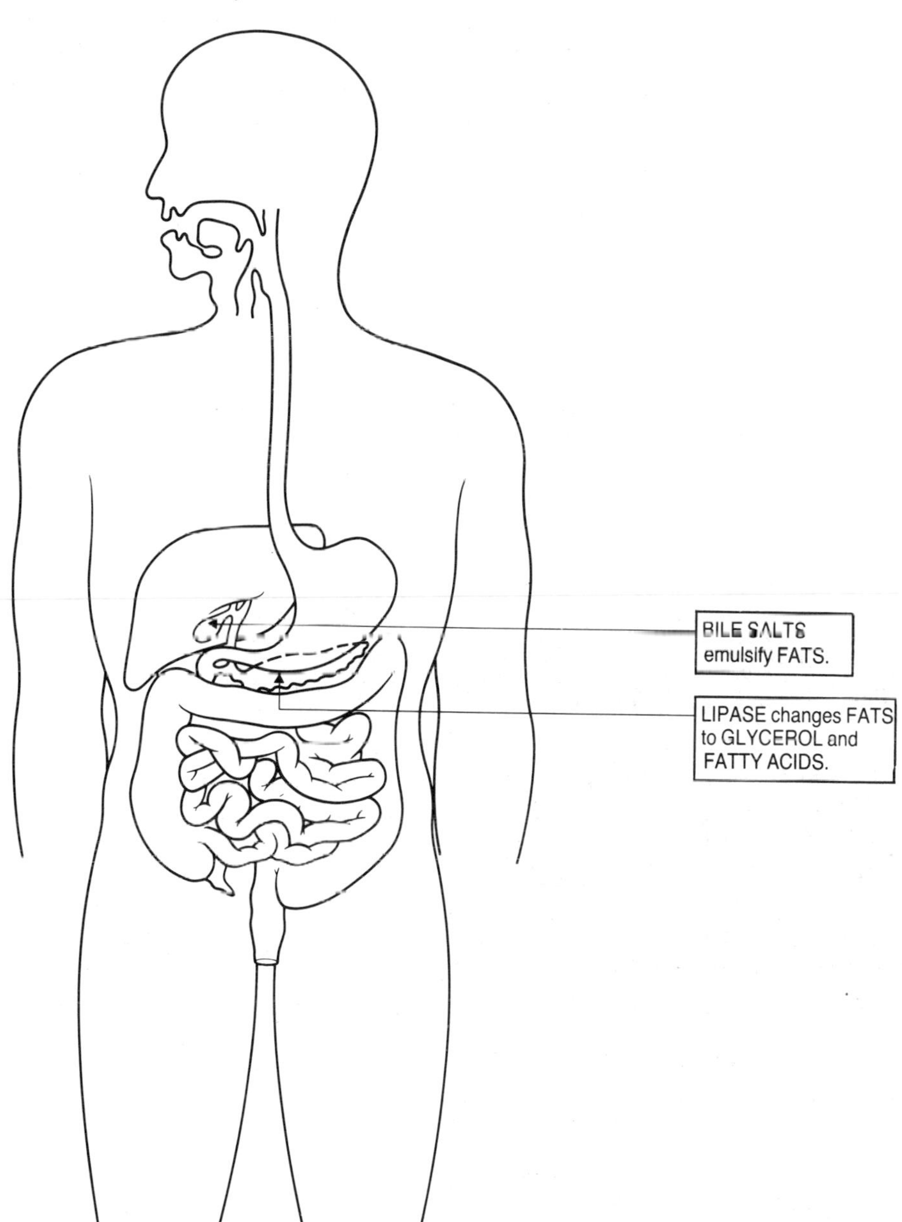

Fig. 1 Digestion of fats

4.13 Nutrient and energy density

Nutrient density

The foods from each of the four main food groups are all rich in nutrients. Each food provides a different combination, and some are richer sources than others. If a food is a good source of a variety of nutrients, it is called **nutrient dense**. This nutrient density is based on the concentration of useful nutrients in a portion of food which provides a specific amount of dietary energy. For example, if we compare the amount and variety of nutrients in a medium slice of wholemeal bread, a medium slice of white bread and a filled biscuit (all of which provide about 400 kJ), we can see that although they provide similar nutrients, the wholemeal bread is the best source of most of them (Fig. 1). It is therefore the most nutrient dense of the three foods. The biscuits have the lowest nutrient density.

Highly refined foods have been purified and most of the nutrients have been removed. Even though there are very few vitamins and minerals, they still provide dietary energy. They therefore have a low nutrient density. Sugar and fat also have low nutrient densities. In general, they provide dietary energy with few or no other nutrients. When they are included in the diet regularly, they dilute the nutrients from other foods. This explains why the biscuits have a much lower nutrient density than the bread. The wholemeal bread is made of the whole wheat grain. The white bread is made from refined flour which has had part of the grain removed, taking with it many of the nutrients. The white flour is also used in the biscuits, but the already depleted nutrients are further diluted by adding sugar and fat to make the biscuits. Avoiding too much sugar and fat and other refined and highly processed foods helps keep up the nutrient density of the diet.

Energy density

A food or diet can also be described in terms of its **energy density**. This is determined by the amount of dietary energy provided by a given weight of the

Fig. 1 Amounts of different nutrients provided by 400 kJ of wholemeal bread, white bread and filled biscuits

Nutrient	*Wholemeal bread* (44 g)	*White bread* (40 g)	*Filled biscuits* (18 g)
Starch (g)	17.5	19.2 ✓	3.8
Dietary fibre (g)	3.7 ✓	1.1	0.3
Protein (g)	3.9 ✓	3.1	0.8
Potassium (mg)	97 ✓	40	29
Calcium (mg)	10	40 ✓	13
Iron (mg)	1.1 ✓	0.7	0.3
Zinc (mg)	0.9 ✓	0.3	0.1
Vitamin A (μg)	0	0	0
Vitamin D (μg)	0	0	0
Thiamin (mg)	0.1 ✓	0.07	0.02
Riboflavin (mg)	0.04 ✓	0.01	0.01
Nicotinic acid (mg)	2.5 ✓	1.2	0.3
Vitamin C (mg)	0	0	0
Vitamin E (mg)	0.09	0	0.3 ✓
Vitamin B6 (mg)	0.06 ✓	0.02	0
Vitamin B12 (μg)	0	0	0
Folic acid (μg)	17 ✓	11	n/a
Pantothenic acid (mg)	0.3 ✓	0.1	n/a
Biotin (μg)	2.6 ✓	0.4	n/a

✓ best source of nutrient n/a figures not available

Fig. 2 Energy densities

Foods with a higher energy density kJ per 100 g food		Foods with a lower energy density kJ per 100 g food	
Digestive biscuits	1981	Wholemeal bread	918
Chips	1065	Boiled potatoes	343
Canned peaches (in syrup)	373	Fresh peaches	156
Avocado pear	922	Tomatoes	60
Fried pork sausages	1317	Roast lean leg of pork	777
Fried beefburger	1099	Grilled lean rump steak	708
Stewed minced beef	955	Cooked haricot beans	396

Fig. 3 Water content of foods and energy densities

Food	Percentage of water	kJ per 100 g
Milk	87.6	272
Cheddar cheese	37.0	1682
Dried apricots	14.7	776
Fresh apricots	86.6	117
Rice krispies	3.8	1584
Boiled rice	69.9	522

food. For example, if a small volume of food provides relatively large amounts of dietary energy, it has a high energy density. If a large volume of food is low in kilojoules, it has a low energy density. See Fig. 2 for examples. In all of the examples, the fat and/or sugar content in each pair of foods is mainly responsible for the differences in energy density. Those foods with a higher proportion of fat and/or sugar have a higher energy density. The energy density of a food can also be affected by the amount of water it contains. See Fig. 3 for examples.

A healthy balanced diet has a much lower energy density than a diet high in fat and sugar. Fat and sugar, being highly refined, provide dietary energy with very little bulk. It is easy to eat too much of them without feeling full up. Fruit, vegetables, starchy vegetables and many high fibre cereal foods are all bulky. They tend to have low energy density. This is particularly useful for people who are trying to lose weight. By eating more of these bulky foods, and less of the energy foods like fat and sugar, it is much easier to cut down the intake of kilojoules while still feeling satisfied after a meal. People who have high dietary energy needs may need to eat more energy dense foods than other people. The bulk of the low energy dense foods may be too much for them. They may not be able to eat enough to satisfy their energy needs.

Summary

- A healthy balanced diet is more nutrient dense than one with a lot of fat and sugar in it.
- The energy density of this type of diet is lower than that of a diet high in fat and sugar.

Questions

1. What is meant by 'nutrient density'?
2. Explain the meaning of high nutrient density and low nutrient density and give examples of three foods from each category.
3. Why is it important for elderly people who have small appetites to eat foods of a high nutrient density?
4. What is meant by energy density?
5. Why are dried apricots more energy dense than fresh ones?

SECTION 5 *Feed the world*

5.1 *Hunger and food aid*

Facts

Total world food production is increasing. In 1981 the world produced approximately 1½ times the amount of food needed to feed its entire population. In 1984 there were record cereal harvests in the USA and Europe, world food production increased by 4% on the previous year and production of staple foods increased by 6%. This is far more than we need to feed the world's growing population. There is no food shortage.

The World Bank estimates that 15 000 people die every day from lack of food. One billion people, one quarter of the world's population, are regularly malnourished (Fig. 1). By the end of 1984, 21 African countries were affected by drought-related food shortage. This means that a population of 200 million people – 40% of the people of Africa – are vulnerable to malnutrition and famine.

It is clear from these two sets of figures that the problem is not food production, but a gross inequality in food distribution. The people who lack food starve because of **poverty**. They are too poor to buy the available food.

Fig. 1 Some of the one quarter of the world's population who are regularly malnourished

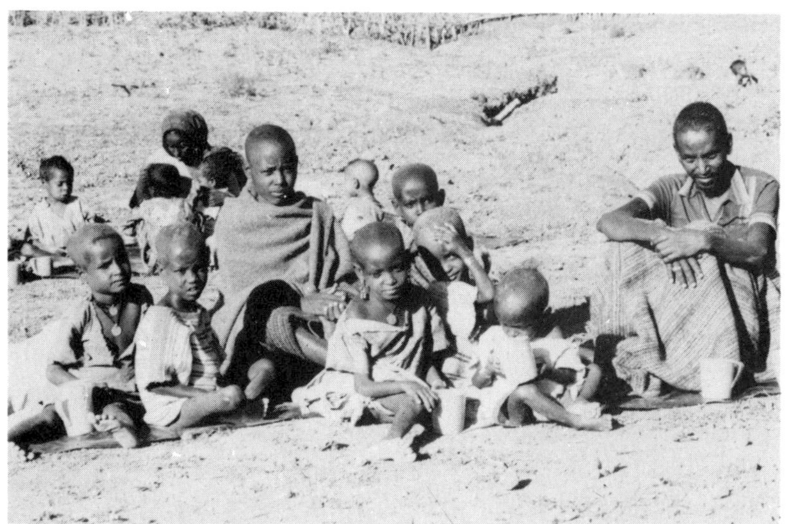

Reasons for local food shortages

There are many reasons for local food shortages. They are complicated and they can build up over a long time. When the local food shortage becomes an acute problem, it is called a **famine**.

Drought The lack of rain causes the harvest to fail (Fig. 2). People eat the stored grain, so there is no seed to plant for the following year.

War/civil disorder Resources (workers, money, etc.) are distracted from food production and distribution. Production is interrupted and the food distribution system fails.

Natural disasters (floods, volcanoes, etc.) Harvest and stores of food are destroyed.

Deforestation (forests being cut down) The climate may be upset and the earth may be eroded (washed or blown away).

Migration (from rural life to the cities) Fewer people are left to produce the food for the same population.

Domestic economic intervention The government of the country needs more money and encourages growth of 'cash crops' (that can be sold abroad). Less food is grown for the local population.

Domestic government intervention This happens when farmers try to raise their prices. This is unpopular with the large numbers of townspeople who blame the government. The government does not want to run the risk of losing support and forces the prices down. It becomes uneconomic for the farmers to work the land and so they stop doing so.

World economic intervention The price of agricultural chemicals and fertilizers increases. Poor farmers cannot afford them. Their production levels drop.

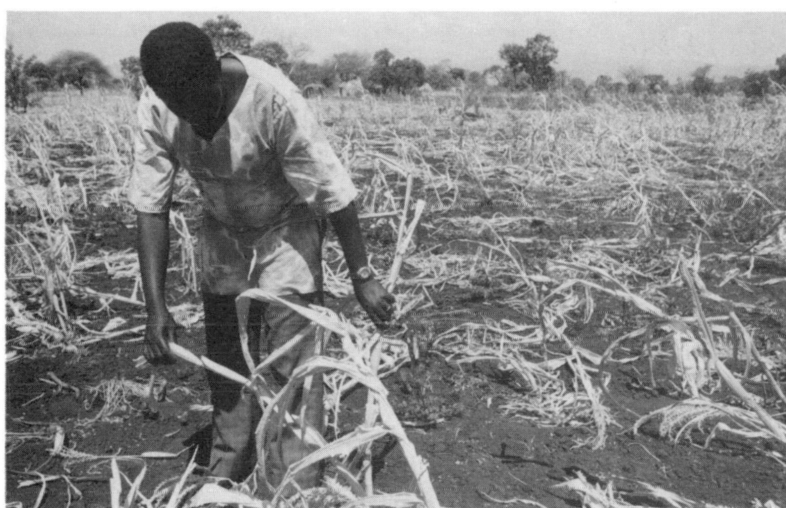
Fig. 2 Drought

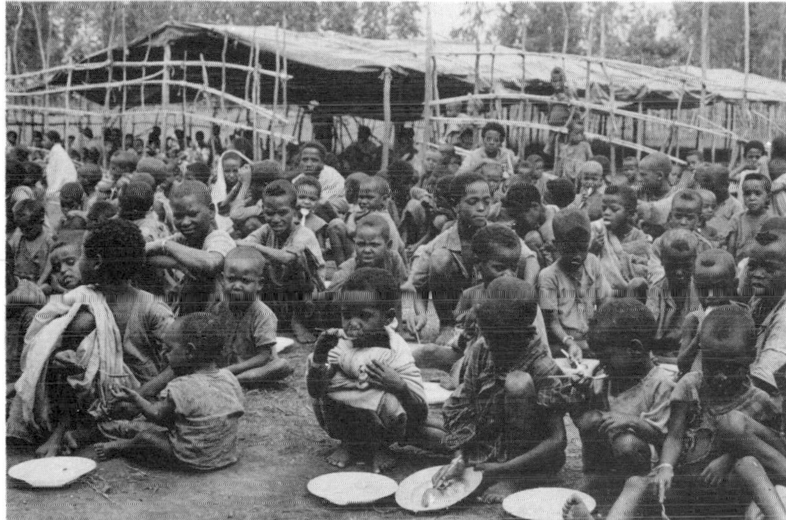
Fig. 3 A feeding centre

These are some of the factors which might, singly or acting together, cause food shortages. They might ultimately cause famine.

Food aid

Food aid is the most obvious answer to the problem of food shortage. 1985 was the year of Live Aid, when TV pictures of the horrific famine in Ethiopia and Sudan caused people around the world to respond. They sent enormous amounts of money to famine relief agencies. In such dire circumstances there is clearly a need for immediate food to stop people dying (Fig. 3). Unfortunately it is a short term answer to a long term famine. The African famine did not suddenly arrive in 1985. It had been predicted for years before. World governments had been warned of it long before 1985. Some governments decided not to send aid because they disapproved of Ethiopia's Marxist government.

If food aid is on a large enough scale, and if it is well managed, it will stop people from dying. However, it might also make worse the problem it is designed to solve (see Fig. 4).

Summary

- There is no overall food shortage in the world.
- Hunger is due to poverty.
- Food aid is only an emergency response.

Questions

1. Explain how any four factors may help cause a famine.
2. List the countries in the world where many people are undernourished.
3. What is wrong with constantly sending food to poor countries?

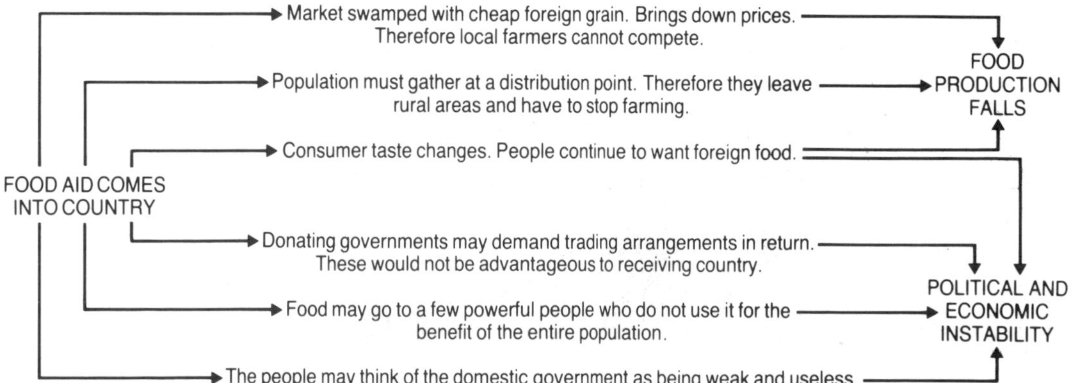

Fig. 4 The problems with food aid

5.2 Long term aid

Short term aid is for immediate problems. Long term development is necessary to help prevent the problems existing in the first place.

The Green Revolution

The Green Revolution was the 1960s' and 1970s' answer to the world food problem. The idea was to improve productivity of the land already in production. This would be done by developing high yielding strains of cereals (Fig. 1). As a result, cereal yields in Turkey have doubled. In Mexico, wheat yields have gone up fourfold. Rice and wheat production in India have also increased dramatically. The biggest success story of the Green Revolution is in the Indian state of Punjab. The new seed varieties there have more than doubled wheat and rice yields. Not only does this mean more food, but the state has become wealthier than any other state in India (Fig. 2).

There are drawbacks to the high yielding varieties:

- New seeds must be bought each year.
- They are less resistant to pests and disease and therefore need more pesticides, herbicides and fungicides.

These factors mean that poorer farmers cannot afford to buy them. Richer landlords invest money in their land and get good profit. They may well decide to work it themselves and not to leave it to landless labourers. This creates more poverty and more inequality among rural people.

In Punjab, conditions were favourable for the new varieties. There was already good irrigation and the state government was prepared to support agricultural investment. When these conditions do not apply, the Green Revolution is no answer.

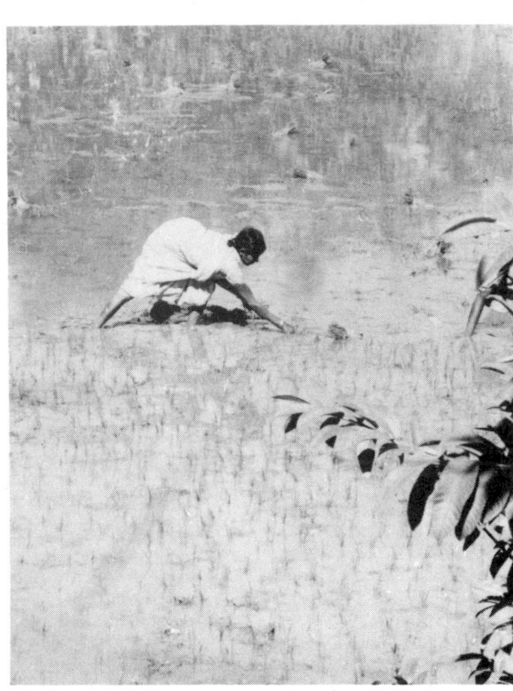

Fig. 1 Short stemmed, high yielding rice is grown in the Punjab

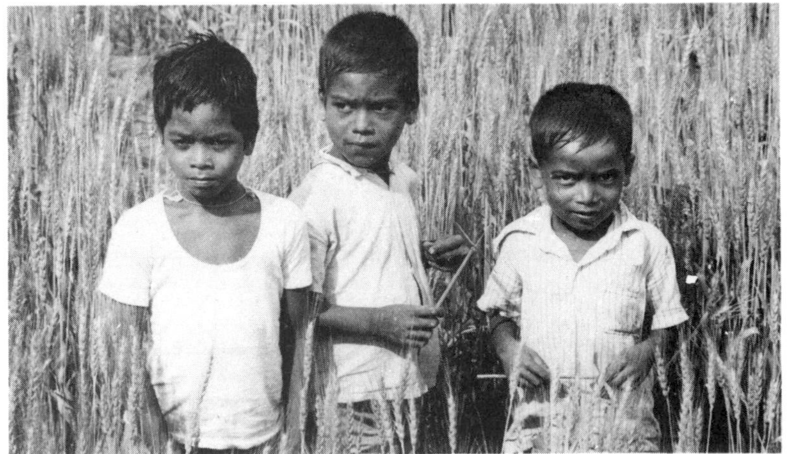

Fig. 2 High yielding wheat is also grown in the Punjab

The Brandt Commission

To overcome the inequality of food resources round the world, there must be worldwide cooperation. This was the idea behind the Brandt Commission. In 1980 it published a report, *North-South: A Programme for Survival*. Little has changed since then, so the recommendations in the report are still relevant. They included the following:

- Rich countries must improve their long term development aid to poorer countries. In the 1970s a target was set of 0.7% of each country's GNP (gross national product – 'earnings') to be spent on such aid. Very few countries have reached this target.

- Hunger should be ended by improving food production in poor countries. A food bank should be established for emergency use.
- Trade reform must give poorer countries a fair return for their goods.
- Energy should be conserved. New sources of energy must be found for poorer countries, because they need energy to develop (Fig. 3).

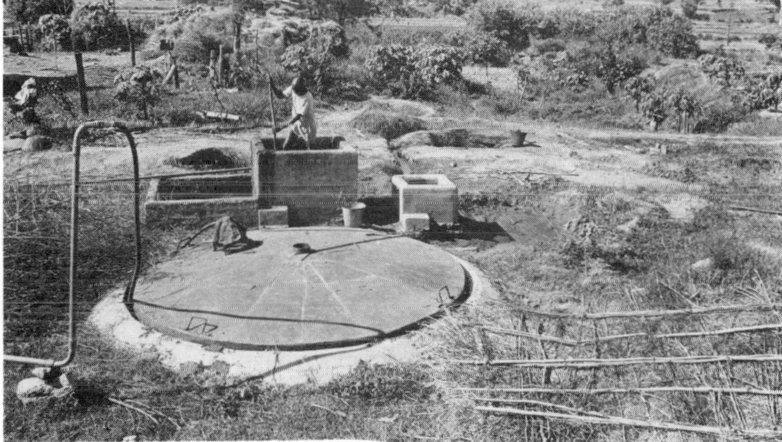

Fig. 3 A biogas plant. Animal manure and human waste are used to provide electricity for the house

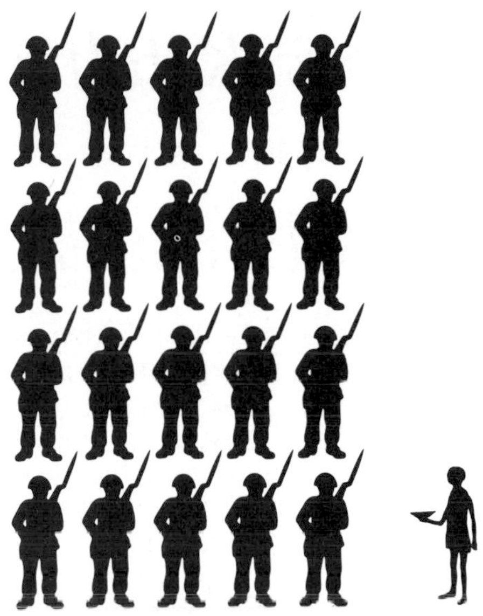

Fig. 4 Defence spending should be diverted to aid

- Technological development must be shared around the world.
- Defence spending must be diverted to development. At the moment, the world spends 20 times more on defence than it does on aid (Fig. 4).

Food for Work

This is a project that has been running for years. Instead of being paid with money, workers are paid with food (Fig. 5). This prevents them from being over-exploited by their employers. Having worked, their wages do actually ensure they and their families can eat. The project also shifts the responsibility for finding food from the worker to the employer, the employer probably being in a better position to do so.

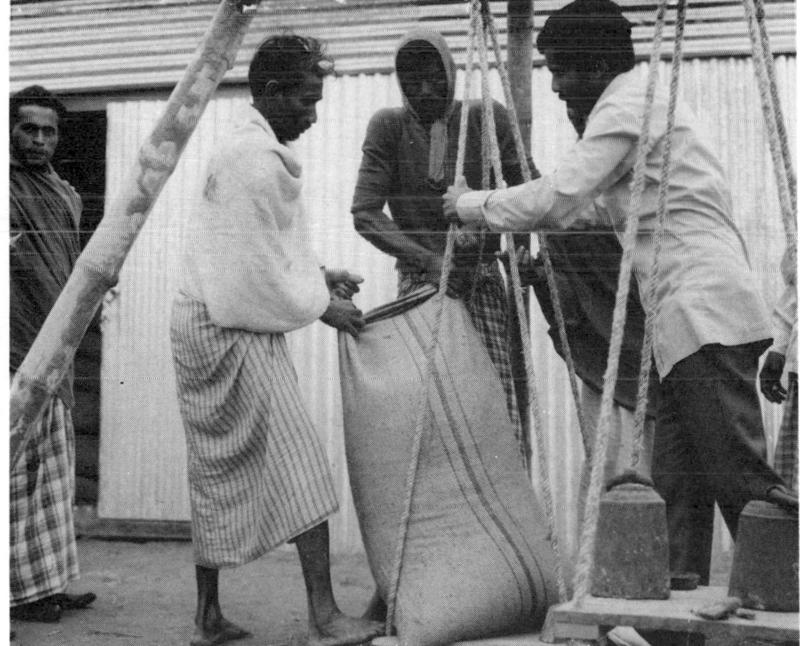

Fig. 5 Food for Work

Summary

- Long term aid for developing countries is essential.

Questions

1. What was the Green Revolution? Where was it most successful?
2. Explain the drawbacks of using high yielding cereal varieties.
3. What did the Brandt Commission recommend?
4. What is Food for Work?

SECTION 6 *Kitchen skills and hygiene*

6.1 *Food hygiene*

In the UK there are **Food Hygiene Regulations**, which are laws that control the production, preparation, manufacture and sale of food. The laws attempt to make food safe to eat. Food Hygiene Regulations apply to commercial kitchens and any other premises where food is handled, like shops, canteens and restaurants (Fig. 1).

If food hygiene is neglected there is the possibility of **food poisoning**. This is the commonest acute disease in the UK and it costs the country about £10 billion a year. The number of food poisoning cases reported is increasing. In 1984 there were 15 500 cases. This rose to 20 000 in 1985. Since it is thought that 90% of the cases of food poisoning are not recorded, the real figure could be 200 000 cases. The fact that food poisoning is such a problem today is due to the rapid increase in commercial catering of all kinds and a lack of attention to hygiene.

The term food poisoning is misleading, since what we understand by this term is not caused by the food itself but by an agent carried by the food. **Food borne disease** is a better term. The agents causing the trouble are **viruses** and **bacteria** (such as **Salmonella**).

Food borne disease is a serious public health problem. Outbreaks must be reported by law, and reports are made by public health laboratories, which investigate the outbreak with the aim of finding the cause and preventing further cases.

The Stanley Royd hospital in Wakefield had an outbreak of Salmonella in 1984. It was traced to cold roast beef which had been contaminated in the kitchen by Salmonella from raw chicken. In 24 hours, 94 people were affected and one person died. The total outbreak resulted in 460 cases and 19 of those people died.

Salmonella was also the causative agent in the outbreak at Farley, the babyfood manufacturers. Forty-three cases among babies were traced to Ostermilk, a formula milk feed. The bacteria was found in dust from a cleaning machine in the factory. Ostermilk, Osterfeed and Complan were all withdrawn from sale. The company lost £4 million as a result of the outbreak. (It is still trading.) Although Salmonella is the commonest cause of food poisoning there are a number of others (Fig. 2).

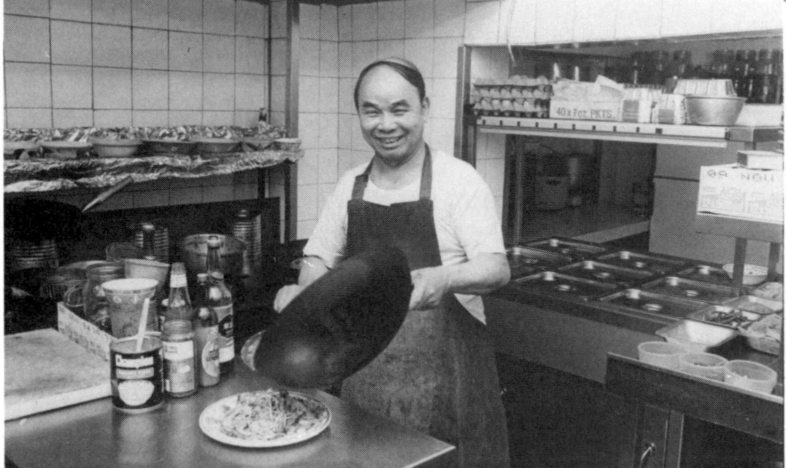

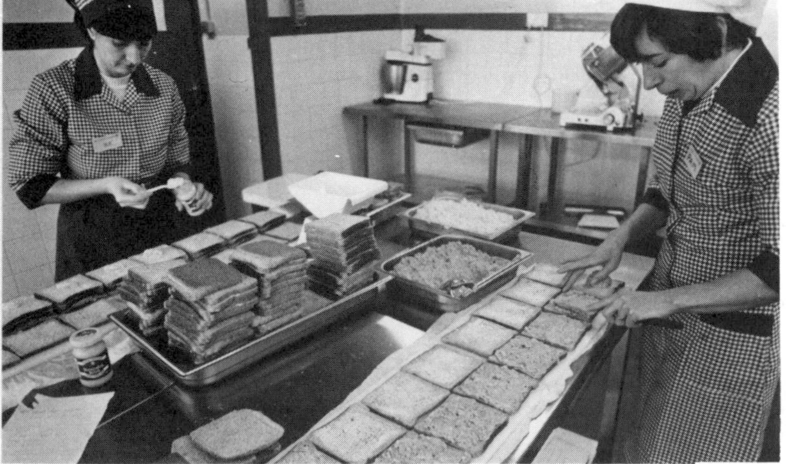

Fig. 1 Two commercial kitchens

Fig. 2 The causes of food poisoning

NAME OF AGENT	*COMMON VEHICLE*	*REPORTED OCCURRENCE*
Salmonella sp.	Raw meat contaminated by faeces during slaughter. Passed to cooked food by unhygienic handling.	98% of occurrences. 20–40 fatal cases per year.
Chlostridium perfingens	Contaminated raw meat. Poultry. Transferred in faeces.	Second most common agent.
Chlostridium botulinum	Fish – uncooked or stale. Faulty canning of fish may give rise to outbreaks.	Spores are heat resistant. Toxin is lethal even in small doses – botulism – which affects the central nervous system.
Staphylococcus	Spread from septic lesions on hands. Commonest cause – unhygienic handling of meat.	10 cases in 1984, all carried by Italian pasta.
Escherichia coli (E. coli)	Normal inhabitant of human gut flora and fauna.	Many strains cause illness, particularly in babies.
Bacillus cereus	Rice which has been reheated.	Cases usually reported from Chinese takeaways. Spores germinate in rice kept warm.
Campylobacter (a relatively new cause of food poisoning)	Chicken and milk.	1300 cases in 1977, 17000 cases in 1983.

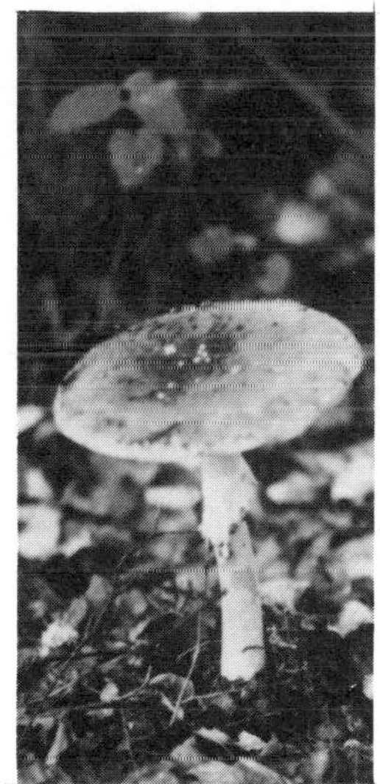

Fig. 3 Fly agaric (*Amarita muscaria*), a poisonous fungus

Natural toxins

Some fruit and vegetables contain natural **toxins**. Toxins are substances which are poisonous to us. One of the best known natural toxins is found in red kidney beans. From 1972 there have been 26 cases of food poisoning caused by eating undercooked red kidney beans. The toxin haemagglutinin is destroyed by boiling for at least 15 minutes.

Potatoes go green if they are left on top of soil in the light before being gathered. Green potatoes contain solanine, which causes a gastrointestinal upset. Another example is cassava, which contains cyanide. This is removed during its preparation for cooking.

There are many fungi which are poisonous (Fig. 3). It is dangerous to gather mushrooms from fields and woods unless you are very familiar with which ones are safe.

Summary

- Food Hygiene Regulations are designed to protect us from contaminated foods.
- Food borne disease is the commonest acute disease in the UK and its incidence is increasing.
- Salmonella is the commonest agent of food borne disease.
- Lack of hygiene is the main reason for the increase in food borne disease.
- Some foods contain natural toxins.

Questions

1. What makes 'food borne disease' a better term than food poisoning?
2. What reasons are given for the current high incidence of food borne disease?
3. Describe what happens during an outbreak of food poisoning. Give an example to illustrate your answer.
4. Write a sentence to describe how each of the following disease agents reaches its victims: (a) Salmonella, (b) Staphylococcus, (c) Bacillus cereus.
5. Describe red kidney bean poisoning.

6.2 Hygienic practices

Since bacteria are the main agents of food poisoning, it is necessary to understand a little of how they live, multiply and spread, in order to prevent them doing so on our food. Bacteria need a source of food, and they favour much of the food we like to eat, particularly meat, milk, eggs and fish. They do not grow well in food containing a lot of salt, sugar, fat or acid. They also need moisture. Some bacteria need oxygen but others, the **anaerobes**, grow without it. Bacteria like warmth and grow best at 37°C – body heat (Fig. 1).

Food may come into the kitchen already contaminated, in which case it needs careful treatment to ensure that the contamination is not spread to other foods and to destroy the source of contamination before the food is eaten. It may be contaminated in the kitchen by handling (bacteria are on human skin, in the nose, mouth and throat, and in the faeces), from the kitchen utensils, or from other animals like flies, vermin or domestic pets (Fig. 2). If simple hygienic practices are always followed, food poisoning can be prevented. These practices are necessary for preparing, cooking, serving and storing food and concern the person handling the food and the environment of the kitchen (Fig. 3).

Fig. 1 Effects of temperature and time on the growth of bacteria

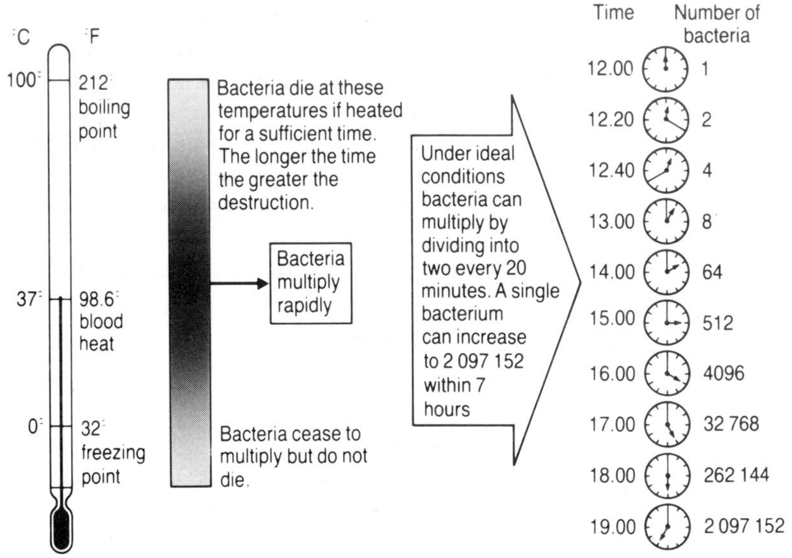

Time	Number of bacteria
12.00	1
12.20	2
12.40	4
13.00	8
14.00	64
15.00	512
16.00	4096
17.00	32 768
18.00	262 144
19.00	2 097 152

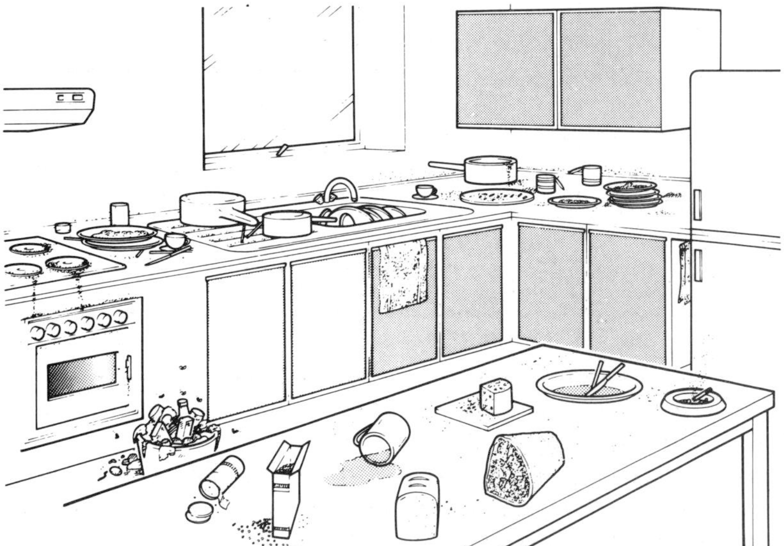

Fig. 2 An unhygienic kitchen

The food handler

Hands must be washed before handling foods and after handling raw meat and fish. Do not touch the face, hair or nose while working with food. Always wash hands after using the WC.

Smoking must not be allowed around food.

Tasting should be done with a clean spoon which is washed afterwards. Do not put fingers into food to taste it.

Hair should be covered and kept tied back while working with foods.

The kitchen

Surfaces should be smooth so that there are no crevices where bits of food can become lodged.

Equipment must be washed with hot soapy water, and that used for raw foods must be washed before being used for cooked foods.

Cleaning is best done with disposable paper or very clean and frequently laundered cloths.

Waste food will go bad very quickly, and may begin to smell. It will also attract flies and vermin. All waste food should be wrapped before being disposed of. Remember that broken glass and other sharp objects should be properly wrapped to prevent accidents.

Preparing and cooking food

Poultry often harbours food poisoning organisms. Do not allow raw poultry to come into contact with any other foods. Wash any surfaces used to prepare the raw bird with hot soapy water. Allow frozen poultry to thaw completely and cook it thoroughly (Fig. 4). Do not put stuffing nor leave the giblets, etc., in the body cavity. Stuffing may be put in under the skin at the neck end. It is important that the centre of the bird reaches a high enough temperature to kill bacteria.

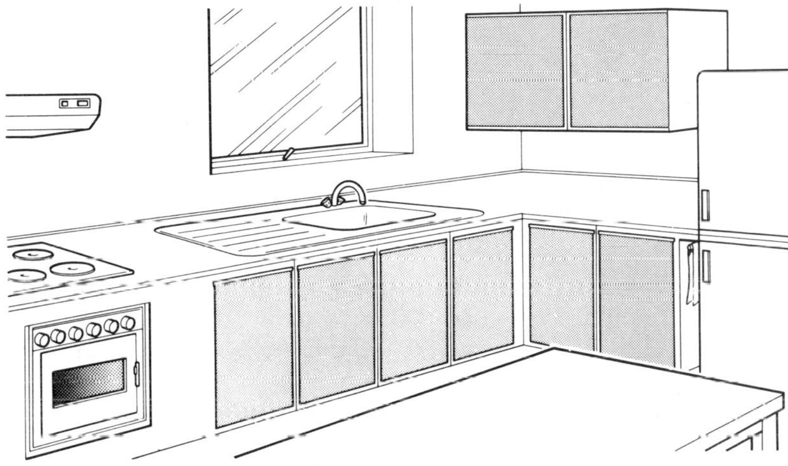

Fig. 3 A clean kitchen

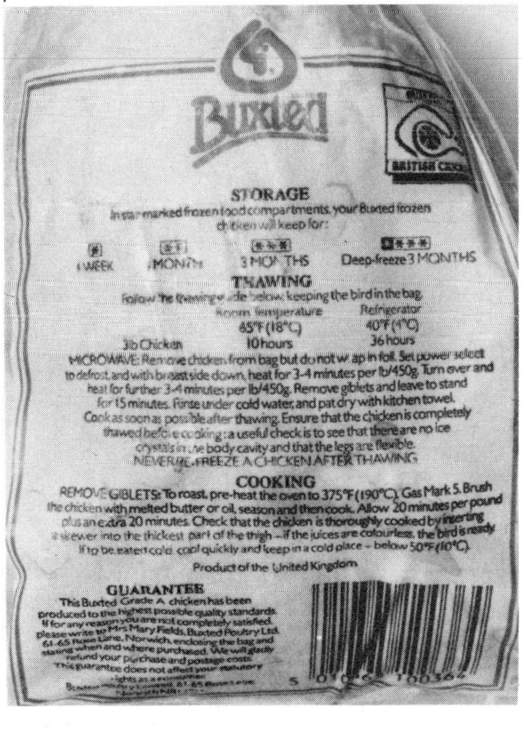

Fig. 4 The label of a frozen chicken. Note the instructions

Raw meat often has bacteria on its surface. Do not allow blood to touch any cooked food and wash any surface or equipment which the meat touches.

Cold cooked meat must be handled carefully. Keep it cool and do not touch it directly with hands.

Shellfish should be bought only from reputable suppliers.

Cooked rice, if kept overnight, must be refrigerated.

Reheating food will provide an ideal way of giving bacteria the warmth they require to reproduce. Always see that food is thoroughly heated and that it boils when being reheated.

Cooked food for eating later must be cooked quickly and stored in a refrigerator. Never keep food warm for long periods.

Refreezing must never be done.

Storing food

Raw and **cooked** meats must be stored separately.

Covering food is essential, and the correct material is important.

Stock rotation is important so that no food is kept for too long.

Summary

- Bacteria are the main agents of food borne disease.
- They need a source of food, moisture and warmth to reproduce.
- Hygienic practices in the handling of food are essential to prevent the spread of the bacteria.

Questions

1. How does temperature affect the rate at which bacteria multiply?
2. As well as warmth, what else do bacteria need to live and reproduce?
3. In what ways might food poisoning be caused by the unhygienic habits of a cook?
4. Explain why it is necessary (a) to allow frozen chickens to thaw properly, (b) to see that ham does not come into contact with raw meat.

6.3 Food storage

Most of the food we eat has a limited **storage life** and begins to deteriorate if kept for too long. The effect of eating food which has begun to 'go off' may be merely that the food is less pleasant or less nutritious than it should be, or much more seriously it may cause food poisoning. Taking care over the way in which food is stored may then preserve it in a reasonable state for as long as possible, and will prevent unnecessary ill health.

In most modern houses and flats, food storage space is limited. The walk-in larder which was once popular is now rare (Fig. 1). Cupboards in centrally heated homes are not cool enough for storing short life foods, and many people keep a great deal of food in refrigerators.

Perishable foods which have a short shelf life, like milk, meat, fish, eggs, cheese, fruit and vegetables, cannot be stored for long. They need to be kept cool and a **refrigerator** is most suitable (Fig. 2).

When many different foods are stored in a confined space like a refrigerator there are several important points to remember:

- Uncooked meat is often contaminated with bacteria and must not be in contact with any food which will be eaten without further cooking (milk, cheese, cooked meat). It must be covered and not allowed to drip onto other foods.
- Strong smelling foods (e.g. onions) give a tainted taste to other foods and must

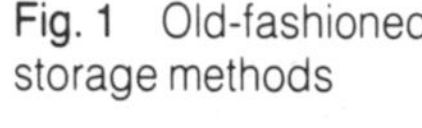

Fig. 1 Old-fashioned storage methods

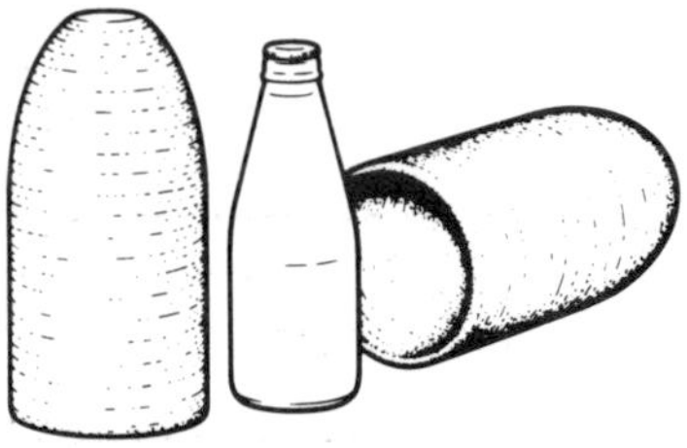

Clay milk saver

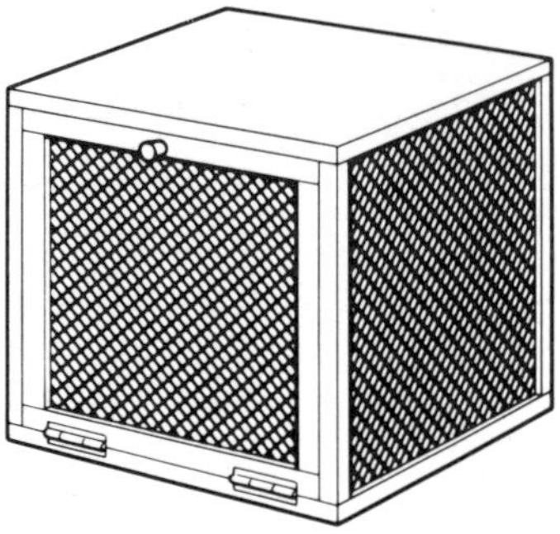

Meat safe

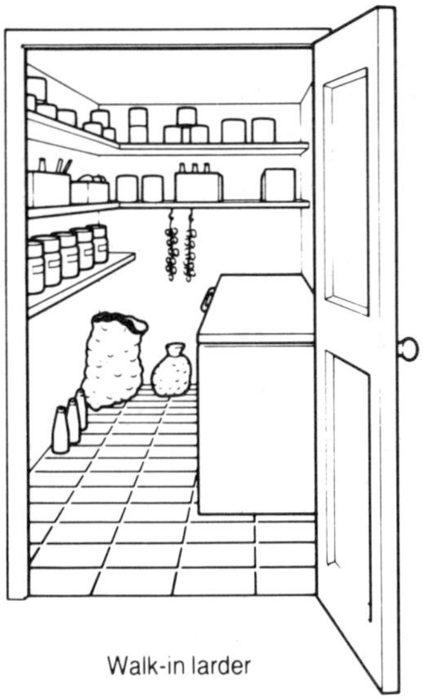

Walk-in larder

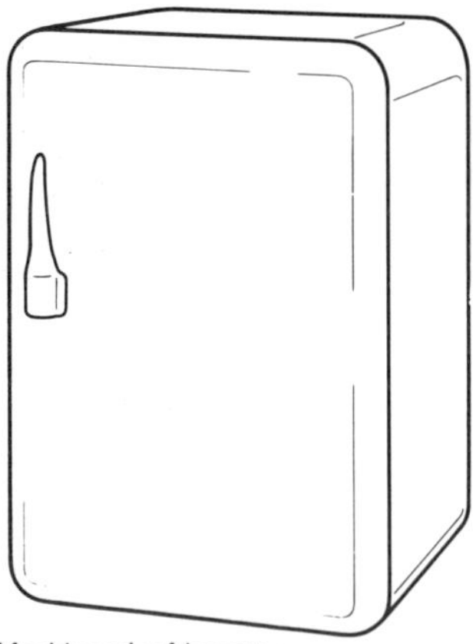

Old fashioned refrigerator

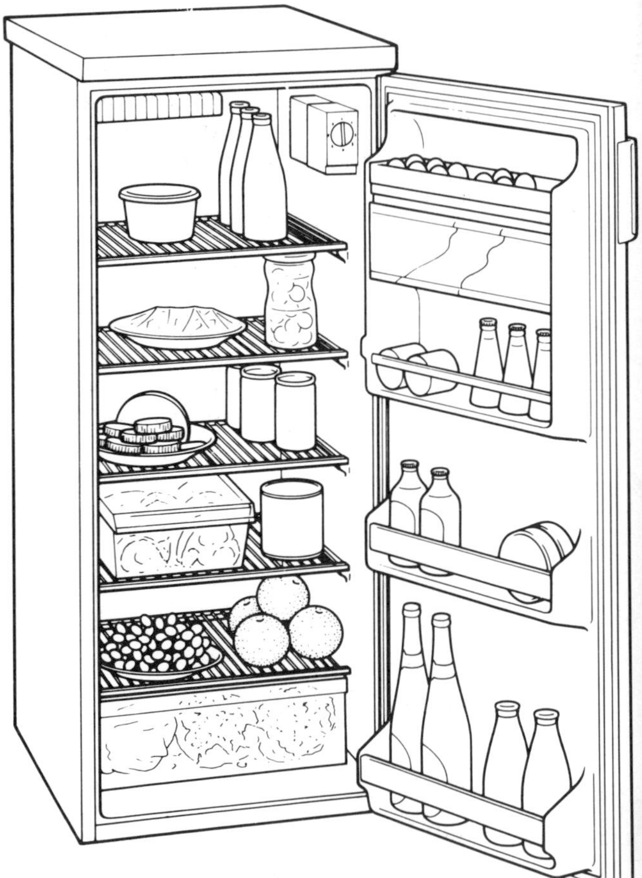

Fig. 2 A modern refrigerator

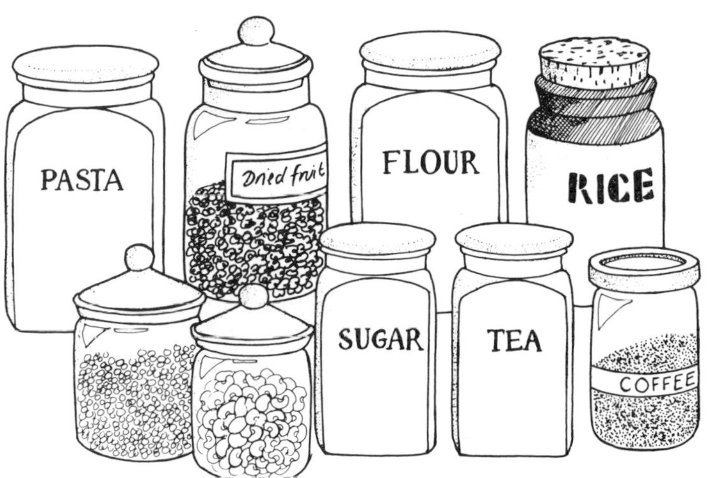

Fig. 3 Dried food containers

be wrapped in an airtight covering.

- Fruit and vegetables will keep well in a crisper tray, but bananas go black and some fruit, like pineapple, have a strong smell.

Bread will go mouldy if kept too long, especially in an airtight tin. It needs a ventilated bin or ceramic container.

Dried goods, like flour and other cereal products, can be stored easily. It is best not to keep them for longer than a month since they may begin to deteriorate. They need to be stored in closed containers or jars. Stored dry foods can become infested with insect pests, like flour beetles. Good containers will prevent this (Fig. 3).

Long life goods, like canned foods and dry pulses, need to be kept correctly and will not last indefinitely. Cans which are dented may cause contamination, and once a can is open it must be emptied and its contents used quickly. All dry goods will deteriorate rapidly if allowed to become damp.

Storing food safely means keeping it in conditions which do not encourage the growth of bacteria and moulds, i.e. cool dry conditions. One of the protections offered to consumers is the 'Sell by . . .' and 'Best before. . .' dates, which many food labels carry (Fig. 4). It is important to take note of these dates and eat food which is fresh. Where food does not carry such information the aim should be to rotate stock – use the older food first and see that no food is eaten when there is a risk of contamination.

Summary

- Most food has a limited 'shelf' life.
- Correct storage is important to safeguard health.

Questions

1. On this diagram of a fridge indicate the places where you would store each of the following foods: (a) fresh meat, (b) eggs, (c) lettuce, (d) cheese, (e) ham. Write a sentence to explain your reasons for each choice.
2. Why should bananas and pineapple not be stored in a fridge?
3. What is the best way to store (a) flour, (b) bread?
4. What is meant by stock rotation?

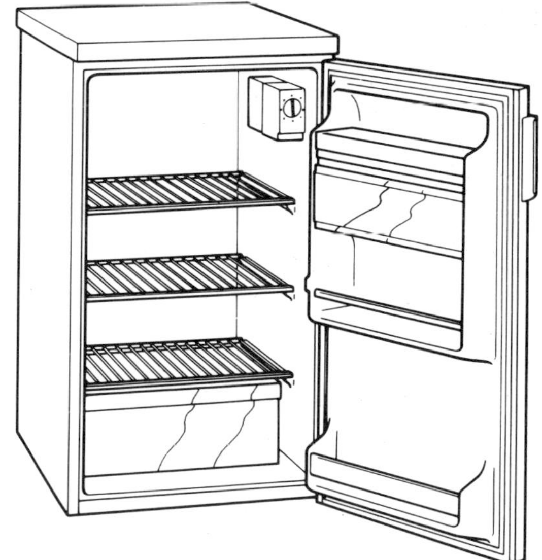

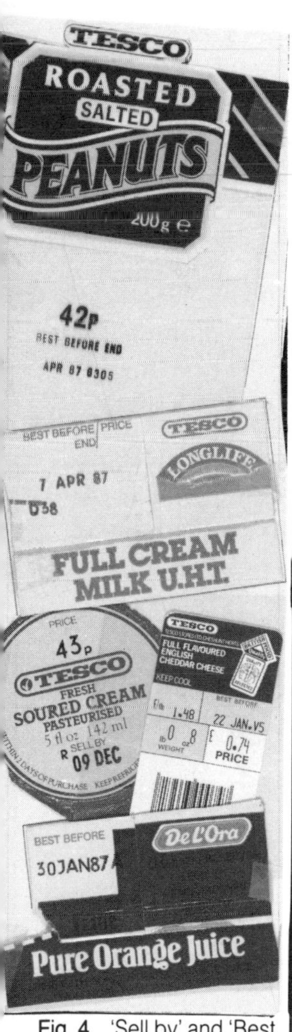

Fig. 4 'Sell by' and 'Best before' dates

6.4 Food spoilage

The aim of preservation is to prevent spoilage and to retain as many of the qualities of the original food as possible. People have been preserving food since ancient times, when the reason for preservation was to make a food store for winter. Now we use preservation as a means of eating foods out of season, using up plentiful cheap stocks of produce and varying our diet by making foods taste different.

Fig. 1 Ripe fruit

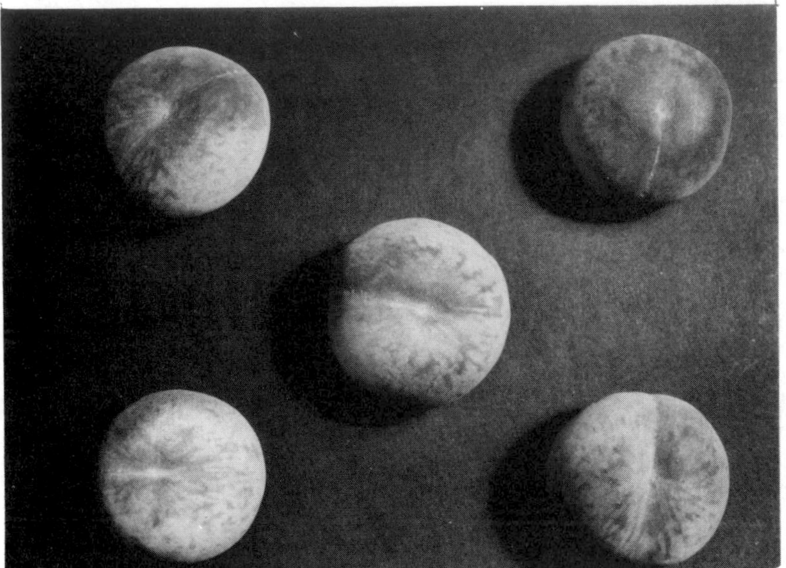

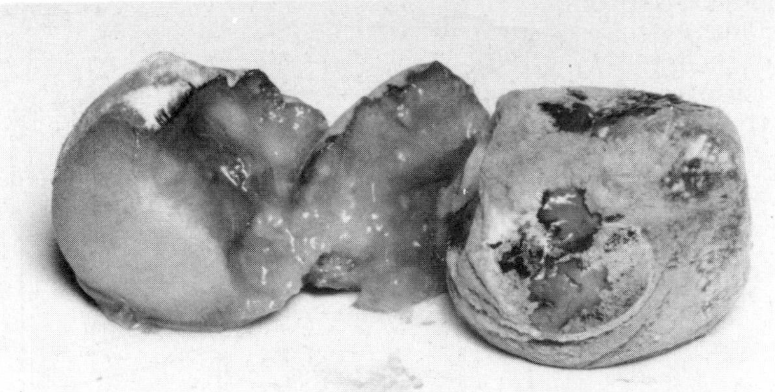

Fig. 2 Rotting fruit

Food spoilage is caused by the activity of enzymes and micro-organisms, like bacteria and fungi. In order to preserve food, enzyme activity must be halted and micro-organisms destroyed. The food must then be protected from further **contamination**.

Enzymes and food spoilage

Enzymes are found in all plant and animal cells. They are there to help the reactions in the cells which are vital for life. The group of enzymes concerned with food spoilage are those which bring about **ripening** of fruit and vegetables (Fig. 1). The changes associated with ripening are changing starch to sugar, breaking down organic acids and softening flesh. They are all dependent on enzyme activity. If the ripening process continues, however, the fruit or vegetables become mushy, go brown and the taste becomes unpleasant (Fig. 2). Breaking cell walls and releasing enzymes (as in bruising) increases the rate of decomposition.

Enzymes can be controlled by:

Heating Enzymes are made of protein and heat will therefore denature (destroy) them and make the enzyme ineffective. **Blanching** (immersing in boiling water) fruit and vegetables before freezing is aimed at controlling enzyme activity (Fig. 3).

Cooling Enzymes may continue to cause spoilage – hence the need for blanching – but the rate of reaction is considerably lowered.

pH change Enzymes, like all proteins, are sensitive to changes in pH. The pH is a measure of the acidity or alkalinity of a substance. pH 1 is very acid; pH 14 is very alkaline.

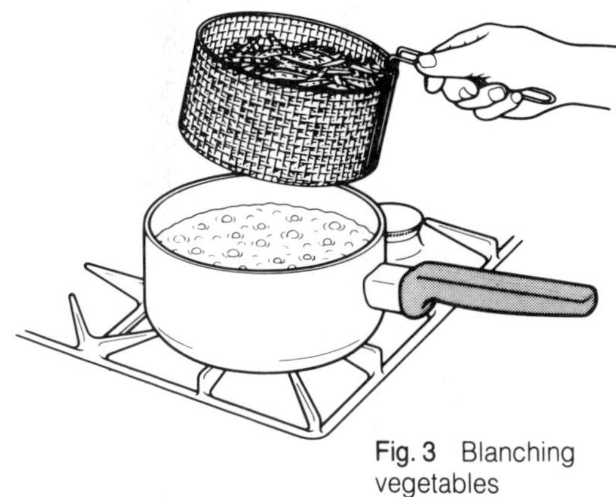

Fig. 3 Blanching vegetables

Cutting off supply of oxygen or moisture Many reactions involve the absorption of oxygen or of moisture. If the supply of either is removed, enzymes cease to be effective (Fig. 4).

Adding preservatives Preservatives like sulphur dioxide (E 220) prevent enzyme activity.

Micro-organisms and food spoilage

Traditional methods of preservation are based on making the food an unsuitable environment for micro-organisms (Fig. 5). Modern food technology uses traditional methods as a basis, but with a larger range of chemicals and more sophisticated equipment the range of foods available has greatly increased.

Summary

- Food spoilage is caused by the action of enzymes or micro-organisms.
- Food preservation aims to prevent the action of both these agents.

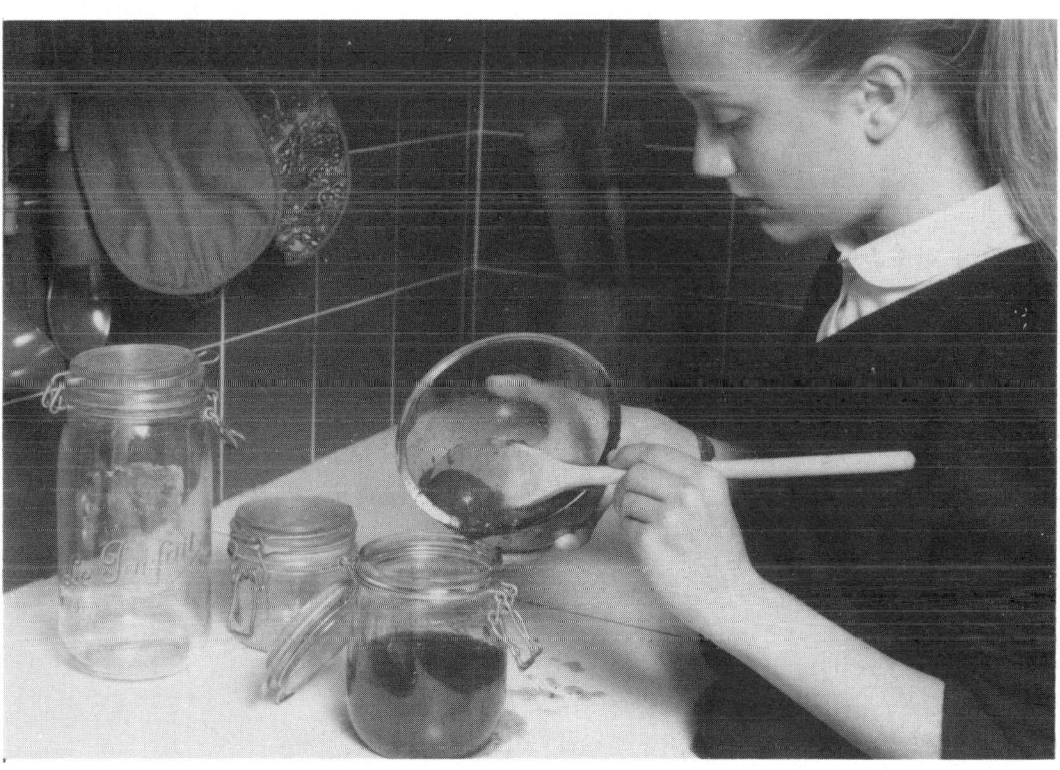

Fig. 4 Kilner jars cut off oxygen

Fig. 5 Unsuitable environments for bacteria

Bacteria need:	Unsuitable environment
warmth	temperatures too high or too low
moisture	conditions too dry
supply of food	too much sugar, salt or fat in the food
neutral pH	pH too low

Questions

1. Explain why we need to preserve foods.
2. What is meant by 'spoilage' and what causes it?
3. Describe 'ripening' in fruit.
4. Explain four ways in which undesirable enzyme activity is controlled.
5. What conditions enable bacteria to thrive?

6.5 Food preservation

Using heat

Although some bacterial spores and toxins are resistant to heat, most micro-organisms are destroyed by temperatures of 100°C.

Sterilizing Milk is sterilized in the bottle by being heated to 113°C in a vacuum for at least 15 minutes (Fig. 1).

Pasteurization Pasteurizing affects the appearance and flavour of food less than sterilization. Milk is commonly pasteurized. This involves heating it to 72°C for 15 seconds then cooling it rapidly. It is now used for many other foods, like fruit juices, cream, beer and wine. It is intended to extend the life of food by killing bacteria, but pasteurized food has a limited shelf life.

Fig. 1 Milk bottling plant

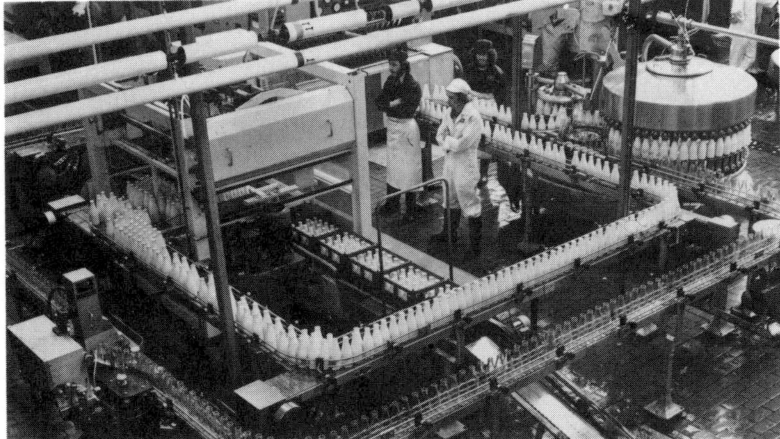

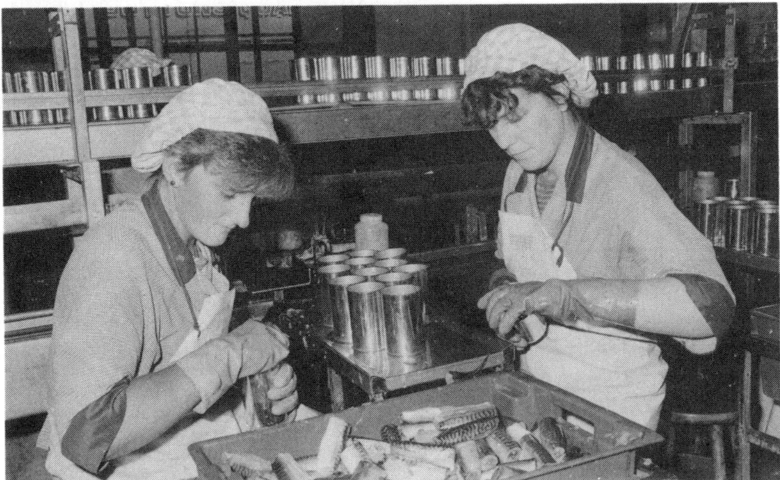

Fig. 2 Inside a canning factory

Ultra heat treatment (UHT) UHT milk is heated to 132°C for 1 second then cooled rapidly and packed in foil lined containers. It can be stored at room temperature until opened.

Bottling This was once a popular method of home preservation, especially for fruit and vegetables. Food is boiled in the jar then sealed to exclude air and micro-organisms.

Canning This grew out of bottling techniques and is today the most used method of preservation. Food is sterilized under pressure in the can, which is then sealed to prevent contamination (Fig. 2). The cans are made of tinned steel. Some are aluminium, but these are expensive. Environmental and economic considerations have encouraged many local authorities to recycle waste cans. Virtually any food can be canned. The recommended shelf life is about one year, although it will keep much longer as long as the can remains undamaged. Once opened the can must be emptied to prevent the contents reacting with metal in an atmosphere containing oxygen, and then it must be treated like fresh food.

Using low temperatures

The domestic **refrigerator** operates at about 4°C. At this temperature microbial activities are slowed down but not stopped. A refrigerator prolongs the shelf life of food but does not preserve it.

Freezers operate at about −18°C. Bacteria become inactive at −10°C. Most foods contain mainly water. When this freezes ice crystals are formed. The quicker the freezing process the smaller the ice crystals and the more satisfactory is the quality of the frozen food.

Commercial freezing methods include:

- Plate freezing. Flat products like fish or beefburgers are frozen on plates by conduction.
- Blast freezing. Cold air blasts are used to freeze vegetables.
- Cryogenic freezing uses liquid nitrogen. This is expensive but ideal for delicate

fruits like raspberries or strawberries which do not freeze well.
– Cook-freeze catering is becoming popular. Meals are cooked in bulk, then frozen in containers. This is used in hospitals and other commercial catering outlets.

Dehydration

Bacteria need moisture to grow and reproduce and are destroyed by dehydration. Food has been preserved by being dried in the sun for thousands of years. In hot sunny countries varieties of meat, fish, vegetables and fruit continue to be dried in this traditional way. Commercial methods of dehydration are carefully controlled and result in a reliable product which keeps well (Fig. 3).

Hot air beds are used to dry solid foods. The food is put on a perforated tray and hot air blown through it, e.g. meat, vegetables, fruit, pulses.

Spray drying is used to dry liquids. A fine spray of the liquid is blown into a chamber of very hot air. The mist turns into powder almost immediately, e.g. soups, desserts, milk.

Accelerated freeze drying is expensive, but the end product retains more taste, e.g. coffee and milk.

Dried foods have the advantage of being lightweight, but they absorb water easily and must be stored dry. For this reason they are often packed in foil.

Fig. 3 Dried foods

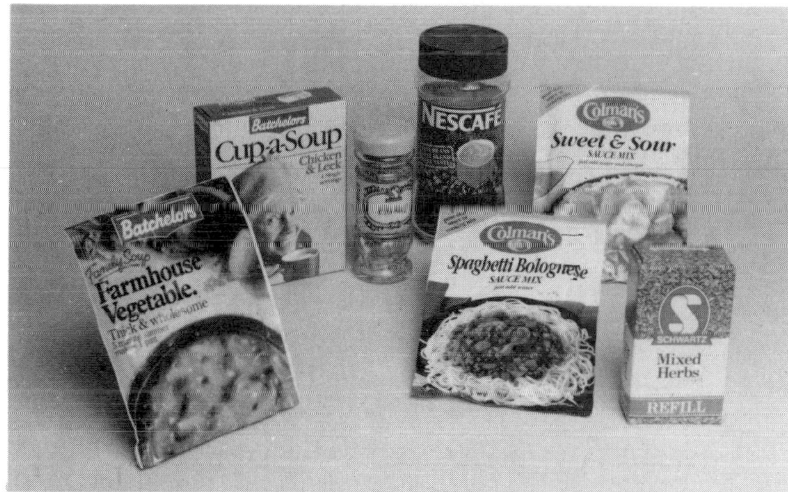

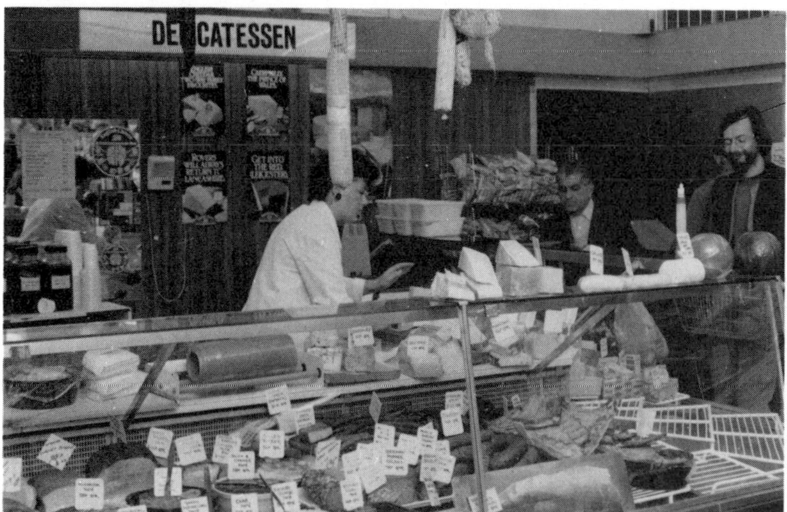

Fig. 4 Foods preserved with sodium or potassium nitrite/nitrate

Use of chemicals

Chemical preservation of foods has been practised for centuries. Traditional methods include salting, smoking, pickling, curing in nitrate salts, and preserving in sugar or alcohol. These traditional methods are still used, although they have been changed by the developments in food technology to increase the scale and decrease the time and expense involved. A large range of chemicals is available for newer methods of preservation. This review includes traditional and modern chemicals.

Sodium chloride (common salt)
Vegetables were once preserved in jars between layers of salt. Now they are commonly canned in brine (salt solution). Fish are preserved in layers of salt. Meat, sausages, cheese and bacon are also preserved in dry salt or brine. As well as preserving, salt adds flavour.

Sodium or potassium nitrite/nitrate
These are used to preserve bacon, ham, sausages, canned meats/meat products and cheeses (Fig. 4). The nitrate salt is changed to the nitrite form by enzyme action. When nitrite combines with haemoglobin it forms a bright red compound familiar in foods preserved in this way. The colour is more pronounced if nitrite is used instead of nitrate and much less need be used. Nitrites inhibit the growth of Chlostridium botulinum.

(Botulism is a fatal kind of food poisoning.) Nitrites, however, may be toxic. They are converted in part to nitrosamines which are carcinogenic (cancer causing). A link between eating nitrites as a food additive and stomach cancer has been suggested. The Government's Food Advisory Committee recommend using the minimum required to control Chlostridium botulinum. But even if we ate none in this way, the amount of nitrates used as fertilizers mean that it would still be present in a variety of foods.

Smoking Food was once preserved by being hung in the smoke from burning firewood. The smoke changed the colour and contained tars, aldehydes and phenols, which have bactericidal action. Because the traditional method takes a long time, modern methods often involve salting and adding chemicals to imitate the taste of smoke. Kippers, for example, are often dyed brown with E154. (BFK, i.e. Brown For Kippers!)

Acids Acetic acid (vinegar) is the commonest acid used for pickling, e.g. onions, eggs, gherkins, olives, walnuts etc. (Fig. 5). The pH of pickling acids is pH2. Tartaric, lactic, benzoic or citric acids are also preservatives.

Alcohol Fruit is often preserved in brandy, rum or gin. Fruit juice when fermented with yeast turns to alcohol, and in controlled conditions it becomes wine, which keeps well. (Wild yeasts are found on the bloom of fruit like grapes and plums. If the skin breaks the fruit begins to ferment.)

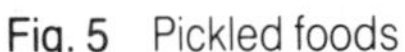

Fig. 5 Pickled foods

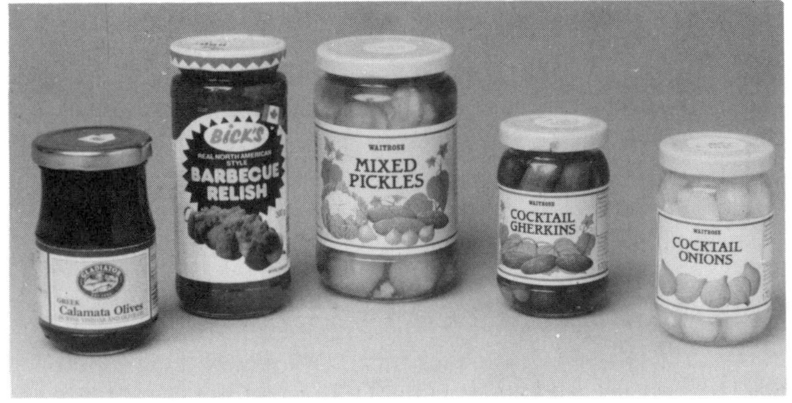

Sugar Sugar has long been used to preserve fruit, as in jam making, crystallizing, bottling and canning. It adds energy to the product. Sugar is used as a preservative in condensed milk.

Fats and oils These are used to preserve fish and vegetables. Potting – covering food with a layer of fat – is used to preserve shrimps and fruit.

Sulphur dioxide Sulphur dioxide was used by the Ancient Greeks to preserve their wine. It is used now in a wide variety of foods, mainly beer, wine, fruit, fruit juices, pickles, sauces, sausages, soft drinks, flour and vegetables.

Other chemicals E numbers 200–290 are all permitted preservatives used to check the growth of micro-organisms. Anti-oxidants are used to prevent changes involving oxidation, e.g. rancidity in fats and oils. Vitamins C and E are both natural anti-oxidants and these are added to a number of foods. E numbers for anti-oxidants are E300–E321.

Antibiotics Antibiotics are chemicals produced by micro-organisms which inhibit the growth of other micro-organisms. They have therapeutic uses, penicillin being the most commonly known antibiotic. They are also used as a food supplement in rearing farm animals. This is an area of possible danger since it encourages the growth of resistant strains of bacteria. Niscin is found naturally in milk and milk products. It has no therapeutic use. It is added to cheeses, clotted cream and canned foods. Tetracyclines have been used to preserve poultry and to add to the ice which preserves fish, but it is no longer permitted in the UK.

Food irradiation

At present, Britain does not allow irradiation of food for general use (Fig. 6). Food for medical purposes, like sterile diets for transplant patients, is exempt. In other European countries the laws controlling irradiation differ. There is no law against irradiation at EEC level, and recommendations have been made to change the law in Britain to

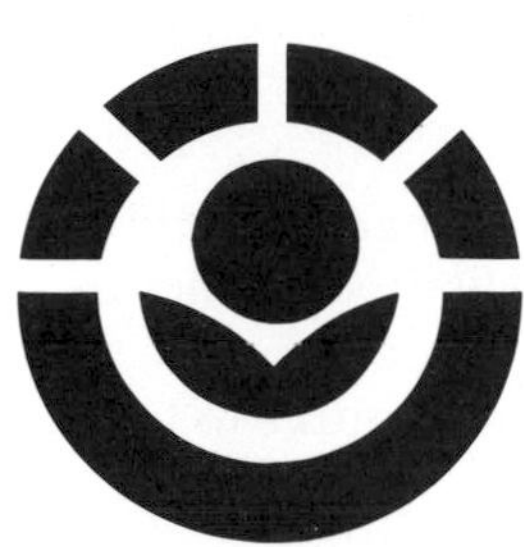

Fig. 6 The food irradiation symbol, not yet in use in Britain

allow it. Irradiating food, that is treating it with large doses of radiation, can
- inhibit (stop) sprouting in vegetables like onions, garlic, shallots and potatoes
- delay ripening of fruit like strawberries
- kill insect pests
- reduce the bacteria which cause food spoilage. (Irradiation can then increase shelf life and make additives less likely to be used.)

Concern has been expressed over several issues:
- the safety of food industry workers
- the loss of nutrients in irradiated food
- the safety of irradiated foodstuffs
- the need for clear labelling of irradiated food
- the possibility of irradiating contaminated food to present further deterioration.

Summary

- Most micro-organisms are destroyed by temperatures of 100°C.
- Bacteria are inactive below −10°C.
- Dehydration destroys micro-organisms.
- A number of chemicals act as preservatives.
- Irradiation of food will preserve it. There is concern over use of radiation for this purpose.

Preserving food at home

Home preserving is used as a means of using a glut of home produced food, usually fruit and vegetables, or of enabling bulk purchasing of perishable food like meat (Fig. 7). Methods have changed over the past 50 years. Home freezing is now the most popular method.

Method	Description	Foods used	Notes
Drying	Suitable for foods with small volumes.	Herbs – mint, sage. Spices – red chillies.	
Bottling	Fruit – heat to 75–88°C. Vegetables – heat to 155°C then seal.	Any suitable fruit or vegetables.	Use kilner jar with sealing tops.
Freezing	Domestic freezers operate at −18–23°C. Food is first blanched to inactivate enzymes and destroy some micro-organisms.	Most raw and cooked food.	Thawed food must never be re-frozen. 'Drip' of frozen foods may cause loss of water soluble vitamins.
Salting	Dry salting – with salt crystals or brine.	Dry – vegetables like runner beans. Brine – olives.	Less popular method now.
Jam making	Fruit is first cooked until tender. Pectin is extracted by cooking. Sugar is added and temperature taken to about 104°C.	Any fruit or mixture of fruit.	Commercial jams are made with less sugar now. Some fruits low in pectin may need extra added.
Pickling	Pickling vinegar contains 5% acetic acid which prevents growth of micro-organisms.	Onions, cabbage, mixed vegetables or fruit.	Chutney is hot sweet pickle. Green tomatoes are suitable.

Fig. 7 Home food preserving

Questions

1. Describe any three methods of preserving food using heat.
2. Food has been preserved for hundreds of years. Write a few sentences about how food was preserved many years ago.
3. Why is sodium nitrite used as a preservative in spite of its carcinogenic nature?
4. Why does pickling preserve food?
5. Describe any five ways in which fruit could be preserved.

6.6 Cooking (heat movement)

Transfer of heat

Heat is a form of energy. When food is subjected to the effects of this energy, it changes. We call this process cooking. When food is cooked it changes in **texture**, **colour** and **palatability**. The chemical and physical changes which occur during cooking make food easier to eat and easier to digest.

Heat is transferred from source to food by one of three methods.

Conduction Molecules within substances absorb heat and begin to

Fig. 1 Convection currents in (a) a liquid and (b) a gas

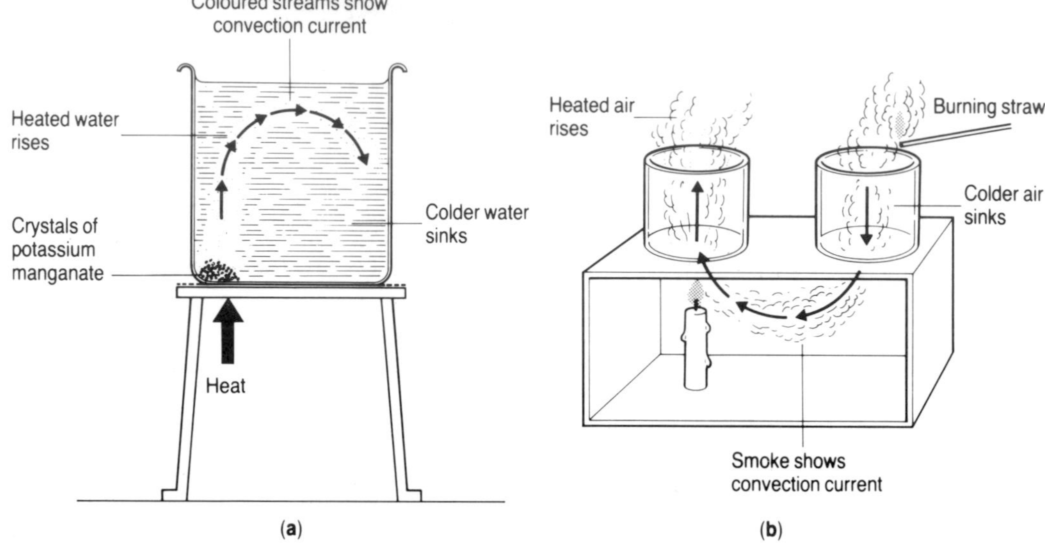

Fig. 2 Cooking methods

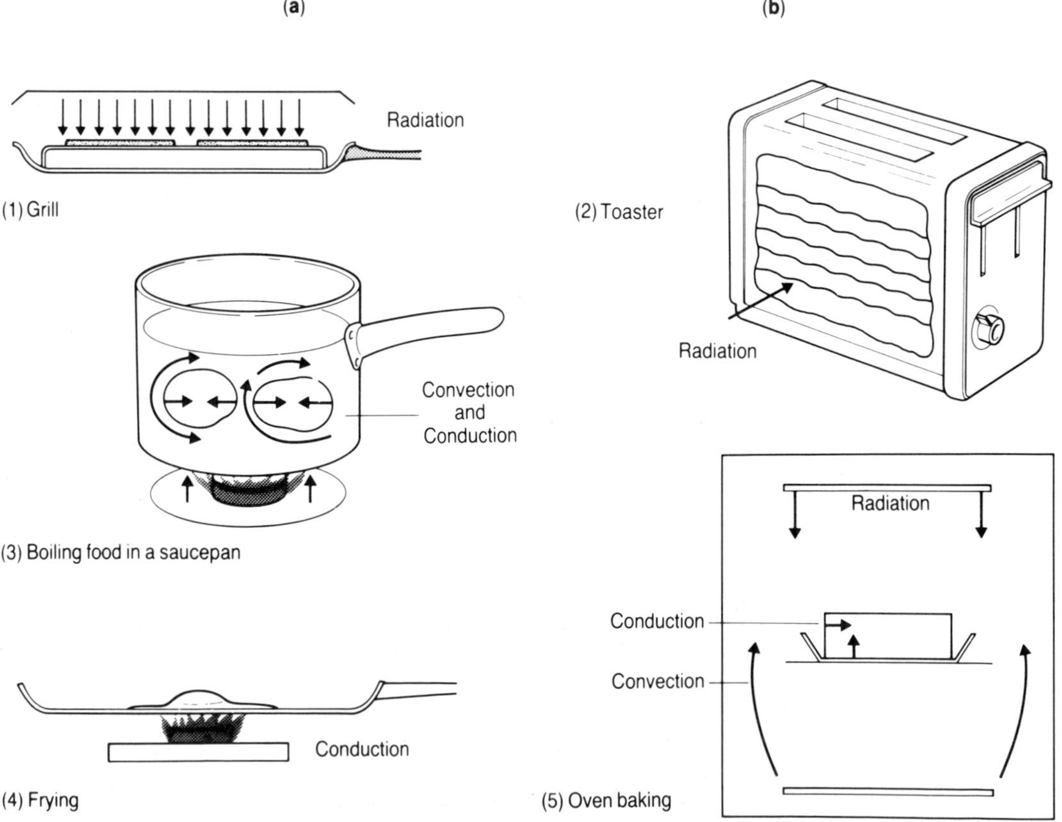

Fig. 3 Uses of insulators

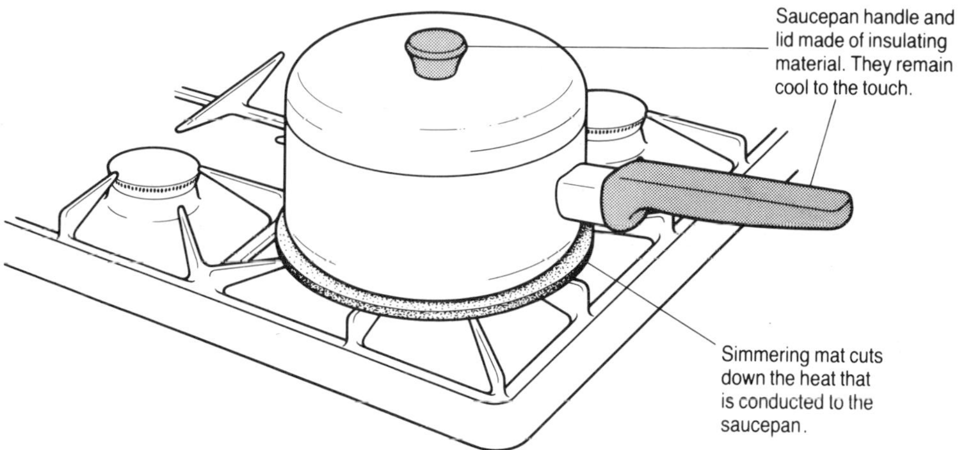

vibrate. This vibration passes from molecule to molecule through the material. Good conductors allow heat to pass through them easily. Metals, because of their structure, are good conductors. Poor conductors do not allow heat to pass through them easily. They are known as insulators.

Convection When liquids or gases are heated they expand, become less dense, therefore lighter, and they rise. This movement causes currents which circulate the heat (Fig. 1).

Radiation Heat energy is radiated in rays which travel in straight lines from hot objects. Radiation energy is reflected by shiny light coloured objects and is absorbed by dark matt surfaces.

When a food is being cooked, one or more of these methods are used (see Fig. 2). Poor conductors do not allow heat to pass through them easily. They are known as **insulators**. Insulating properties are used for some saucepan handles and for simmering mats (Fig. 3).

Food may be cooked dry, with water or with other liquid, or with fat. When it is dry cooked, as in baking potatoes, and when the food is fat-free grilled, the heat reaches the food through radiation or convection and passes into the food by conduction. Water and other liquids are used to cook foods in boiling, steaming and poaching methods, for example. In these cases the heat reaches the food by convection and conduction and passes through the food by conduction.

When fat is used in the cooking process it adds to the energy value of food. Since healthy eating requires a reduction in fat consumption, it is best to use methods which require only a little fat. Grilling, frying and roasting use fat, but the quantities used can be reduced. The heat is transferred to the food by radiation, convection and conduction. It then enters the food by conduction.

Summary

- Heat is transferred into food by conduction, convection and by radiation.

Questions

1. Explain how heat is transferred by each of the following: (a) conduction, (b) convection, (c) radiation.
2. Describe which methods of heat transference are used in the following cooking methods: (a) boiling, (b) frying, (c) grilling, (d) baking.
3. Explain why frying should be avoided as a cooking method.

6.7 Cooking methods

Methods of cooking without adding fat

Baking Foods cooked by this method include meat, fish, potatoes, pastry and cakes. Baked food has a crisp brown surface. Cooking is by radiation and convection, and is done in an oven. Materials such as cooking bags and foil can be used to keep food moist during cooking. Foil has to be taken off before the end of the cooking time to allow browning. A tandoor is a clay oven used to bake tandoori chicken. Clay pots can be used in a gas or electric oven to produce a similar effect. Electric frying pans can also be used to bake foods.

Boiling Foods cooked by this method are vegetables (food group 2), potatoes, pulses and rice. The amount of water used should be just enough to cover the food and the saucepan should be big enough to cover the source of heat (electric or gas ring). Cooking is by conduction. Foods are brought to boiling point for a few minutes, then the heat reduced so the temperature is between 90 and 100°C (190–212°F).

Braising This method is used for meat, fish and vegetables. The food can be in large pieces, e.g. joints of meat or a head of celery. It is a slow method of cooking which makes food tender. The cooking liquid should be served with the food as it contains many of the nutrients by the end of cooking time. Cooking is by conduction. Braising can be done on a hob or in an oven.

Fig. 1 Cooking vegetables in a steamer

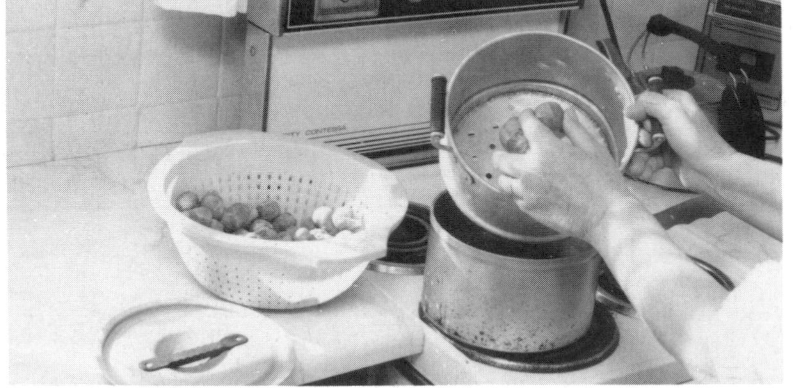

Grilling Foods cooked by this method include meat, fish, cheese and bread. These foods can be protected with foil or cooking bags for part of the time. Cooking is by radiation.

Poaching This method of cooking can be used for fish, fruit and eggs. It is a gentle method of cooking in liquid. The cooking liquid from fish or fruit can be used to make a sauce. The cooking temperature is less than 90°C (190°F) so the cooking liquid hardly bubbles. Cooking is by conduction. Poaching can be done in an oven or on a hob.

Pressure cooking This method of cooking is suitable for meat, pulses, potatoes and vegetables (from group 2), and fruit. It is similar to boiling but is quicker (usually half the cooking time), because the cooking is done under pressure. A small amount of liquid is used. The cooking liquid can be used for sauces. Cooking is by conduction. Pressure cooking is done on a hob.

Steaming Foods suitable for cooking by this method are fish, new vegetables (e.g. green beans, courgettes, potatoes) and flour mixtures (e.g. Chinese pancakes, dim sum, suet pastry, cake mixture puddings) (Fig. 1). Cooking is by conduction. Steaming is done on a hob.

Stewing/casserole This method of cooking uses just enough liquid to cover the food. The cooking liquid is always served with the food. It is a long slow method of cooking suitable for meat, pulses, vegetables, fruit and some fish. A casserole is a cooking pot which can be used on a hob or in the oven.

Dry frying This method is suitable for foods which naturally contain a large amount of fat, e.g. bacon, sausages, beefburgers. Cooking is by radiation and conduction.

Simmering Soups, stews/casseroles and braised foods are all simmered. Simmering is cooking at temperatures of 90°C (190°F). Slow cookers maintain this kind of temperature. They are not suitable for foods which require boiling first, e.g. red kidney beans, potatoes. You can boil them in another pan first and then transfer them to a slow cooker.

Microwave Microwave ovens are a recent development. Food is cooked very quickly by the microwave energy which makes the molecules of water in the food vibrate. The fast movement of the molecules makes the food hot. Microwaves can pass through air, glass and plastic without heating them. Microwave ovens are much smaller than conventional ovens and do not need any special installation, only a 13 amp electric socket.

Methods of cooking adding a little fat

Popping This is a method of cooking seeds and spices to flavour dishes. A small amount of oil (1 teaspoon or less) is heated and the seeds added and cooked until they pop. The method of cooking uses radiation and conduction.

Roasting This method of cooking is by radiant heat in front of or over a glowing heat. Spit roasters or rotisserie and barbecue are examples of this method. A very small amount of oil is used to protect fat free foods (e.g. potatoes and vegetables) during cooking. It is suitable for potatoes, vegetables (group 2), meat, fish and nuts (e.g. chestnuts). A gas or electric oven can be used for joints of meat and vegetables.

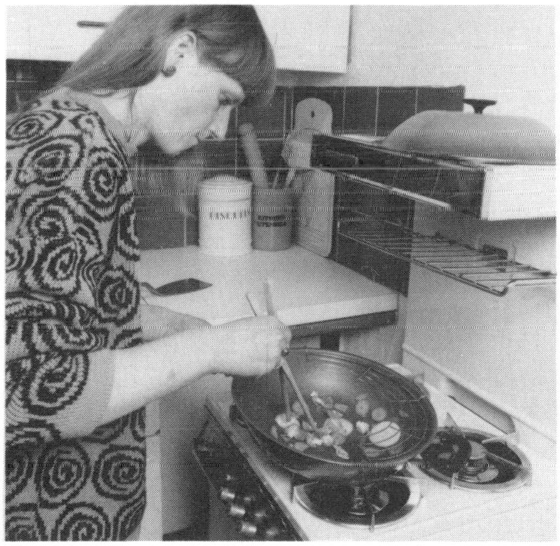

Fig. 2 Stir frying in a wok

Stir frying Foods suitable for this method of cooking are vegetables (food group 2), meat and fish. It is a quick method of cooking, so fresh tender vegetables and tender meat (e.g. steak, chicken, ham) should be used. A small amount of oil is heated in a wok or a frying pan (Fig. 2). Cooking is by radiation and conduction.

Frying Cooking food by frying greatly increases the energy value (i.e. calorie content) of foods. The amount of fat absorbed during cooking depends upon the food being cooked. Shallow frying and deep fat frying both add extra fat to foods. If the fat is hot before foods are added, less fat is absorbed as the hot fat seals the foods. Frying is a fairly quick method of cooking. It is suitable for tender cuts of meat, fish, vegetables and some flour mixtures (e.g. pakoras, doughnuts). Hot fat catches fire very easily. Do not leave a frying pan unattended. Fat is highly combustible. Nutritionally, fried foods should be avoided or eaten only occasionally.

Summary

- Boiling, baking, braising, grilling, poaching, pressure cooking, steaming, stewing and dry frying are all methods of cooking which do not require fat.
- Roasting and frying require the use of fat.

Questions

1. For each of these foods, name two suitable cooking methods which do not require fat: rice, chicken, potatoes, green vegetables, stewing beef, bread, fish.
2. Describe fully how to 'simmer' foods. Which foods are commonly cooked in this manner?
3. For each of these methods of cooking, name a dish you have cooked using this method and explain why it is a suitable means of cooking: baking, stewing, grilling, stir frying.

6.8 Equipment and safety

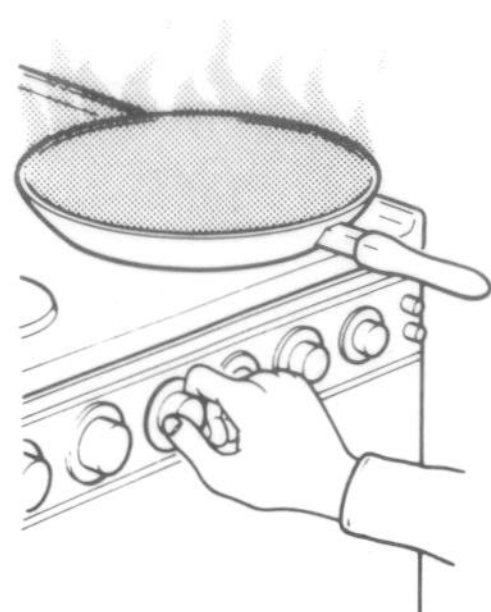

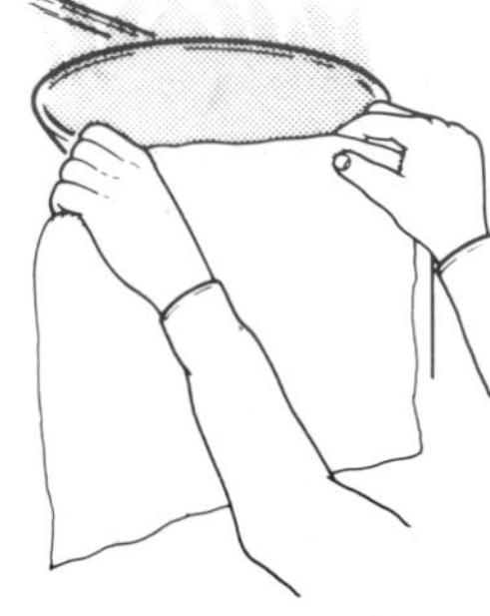

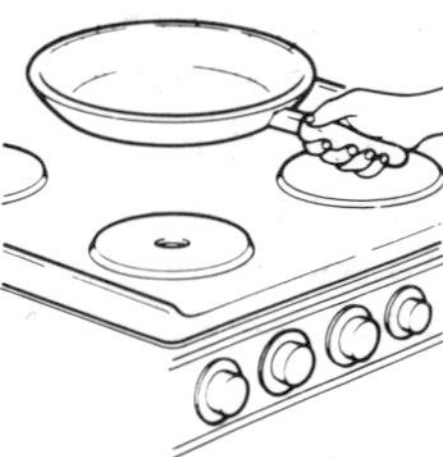

Fig. 1 Coping with a frying pan fire

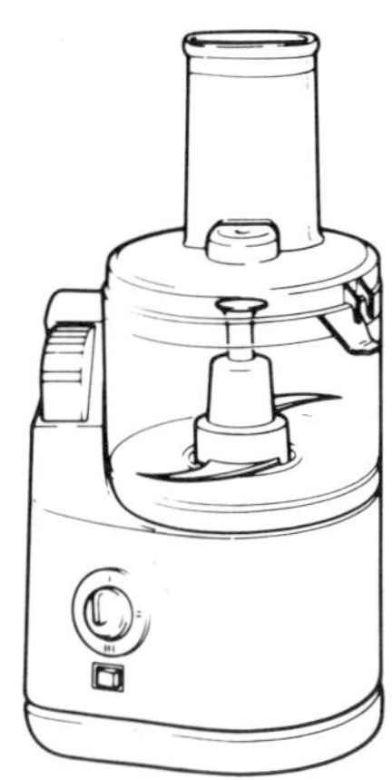

Fig. 2 A food processor

Saucepans, woks, karhais and casseroles

Cooking pans need to have a flat base so that they have even contact with the source of heat and cannot be toppled over. Pans such as woks and karhais with a curved base have to be used with the ring provided with them to sit them over the heat. The base is curved to allow as much of the large surface area as possible to get hot so that foods cook quickly.

A **wooden spoon**, or a spatula or metal spoon with a wooden handle, is best for stirring food in a saucepan or wok, because wood is a poor heat conductor (i.e. it takes longer to get hot).

Oven gloves protect hands and arms from heat and are used to hold a cooking pan whilst stirring, or removing lids.

Any kind of saucepan should be allowed to cool before washing up. Putting cold water into a hot pan can distort metal and crack Pyrex, etc.

Frying pans

It is most important that frying pans have a flat base, to make even contact with the heat and to stop them falling over. Frying can be dangerous. Fats and oils are highly inflammable. Many house fires are started by frying pans. Overheating the oil or fat is usually the cause. Most foods cook at temperatures of 170–185°C. Once the oil/fat has reached this temperature, reduce the heat so that the temperature is maintained but does not get any hotter. For this reason, frying is a method of cooking where you need to be there all the time. If you are interrupted, **take the frying pan off the heat**. Should the oil/fat catch fire (Fig. 1):

- Turn off the heat.
- Smother the flames (use the frying pan lid, a baking tray, large meat tin or wet towel.
- Move the pan over on to a cooler part of the cooker.

To prevent fat/oil splashing over the pan whilst cooking, only fill the pan ⅔ full with oil/fat and not more than ¾ full when the food is put in. A fish slice is useful to lower food into the fat to prevent splashing. Many deep fat frying pans have a basket to place foods in.

Each time oil or fat is heated it becomes less stable. It can be used for a longer time if strained between each use to remove bits of food and sediment. This is done once the oil/fat has cooled. Once the oil/fat is a deep golden colour it is past its best and should be thrown away.

Steamers

Steamers are useful cooking pans because they cook foods quickly and save fuel if placed over another pan of cooking food. The steamer should fit into the saucepan firmly so it cannot be toppled over. Steamers are usually aluminium, enamelled steel, brushed steel or bamboo. They all get hot and you need oven gloves to handle them. After lifting the steamer off, place a plate underneath to prevent dripping boiling water.

Food processors, mixers and blenders (Fig. 2)

The blades in this type of equipment are very sharp and revolve at very high speed. For this reason, a 'pusher' is part of the appliance to push food down on to the blade, usually through a tunnel. A plastic or rubber spatula is useful to scrape food from the sides of the bowl when mixing or blending. Always remember to put the lid on before blending or mixing. If you forget, the mixture will be all over you and the walls. This is inconvenient if the mixture is cold, but dangerous if it is hot.

Knives

Sharp knives are much safer to use than blunt ones. Very skilled people are able to use one tool, e.g. a cleaver or chopper, for a wide range of cutting and chopping tasks, but most of us need different knives for different purposes.

Serrated knives are used for chopping parsley or cutting meat and skinning fish. Blades can be 15–30 cm (6–12 ins).

Filleting/boning knives have a narrow blade to remove bones from meat and fillet fish and meat.

Vegetable knives are small-bladed pointed knives, approximately 20 cm (4 ins), used for vegetable preparation.

Vegetable peelers enable thin peelings to be cut and are faster and safer than knives for most people.

Round blade/table knives are for spreading fats and mixing pastry.

Palette knives have the same uses as table knives, but are available in a variety of sizes – 10–30 cm (4–12 ins).

A chopping board should be used for any cutting or chopping process, to prevent marking the work surface and provide a firm, hard surface to work on. The positioning of the hands and fingers is important to be efficient in using knives and to prevent cuts. For chopping, make a bridge with the hand to hold the food. Cut under the bridge (Fig. 3). For slicing, move the fingers back in front of the knife (Fig. 4). Always wash sharp, pointed knives separately. Do not put them into the washing-up bowl.

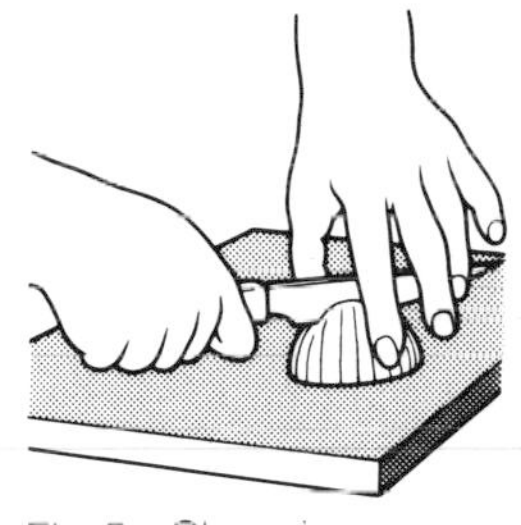
Fig. 3 Chopping

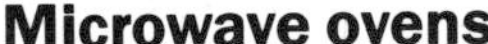

Microwave ovens

Microwaves will pass through most materials except metal. Metal dishes, including enamel-coated ones, and aluminium foil cannot be used in a microwave oven. Suitable coverings for food are clear plastic cook bags and greaseproof paper. Microwaves are dangerous to living flesh. Ovens have a built-in safety device which prevents them operating when the door is opened. The door seal on the oven should be checked periodically to prevent leakage. Check manufacturer's instructions for recommended times. Wipe over the inside of the microwave after use with a soft cloth and washing-up liquid.

Cookers

The outside case of split-level and conventional cookers is not well insulated and therefore gets hot. This can be a hazard, particularly to young children, when the oven door is on the same level as they are.

Saucepan guards can be bought for most cooker hobs to prevent saucepans being knocked or pulled off the hob, handles should be turned so that they do not overhang the edge of the cooker.

To prevent explosion when lighting a gas oven, whatever the ignition system, the door should always be open until you see that all the gas jets are alight. Gas and electric ovens should be pre-heated for 10–15 minutes to make sure they reach the correct temperature before putting the food in. Frozen foods should always be cooked in a pre-heated oven to prevent bacterial growth.

Electric ignition systems on gas cookers use 13 amp sockets and plugs. An electric cooker must be connected to its own 30 amp box and be separately earthed.

Questions

1. Write a sentence to explain each of the following:
   (a) why cooking pans need a flat base
   (b) why woks and karhais have a curved base
   (c) why a wooden spoon is used to stir food in a saucepan
   (d) when oven gloves are needed to handle saucepans and why
   (e) why a flat base is needed for frying pans
   (f) how the temperature of oil/fat is maintained once it is hot enough
   (g) what action to take if a frying pan catches fire
   (h) three things you can do to prevent frying pan fires.
2. Draw four knives used in food preparation. Give a use for each knife.
3. What kind of cooking dishes cannot be used in a microwave oven?
4. Describe what actions you would take to prevent accidents to young children and others near the cooker.

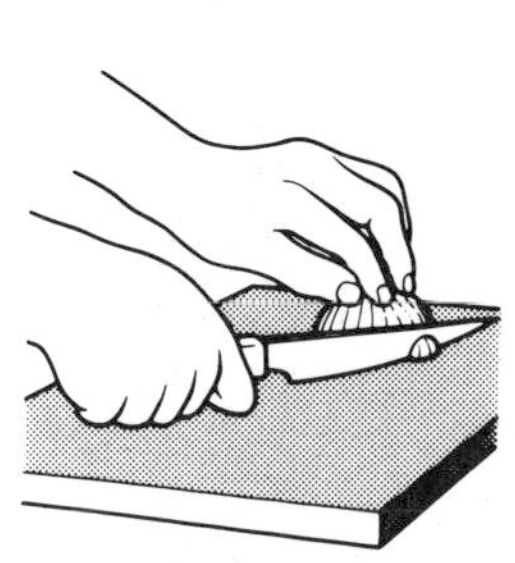
Fig. 4 Slicing

6.9 Aesthetics and food

We have to eat food to live. Ensuring a supply of food, preparing it, cooking it, preserving it, serving it and eating it are experiences all people have in common. But food is much more significant to us than a means of maintaining life. Food is eaten for pleasure and to celebrate happy and sad events, such as birthdays, funerals, religious festivals, harvest festivals, marriages, to make friendship, share good fortune, show off wealth, etc. (Fig. 1).

In countries where an adequate supply of food is ensured, a great deal of time and skill is used in preparing, cooking and preserving food to make it attractive to eat. It is a vast industry employing millions and a domestic occupation which many people enjoy.

The kinds of foods we eat depend upon many factors. The importance and combination of each of these factors varies with individuals. Some of the factors are cultural and religious custom, ethical beliefs, past experience, current fashions, cooking methods available, the skill of the cook, money available, foods available, time available, state of mind, state of physical health and personal tastes. These points help to determine how the food we choose to eat looks, smells, tastes and feels, and our enjoyment of it.

Some fresh foods look attractive, taste good and have a texture that is edible and pleasant without any cooking, e.g. most fruit (kiwi fruit, strawberries, raspberries, mangoes, apples, pineapples, pears, oranges, bananas, peaches, etc.), many vegetables (lettuce, carrots, cucumber, tomatoes, celery, radishes, courgettes, green and red peppers, onions, shredded white or red cabbage, Chinese leaf, etc.) and most cheeses and yoghurt. Other fresh foods need only simple cooking or preservation methods, such as boiling or grilling, smoking or pickling to destroy bacteria. These foods are delicious eaten on their own, e.g. shellfish (prawns, mussels,

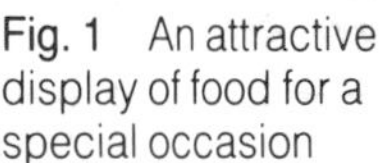

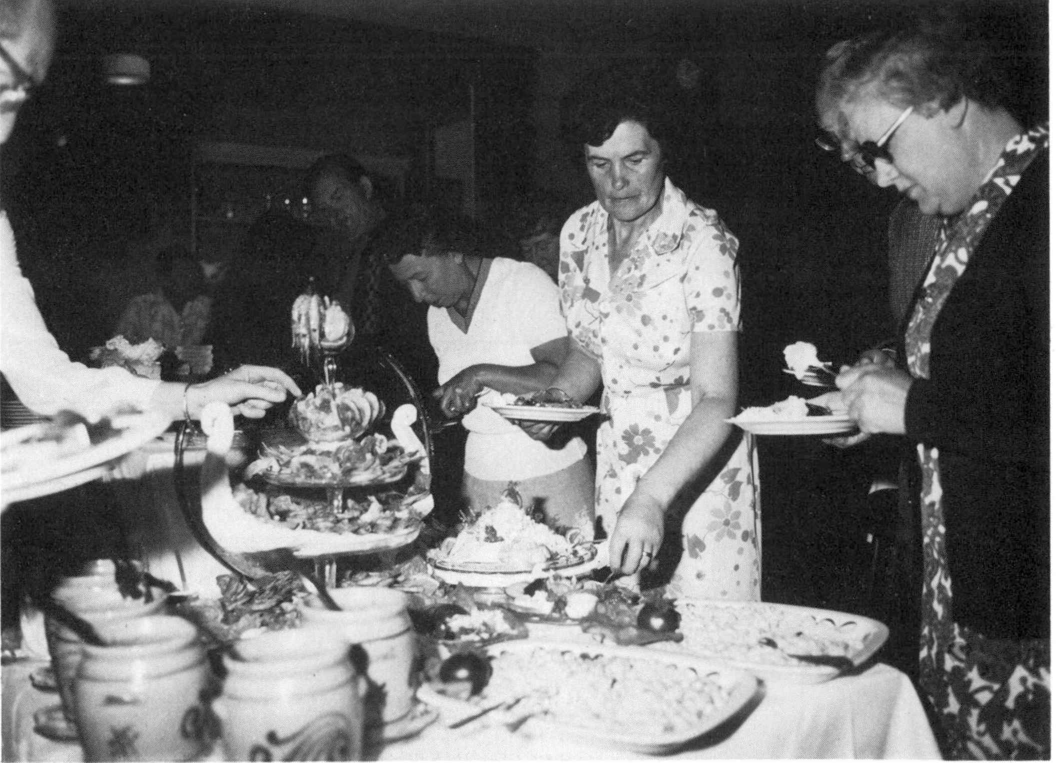

Fig. 1 An attractive display of food for a special occasion

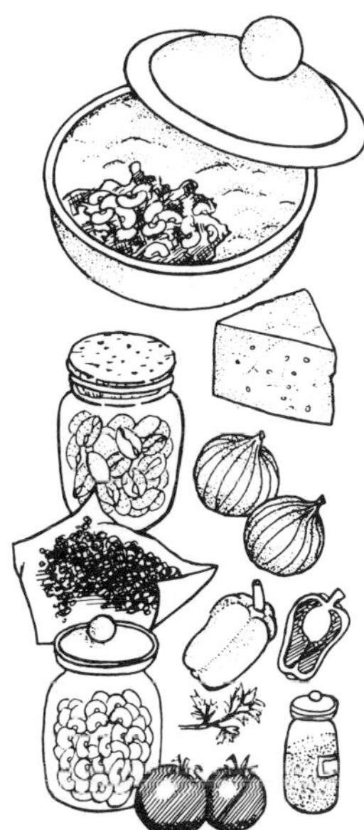

Fig. 2 A staple food cooked using a complicated recipe

etc.), fish (eels, trout, bass, snapper, sardines, herrings, etc.) and smoked mackerel, haddock or salmon, or pickled herrings. However, the majority of foods require more complicated preparation and cooking to make them edible and attractive. Some foods, such as potatoes, yam, rice, pulses and bread, can be simply cooked and are pleasant to eat, but because they are staple foods and eaten daily, they can be prepared in complicated recipes to provide variety (Fig. 2).

Herbs, spices, peppers, roots, seeds, bulbs and leaves are not foods themselves, but they are used to change the flavour and sometimes the texture and colour of other foods and are therefore important in food preparation (Fig. 3). A bland food like potato can be made sweet, sour, hot, spicy or aromatic.

Food which is pleasant to eat usually combines complementary textures as well as colours and flavours, e.g. chewy or firm textures with soft and crisp ones. The consistency of foods adds to the overall texture so a combination of dry and wet foods are used to make a meal.

Almost as important as the food itself is how the food is served (Fig. 4). Using different types of serving dish (e.g. glass, metal, wood, china, ceramic, rush, bamboo) or different finishes (shiny, smooth, glazed, unglazed, etc.) in different colours can greatly alter the appearance of the same food. The shape of the serving dish also affects the appearance of food, and the type of cutlery contributes to the experience of eating and enjoyment of the food.

Summary

- Food gives pleasure as well as being a basic necessity.
- The appearance of food is important, as is its taste.

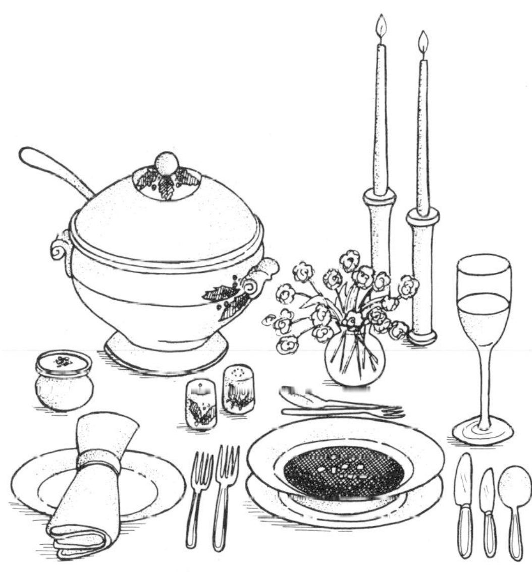

Fig. 4 Attractively served food

Fig. 3 Herbs and spices

Leaves	*Stem*	*Fruit*	*Seed*	*Flower*	*Underground Stem*	*Root*
Sage Tarragon Coriander Bay Mint Rosemary	Cinnamon (Bark) Angelica	Tamarind Juniper Chilli Star Anise Vanilla	Sesame Fennel Pepper Cumin Mustard Caraway	Cloves (Bud) Saffron (stigmas)	Ginger Turmeric	Liquorice Yarrow

Questions

1. What 'food experiences' do all people have in common?
2. List four occasions where food is an important part of the event.
3. Choose one of the following occasions and make a list of the kinds of foods served (from your experience or imagined). Explain the circumstances of the occasion (e.g. ages of people there, where it took place) and say why these particular foods were served and the traditions behind them, if any.
   Birthday, a religious festival, marriage, harvest festival.
4. What is meant by 'garnish'? Why is it important?

Section 7. Food tables

Some typical nutritional values per 100 g of food

	kJ	Carbo-hydrate (g)	Starch (g)	Sugars (g)	Dietary fibre (g) (see note)	Protein (g)	Fat (g)	Saturated fat (g)	Sodium (mg)
FOOD GROUP 1									
Cereal foods									
Bread White	991	49.7	47.9	1.8	2.7	7.8	1.7	0.3	540
Wholemeal	918	41.8	39.7	2.1	8.5	8.8	2.7	0.5	540
Chapatti (no fat)	860	43.7	42.1	1.6	3.4	7.3	1.0	0.2	120
Pitta (white)	1127	57.9	n/a	n/a	4.3	9.2	1.2	0.2	520
Flour White	1493	80.1	78.4	1.7	3.4	9.8	1.2	0.2	2
Wholemeal	1351	65.8	63.5	2.3	9.6	13.2	2.0	0.4	3
Rice White (raw)	1536	86.8	86.8	0	2.4	6.5	1.0	0.3	6
boiled	522	29.6	29.6	0	0.8	2.2	0.3	0.1	2
Brown (raw)	1518	81.3	81.3	0	4.2	6.7	2.8	0.8	3
Pasta White (cooked)	499	26.0	25.2	0.8	n/a	4.2	0.3	0.1	2
Breakfast cereals									
All Bran	1055	44.9	27.6	15.4	28.6*	15.1	2.2	0.4	1470
Cornflakes	1460	84.4	77.7	7.4	1.4*	7.9	0.3	n/a	1110
Rice Krispies	1500	86.1	79.1	9.0	0.9*	6.2	0.4	0.1	1270
Puffed Wheat	1386	68.5	67.0	1.5	15.4	14.2	1.3	0.3	4
Weetabix	1444	70.3	66.5	6.1	12.7	11.4	3.4	0.7	360
Shredded Wheat	1378	67.9	67.5	0.4	12.3	10.6	3.0	0.6	8
Starchy vegetables									
Potatoes (boiled)	343	19.7	19.3	0.4	1.0	1.4	0.1	Tr	3
(chips)	1065	37.3	n/a	n/a	n/a	3.8	10.9	depends on oil used	12
(crisps)	2224	49.3	48.6	0.7	11.9	6.3	35.9	depends on oil used	550
Sweet potato (boiled)	363	20.1	11.0	9.1	2.3	1.1	0.6	0.3	18
Yam (boiled)	508	29.8	29.6	0.2	1.6	1.6	0.1	Tr	17
Plantain (green, boiled)	518	31.1	30.2	0.9	6.4	1.0	0.1	Tr	4
(ripe, fried)	1126	47.5	36.0	11.5	5.8	1.5	9.2	depends on oil used	3
FOOD GROUP 2									
Vegetables									
Ackee (canned)	625	0.8	0	0.8	2.7	2.9	15.2	n/a	240
Aubergine/eggplant/brinjal (raw)	62	3.1	2.9	0.2	2.5	0.7	Tr	Tr	3
Bamboo shoots (canned)	113	4.2	n/a	n/a	n/a	2.6	0.3	Tr	n/a
Beans, French (boiled)	31	1.1	0.3	0.8	3.2	0.8	Tr	Tr	3
Beansprouts (canned)	40	0.8	0.4	0.4	3.0	1.6	Tr	Tr	80
Brussels sprouts (boiled)	75	1.7	0.1	1.6	2.9	2.8	Tr	Tr	2
Cabbage, spring (boiled)	32	0.8	Tr	0.8	2.2	1.1	Tr	Tr	12
white (raw)	93	3.8	0.1	3.7	2.7	1.9	Tr	Tr	7

Note Figures given for dietary fibre are those in current use, and may change as new methods of measurement are developed.

	kJ	*Carbo-hydrate* (g)	*Starch* (g)	*Sugars* (g)	*Dietary fibre* (g)	*Protein* (g)	*Fat* (g)	*Saturated fat* (g)	*Sodium* (mg)
Carrots (boiled)	79	4.3	0.1	4.2	3.1	0.6	Tr	Tr	50
Cauliflower (boiled)	40	0.8	Tr	0.8	1.8	1.6	Tr	Tr	4
Cho-cho/christophene/ chayote (raw)	79	4.0	n/a	n/a	n/a	0.7	0.1	Tr	2
Courgette/zucchini/squash (raw)	105	4.5	n/a	n/a	n/a	1.6	0.4	Tr	1
Cucumber/khira/kakdi (raw)	43	1.8	0	1.8	0.4	0.6	0.1	Tr	13
Leeks (boiled)	104	4.6	0	4.6	3.9	1.8	Tr	Tr	6
Marrow (boiled)	29	1.4	0.1	1.3	0.6	0.4	Tr	Tr	1
Mushrooms (raw)	53	0	0	0	2.5	1.8	0.6	0.2	9
Okra/lady's fingers/bhindi (raw)	71	2.3	Tr	2.3	3.2	2.0	Tr	Tr	7
Onions (boiled)	53	2.7	0	2.7	1.3	0.6	Tr	Tr	7
Peas, frozen (boiled)	175	4.3	3.3	1.0	12.0	5.4	0.4	0.2	2
Pepper, green (raw)	65	2.2	Tr	2.2	0.9	0.9	0.4	0.1	2
Pumpkin (raw)	65	3.4	0.7	2.7	1.5	1.6	Tr	Tr	1
Spinach (boiled)	128	1.4	0.2	1.2	6.3	5.1	0.5	0.1	120
Swede (boiled)	76	3.8	0.1	3.7	2.8	0.9	Tr	Tr	14
Tomatoes (raw)	60	2.8	Tr	2.8	1.5	0.9	Tr	Tr	3
(canned)	51	2.0	Tr	2.0	0.9	1.1	Tr	Tr	29
(purée)	286	11.4	Tr	11.4	n/a	6.1	Tr	Tr	420
Turnip (boiled)	60	0.3	0	2.3	2.2	0.7	0.3	Tr	28
Water chestnuts (canned)	205	12.5	n/a	n/a	n/a	0.9	Tr	Tr	14
Watercress (raw)	61	0.7	0.1	0.6	3.3	2.9	Tr	Tr	60
Fruit (weighed as bought unless stated)									
Apples (eating)	151	9.2	0.1	9.1	1.5	0.2	Tr	Tr	2
Avocado pear	922	1.8	Tr	1.8	2.0	4.2	22.2	2.7	2
Banana	202	11.4	1.8	9.6	2.0	0.7	0.2	0.1	1
Cherries	175	10.4	0	10.4	1.5	0.5	Tr	Tr	2
Grapefruit	45	2.5	0	2.5	0.3	0.3	Tr	Tr	1
Grapes	217	13.0	0	13.0	0.3	0.5	Tr	Tr	1
Guavas (fresh)	259	9.4	n/a	n/a	n/a	0.8	0.6	n/a	4
Lemons	65	3.2	0	3.2	5.2	0.8	Tr	Tr	6
Lychees (canned)	290	17.7	0	17.7	0.4	0.4	Tr	Tr	2
Mango (flesh only)	253	15.3	Tr	15.3	1.5	0.5	Tr	Tr	7
Melon, honey dew	56	3.1	0	3.1	0.6	0.4	Tr	Tr	12
Water melon	47	2.7	0	2.7	n/a	0.2	Tr	Tr	2
Nectarines	198	11.4	0	11.4	2.2	0.9	Tr	Tr	8
Orange juice	161	9.4	0	9.4	0	0.6	Tr	Tr	2
Oranges	113	6.4	0	6.4	1.5	0.6	Tr	Tr	2
Passion fruit	60	2.6	0	2.6	6.7	1.1	Tr	Tr	12
Paw-paw/papaya (fresh)	188	11.3	0	11.3	n/a	0.5	0.1	Tr	4
Peaches	137	7.9	0	7.9	1.2	0.6	Tr	Tr	2
Pears	125	7.6	0	7.6	1.7	0.2	Tr	Tr	1
Pineapple (fresh)	194	11.6	0	11.6	1.2	0.5	Tr	Tr	2
Plums	153	9.0	0	9.0	2.0	0.5	Tr	Tr	2
Pomegranate	301	16.6	0	16.6	n/a	1.0	0.6	n/a	1
Raspberries	105	5.6	0	5.6	7.4	0.9	Tr	Tr	3
Strawberries	109	6.2	0	6.2	2.2	0.6	Tr	Tr	2
Tangerines	100	5.6	0	5.6	1.3	0.6	Tr	Tr	2

	kJ	Carbo-hydrate (g)	Starch (g)	Sugars (g)	Dietary fibre (g)	Protein (g)	Fat (g)	Saturated fat (g)	Sodium (mg)
FOOD GROUP 3									
Meat									
Bacon									
1 boiled gammon (lean and fat)0	1119	0	0	0	0	24.7	18.9	8.2	960
(lean only)	703	0	0	0	0	29.4	5.5	2.4	1110
grilled gammon rashers									
(lean and fat)	953	0	0	0	0	29.5	12.2	5.3	2140
(lean only)	726	0	0	0	0	31.4	5.2	2.3	2210
Beef									
rump steak grilled (lean and fat)	912	0	0	0	0	27.3	12.1	5.4	55
(lean only)	708	0	0	0	0	28.6	6.0	2.7	56
Lamb									
breast, roast (lean and fat)	1697	0	0	0	0	19.1	37.1	19.3	73
(lean only)	1049	0	0	0	0	25.6	16.6	8.6	86
chops, weighed with bone									
(lean and fat)	1147	0	0	0	0	18.3	22.6	6.4	56
(lean only)	512	0	0	0	0	15.3	6.8	3.5	41
Pork									
chops, weighed with bone									
(lean and fat)	1073	0	0	0	0	22.2	18.8	8.0	66
(lean only)	558	0	0	0	0	19.1	6.3	2.7	50
leg, roast (lean and fat)	1190	0	0	0	0	26.9	19.8	8.4	79
(lean only)	777	0	0	0	0	30.7	6.9	2.9	79
Various meats									
Chicken, roast (all)	902	0	0	0	0	22.6	14.0	4.9	72
Duck, roast (all)	1406	0	0	0	0	19.6	29.0	8.8	76
Turkey, roast (all)	717	0	0	0	0	28.0	6.5	2.4	52
Rabbit, stewed	749	0	0	0	0	27.3	7.7	3.3	32
Heart (lamb), raw	498	0	0	0	0	17.1	5.6	3.8	140
Kidney (pig), stewed	641	0	0	0	0	24.4	6.1	2.7	370
Liver (pig), stewed	793	3.6	n/a	n/a	0	25.6	8.1	3.4	130
Trotters and tails (pig), salted and boiled	1162	0	0	0	0	19.8	22.3	n/a	1615
Corned beef	905	0	0	0	0	26.9	12.1	5.4	950
Luncheon meat	1298	5.5	n/a	n/a	n/a	12.6	26.9	10.9	1050
Sausage (beef), grilled	1104	15.2	n/a	n/a	n/a	13.0	17.3	7.7	1100
(pork), grilled	1320	11.5	n/a	n/a	n/a	13.3	24.6	10.2	1000
Beefburgers, fried	1099	7.0	n/a	n/a	n/a	20.4	17.3	7.8	880
Cornish pastie	1388	31.1	n/a	n/a	n/a	8.0	20.4	n/a	590
Pork pie	1564	24.9	n/a	n/a	n/a	9.8	27.0	11.6	720
Individual steak pie	1349	25.6	n/a	n/a	n/a	9.1	21.2	n/a	510
Fish									
Haddock fillet (steamed)	417	0	0	0	0	22.8	0.8	0.2	120
Smoked haddock (steamed)	429	0	0	0	0	23.3	0.9	0.3	1220
Plaice (fried in batter)	1165	14.4	n/a	n/a	n/a	15.8	18.0	n/a	220
Cod (dried and salted)	586	0	0	0	0	32.5	0.9	0.2	400
Red snapper/Malabar	414	0	0	0	0	18.7	2.1	n/a	120
Herring, weighed with bone (grilled)	562	0	0	0	0	13.9	8.8	2.0	120
Mackerel, weighed with bone (fried)	574	0	0	0	0	15.7	8.3	2.2	110

	kJ	Carbo-hydrate (g)	Starch (g)	Sugars (g)	Dietary fibre (g)	Protein (g)	Fat (g)	Saturated fat (g)	Sodium (mg)
Pilchards in tomato sauce	531	0.7	n/a	n/a	0	18.8	5.4	1.9	370
Sardines in oil (fish only)	906	0	0	0	0	23.7	13.6	2.8	650
Tuna in oil	1202	0	0	0	0	22.8	22.0	4.1	420
Octopus (raw)	285	0	0	0	0	13.5	1.1	n/a	n/a
Prawns (boiled)	451	0	0	0	0	22.6	1.8	0.4	1590
Eggs									
Hen eggs	612	Tr	0	0	0	12.3	10.9	4.1	140
Duck eggs	787	0.7	n/a	n/a	0	13.2	14.2	n/a	191
Pulses									
Most beans (boiled) approx.	405	17.1	15.6	1.5	5.1	7.1	0.3	0.1	16
Soya beans (boiled)	562	9.5	n/a	n/a	n/a	11.4	5.9	0.9	2
Nuts									
Almonds	2336	4.3	0	4.3	14.3	16.9	53.5	4.4	6
Brazil nuts	2545	4.2	2.4	1.7	9.0	12.0	61.5	16.4	2
Coconut (fresh)	1446	3.7	0	3.7	13.6	3.2	36.0	29.9	17
Hazel nuts	1570	6.8	2.1	4.7	6.1	7.6	36.0	2.7	1
Peanuts	2364	8.6	5.5	3.1	8.1	24.3	49.0	7.4	6
Walnuts	2166	5.0	1.8	3.2	5.2	10.6	51.5	5.9	3
FOOD GROUP 4									
Milk									
Whole	272	4.7	0	4.7	0	3.3	3.8	2.3	50
Skimmed	142	5.0	0	5.0	0	3.4	0.1	Tr	52
Evaporated	660	11.3	0	11.3	0	8.6	9.0	5.5	180
Condensed	1362	55.5	0	55.5	0	8.3	9.0	5.5	130
Soya milk	164	9.0	0	9.0	0	1.2	n/a	n/a	54
Cheese									
Camembert type	1246	Tr	0	0	0	22.8	23.2	14.2	1410
Cheddar type	1682	Tr	0	0	0	26.0	33.5	20.5	610
Edam type	1262	Tr	0	0	0	24.4	22.9	14.0	980
Fetta	1017	Tr	0	0	0	16.5	19.9	12.2	1260
Cottage low fat	266	1.4	0	1.4	0	13.6	0.4	0.2	450
Cream	1807	Tr	0	0	0	3.1	47.4	29.0	300
Processed	1291	Tr	0	0	0	21.5	25.0	15.3	1360
Yoghurt									
Natural	216	6.2	0	6.2	0	5.0	1.0	0.6	76
FOOD GROUP 5									
Chocolate biscuits	2197	67.4	24.0	43.4	3.1	5.7	27.6	17.4	160
Sandwich biscuit	2151	69.2	39.0	30.2	1.2	5.0	25.9	14.8	220
Shortbread	2115	65.5	48.3	17.2	2.1	6.2	26.0	13.6	270
Fruit cake	1490	57.9	14.8	43.1	2.8	5.1	12.9	6.1	250
Jam sponge	1280	64.2	16.5	47.7	1.2	4.2	4.9	2.0	420
Jam tart	1616	62.8	25.3	37.5	1.7	3.5	14.9	n/a	230
Eclairs	1569	38.2	11.9	26.3	n/a	4.1	24.0	n/a	160
Gulab jamen	1500	50.5	n/a	n/a	0.5	8.3	14.9	n/a	123
Chinese rice cakes	1230	58.8	n/a	n/a	n/a	3.5	6.2	n/a	8
Greek halva	2569	54.2	n/a	n/a	n/a	14.8	39.2	n/a	195
Sugar	1680	100.0	0	100.0	0	Tr	0	0	Tr
Golden syrup	1269	79.0	0	79.0	0	0.3	0	0	270

	kJ	*Carbo-hydrate* (g)	*Starch* (g)	*Sugars* (g)	*Dietary fibre* (g)	*Protein* (g)	*Fat* (g)	*Saturated fat* (g)	*Sodium* (mg)
Black treacle	1096	67.2	0	67.2	0	1.2	0	0	96
Honey	1229	76.4	0	76.4	0	0.4	Tr	0	11
Jam	1114	69.0	0	69.0	1.1	0.6	0	0	16
Boiled sweets	1397	87.3	0.4	86.9	0	Tr	Tr	0	25
Milk chocolate	2214	59.4	2.9	56.5	n/a	8.4	30.3	18.3	120
Toffees	1810	71.1	1.0	70.1	n/a	2.1	17.2	10.5	320
Cola	168	10.5	Tr	10.5	0	Tr	0	0	8
Lemonade	90	5.6	0	5.6	0	Tr	0	0	7
Orange squash (undiluted)	456	28.5	0	28.5	0	Tr	0	0	21
FOOD GROUP 6									
Butter	3041	Tr	0	0	0	0.4	82.0	50.1	870
Coconut oil	3694	Tr	0	0	0	Tr	99.9	75.8	n/a
Dripping	3663	0	0	0	0	Tr	99.0	42.7	5
Lard	3663	0	0	0	0	Tr	99.0	43.6	2
Ghee (butter)	3693	Tr	0	0	0	Tr	99.8	61.0	2
Margarine									
hard								30.4	
soft	3000	0.1	0	0	0	Tr	81.0	24.9	800
pufa's								20.0	
Olive oil	3696	0	0	0	0	Tr	99.9	14.7	0
Red palm oil	3661	0.3	n/a	n/a	0	0	98.9	46.9	n/a
Sesame oil	3686	0.1	n/a	n/a	0	0.2	99.7	n/a	2
Soya oil								14.7	
Sunflower oil	3696	0.1	n/a	n/a	0	0.2	99.9	13.7	n/a
Corn oil								17.2	

Tr = a trace
n/a = information not available
* = manufacturer's data, main source

Source: McCance and Widdowson's *The Composition of Food* by A.A. Paul and D.A.T. Southgate (4th Edition, 1978, HMSO) and second supplement *Immigrant Food* by S.P. Tan, R.W. Wenlock and D.H. Buss (1985, HMSO).

Recommended daily amounts of food energy and some nutrients for population groups in the UK

Age range[a]	Occupational category	Energy[b]		Protein[c]	Thiamin	Riboflavin	Nicotinic acid	Ascorbic acid	Vitamin A	Vitamin D[f]	Calcium	Iron
years		MJ	Kcal	g	mg	mg	equivalents mg[d]	mg	retinol equivalents μg[e]	cholecalciferol μg	mg	mg
BOYS												
under 1					0.3	0.4	5	20	450	7.5	600	6
1		5.0	1200	30	0.5	0.6	7	20	300	10	600	7
2		5.75	1400	35	0.6	0.7	8	20	300	10	600	7
3–4		6.5	1560	39	0.6	0.8	9	20	300	10	600	8
5–6		7.25	1740	43	0.7	0.9	10	20	300	(f)	600	10
7–8		8.25	1980	49	0.8	1.0	11	20	400	(f)	600	10
9–11		9.5	2280	57	0.9	1.2	14	25	575	(f)	700	12
12–14		11.5	2640	66	1.1	1.4	16	25	725	(f)	700	12
15–17		12.0	2880	72	1.2	1.7	19	30	750	(f)	600	12
GIRLS												
under 1					0.3	0.4	5	20	450	7.5	600	6
1		4.5	1100	27	0.4	0.6	7	20	300	10	600	7
2		5.5	1300	32	0.5	0.7	8	20	300	10	600	7
3–4		6.25	1500	37	0.6	0.8	9	20	300	10	600	8
5–6		7.0	1680	42	0.7	0.9	10	20	300	(f)	600	10
7–8		8.0	1900	47	0.8	1.0	11	20	400	(f)	600	10
9–11		8.5	2050	51	0.8	1.2	14	25	575	(f)	700	12[h]
12–14		9.0	2150	53	0.9	1.4	16	25	725	(f)	700	12[h]
15–17		9.0	2150	53	0.9	1.7	19	30	750	(f)	600	12[h]
MEN												
18–34	Sedentary	10.5	2510	63	1.0	1.6	18	30	750	(f)	500	10
	Moderately active	12.0	2900	72	1.2	1.6	18	30	750	(f)	500	10
	Very active	14.0	3350	84	1.3	1.6	18	30	750	(f)	500	10
35–64	Sedentary	10.0	2400	60	1.0	1.6	18	30	750	(f)	500	10
	Moderately active	11.5	2750	69	1.1	1.6	18	30	750	(f)	500	10
	Very active	14.0	3350	84	1.3	1.6	18	30	750	(f)	500	10
65–74	Assuming a	10.0	2400	60	1.0	1.6	18	30	750	(f)	500	10
75+	sedentary life	9.0	2150	54	0.9	1.6	18	30	750	(f)	500	10
WOMEN												
18–54	Most occupations	9.0	2150	54	0.9	1.3	15	30	750	(f)	500	12[h]
	Very active	10.5	2500	62	1.0	1.3	15	30	750		500	12[h]
55–74	Assuming a	8.0	1900	47	0.8	1.3	15	30	750	(f)	500	10
75+	sedentary life	7.0	1680	42	0.7	1.3	15	30	750	(f)	500	10
Pregnancy		10.0	2400	60	1.0	1.6	18	60	750	10	1200[g]	13
Lactation		11.5	2750	69	1.1	1.8	21	60	1200	10	1200	15

Notes:

(a) Since the recommendations are average amounts, the figures for each age range represent the amounts recommended at the middle of the range. Within each age range, younger children will need less, and older children more, than the amount recommended.

(b) Megajoules (10^4 joules) Calculated from the relation 1 kilocalorie = 4,184 kilojoules, that is to say, 1 megajoule = 240 kilocalories.

(c) Recommended amounts have been calculated as 10% of the recommendations for energy.

(d) 1 nicotinic acid equivalent = 1 mg available nicotinic acid for 60 mg tryptophan.

(e) 1 retinol = 1 μg retinol or 6 μg β carotene or 12 μg other biologically active carotenoids.

(f) No dietary sources may be necessary for children and adults who are sufficiently exposed to sunlight, but during the winter children and adolescents should receive 10 μg (400 i.u.) daily by supplementation. Adults with inadequate exposure to sunlight for example those who are housebound, may also need a supplement of 10 μg daily.

(g) For the third trimester only.

(h) This intake may not be sufficient for 10% of girls and women with large menstrual losses.

Source: *Nutrition Guidelines*

Summary of the importance and dietary sources of different nutrients

Nutrient	*Function*	*(i) Deficiency/ (ii) Excess intake*	*Main sources*	*Proportion supplied by each food group in the 'average' UK diet*	*Effects of cooking and processing and storage*	*Other comments*
DIETARY ENERGY	Fuel for all the body's activities. *RDA* Depends on age, sex and activity. Varies from 4.5 MJ (girls 1 year) to 14.0 MJ (very active men, 18–64 years). Boys 12–14 years: 11.0 MJ. Girls 12–14 years: 9.0 MJ.	(i) Weight loss and, in extreme cases, death. (a) Protein energy malnutrition. Kwasiorkor and marasmus occur in children when there is insufficient food available, usually in economically deprived countries. Kwasiorkor: poor growth, distended stomach, diarrhoea, infections. Marasmus: wasting of muscle, pot belly, emaciated appearance. (b) Anorexia nervosa: needs medical attention. (ii) Weight gain. Obesity and higher risk of high blood pressure, heart disease, respiratory illness, varicose veins, and diabetes.	All foods. Most concentrated sources are those foods with a high percentage of fat and sugar, e.g. fats and oils (food group 6), sugar and sugary foods (food group 5), hard cheeses (food group 4), meat products (food group 3). Least concentrated sources are those with a high percentage of water and dietary fibre, e.g. fruit and vegetables (food group 2).	(This column on all sheets only applies to food brought into the home, nothing eaten out is included.) Average intake: 8.7 MJ.	The energy content of a food can be increased dramatically if the cooking process involves the addition of fat, e.g. frying or roasting.	Fat provides 38 kJ per g. Carbohydrate provides 16 kJ per g. Protein provides 16 kJ per g. Alcohol provides 29 kJ per g.

CARBO-HYDRATES Starch	Provides dietary energy. *RDA* No specific recommendation.	(i) Insufficient dietary energy or over consumption of protein, sugars and fat (see below). (ii) Excess dietary energy intake leading to obesity.	Food group 1 – all foods, including bread, flour, rice, yam, plantain, couscous, pasta. Food group 3 – pulses.		Starch grains swell and burst when heated with water and so can be used as a thickening agent.	
Sugars	Provide dietary energy. *RDA* Added sucrose. Not more than 20 kg a year, i.e. average for the whole population or not providing more than 10% of dietary energy from added sucrose and glucose.	(i) Could indicate low fruit intake. (ii) Frequent intake of refined sugars, e.g. sucrose and glucose, is associated with tooth decay (dental caries). Excess dietary energy intake leading to obesity.	Food group 5 – sugar, treacle, honey, syrup sweets, chocolate, fruit squash and cordial, fizzy drinks, biscuits, cakes (sucrose and glucose). Food group 2 – fruit (fructose). Food group 4 – milk and yoghurt (lactose).	Average intake: 246 g.	Sucrose and glucose syrups are added to many processed foods. If heated, dry sugar melts and turns to caramel.	Fructose in whole fruit and lactose in milk are not thought to be associated with tooth decay.
Dietary fibre	Maintaining healthy bowel function by forming a bulky, easily passed stool. *RDA* Average for whole population 30 g. May be related to RDA for energy intake. No specific individual recommendation.	(i) Constipation, haemorrhoids, diverticular disease, cancer of the colon (possibly varicose veins, hiatus hernia). (ii) Little is known. Possibly reduced absorption of some vitamins and minerals, also excessively bulky diet which is unpalatable and does not provide enough dietary energy especially in young children.	Food group 1 – whole grain cereal foods, some breakfast cereals. Food group 2 – most fruit and vegetables. Food group 3 – pulses, nuts.	Information not available.	Pectin (found in some fruits) when heated thickens and sets and can be used as a 'jelling' agent.	Bran should only be used as a medicine when medically prescribed. It is important to eat different types of fibre found in cereals, pulses and fruit and vegetables.

Food group 1 Food group 2 Food group 3 Food group 4 Food group 5 Food group 6

Nutrient	*Function*	*(i) Deficiency/ (ii) Excess intake*	*Main sources*	*Proportion supplied by each food group in the 'average' UK diet*	*Effects of cooking and processing and storage*	*Other comments*
PROTEIN	Growth, production, repair and maintenance of all the body's tissues, fluids, hormones and enzymes. *RDA* Depends on age, sex and physical activity. Varies from 27 g (girls 1 year) to 84 g (very active men 18–64 years). Boys 12–14 years: 66 g. Girls 12–14 years: 53 g.	(i) In young children growth slows down or stops. Failure to digest and absorb foods properly, diarrhoea, loss of fluid, dehydration. Muscle wasting and anaemia. (ii) Little is known. May put excess load on the kidneys.	Food group 1 – cereal foods, e.g. flour, bread, rice, couscous, pasta. Food group 3 – all foods, i.e. meat, fish, eggs, pulses, nuts. Food group 4 – all foods, i.e. milk, cheese, yoghurt.	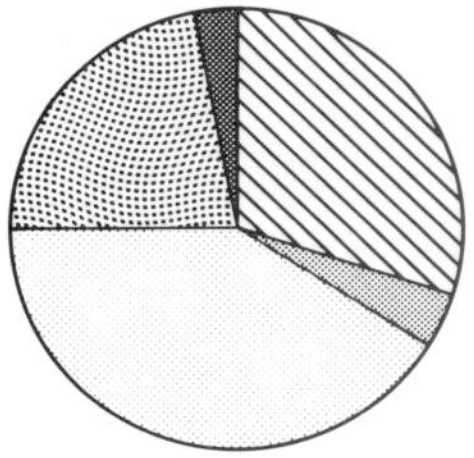 Average intake: 68 g.	When heated dry and quickly can toughen and harden. Gluten in wheat is elastic when kneaded allowing bread to hold its shape when baked.	If a diet contains only protein from vegetable sources the combination of foods eaten is very important.
FAT	Provides dietary energy: some contain fat soluble vitamins. *RDA* Provides 30–35% dietary energy.	(i) See below (polyunsaturated fats). Low energy dense diets which can be very bulky and unpalatable leading to inadequate dietary energy intakes in children. (ii) Excess dietary intakes leading to obesity. See below (saturated fats).	Food group 1 – starchy vegetables which have been fried, e.g. chips, crisps, fried plantain. Food group 3 – fatty meats and meat products, e.g. sausages, pies, burgers, pâtés, oily fish, nuts. Food group 4 – whole milk, most cheeses. Food group 5 – chocolate, biscuits, cakes.	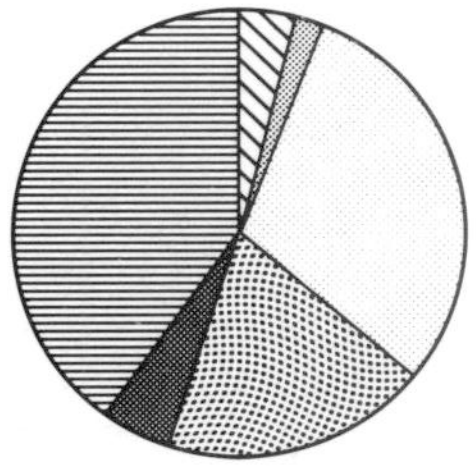 Average intake: 97 g.	Prolonged storage can lead to rancidity.	

			Food group 6 – all foods including butter, margarine, oil, lard, suet, ghee, coconut cream.			
Polyunsaturated fats	Essential fatty acids, crucial for brain growth and metabolism. Cannot be produced in the body. May play a role in preventing heart disease. *RDA* No specific RDA.	(i) Restricted growth, development and repair of the brain. Possibly a greater risk of cardiovascular disease. (ii) Little is known. Possibly connected with increase in some types of cancer.	Food group 1 – whole grain cereals. Food group 2 – fruit and vegetables (very small amounts). Food group 3 – pulses (especially soya beans), nuts, oily fish. Food group 6 – corn oil, sunflower and safflower seed oil, soya oil, 'polyunsaturated' margarines	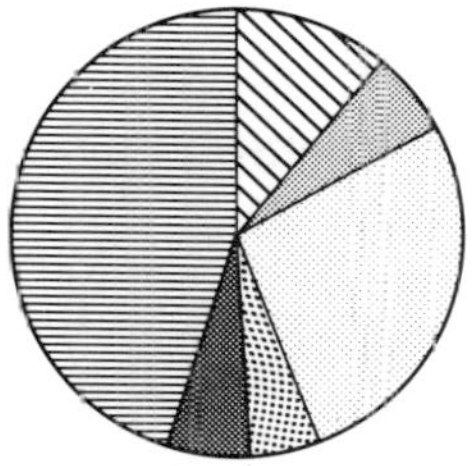 Average intake: 13 g.	Converted to saturated fats after repeated heating.	Liquid at room temperature unless processed in some way.
Monounsaturated fats	Little is known. *RDA* No specific RDA.	Little is known.	Food group 4 – oily fish, nuts. Food group 6 – olive oil. Most fat containing foods.	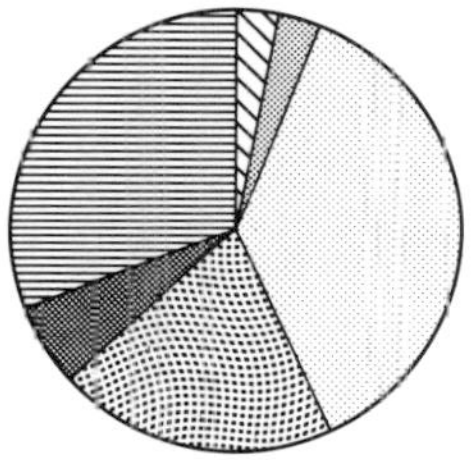 Average intake: 35 g.	Converted to saturated fats after repeated heating.	

Food group 1 · Food group 2 · Food group 3 · Food group 4 · Food group 5 · Food group 6

Nutrient	*Function*	*(i) Deficiency/ (ii) Excess intake*	*Main sources*	*Proportion supplied by each food group in the 'average' UK diet*	*Effects of cooking and processing and storage*	*Other comments*
Saturated fats	Not essential in the diet and can be manufactured in the body from essential fatty acids. *RDA* Provides not more than 10–15% dietary energy.	(i) Little is known. (ii) Seems to be connected with higher risk of cardiovascular disease and also breast cancer in women.	Food group 3 – meat, meat products, eggs. Food group 4 – whole milk, most cheeses, yoghurt. Food group 5 – cakes, biscuits. Food group 6 – lard, suet, butter, most margarines, vegetable oils containing palm oil, coconut oil/ cream, ghee.	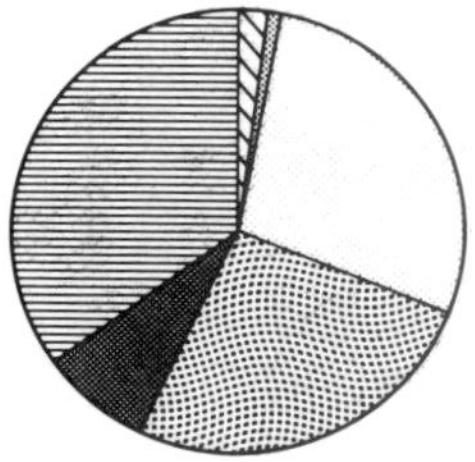 Average intake: 42 g.		Solid at room temperature unless processed in some way.
FAT SOLUBLE VITAMINS Vitamin A (retinol and β carotene)	May play a role in preventing some types of cancer. Maintenance of moist surface tissues, e.g. at the front of the eyes and the lining of the gut and respiratory passages. Helps regulate growth. Needed to manufacture visual purple in the retina of the eye enabling night vision. β carotene from plant foods is converted to retinol in the body. *RDA* Depends on age.	(i) Reduced vision in dim light followed by the eyes becoming dry, grey and opaque (xeropthalmia). Possibly increased risk of some types of cancer. (ii) May be toxic. Excess consumption of fruit and vegetables high in β carotene can lead to yellow colouring of the skin. Little is known about the effects of this although it is thought to be harmless.	Food group 1 – yellow starchy vegetables, e.g. sweet potato, yellow yam. Food group 2 – bright green, red, yellow and orange fruit and vegetables. Food group 3 – liver, egg yolk, green, yellow and orange pulses, oily fish. Food group 4 – milk, cheese. Food group 6 – butter, margarine.	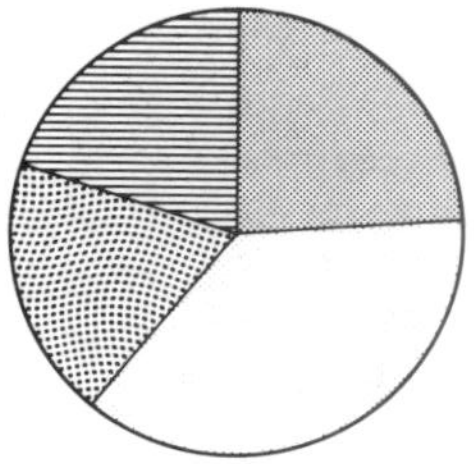 *Nearly 80% of this comes from liver. For those who do not eat liver, food group 3 is not such a major source. Average intake: 1380 μg.	Relatively stable in cooking and storage.	2 μg β carotene produce 1 μg retinol in the body.

	Varies from 450 μg (children under 1 year) to 1200 μg (women who are breast-feeding). 12–14 years: 725 μg.					
Vitamin D	Required for the absorption of calcium and phosphorus in the small intestine and with their utilization in the formation, growth and repair of bones and teeth. *RDA* Depends on likely exposure to sunlight and rate of growth. Varies from 0 in most people to 10 μg in children and breastfeeding or pregnant women.	(i) Rickets in children and osteomalacia in adults. Rickets – poor bone development leading to short, soft, deformed bones. Osteomalacia – bones become weak and joints painful. (ii) Toxic: can lead to nausea, vomiting, thirst, pain, weight loss, irritability and can be fatal.	Exposure of the skin directly to the sun's rays especially in summer. Food group 1 – some fortified breakfast cereals. Food group 3 – liver, oily fish, egg yolk. Food group 6 – margarine (fortified).	Average intake: 3.0 μg.	Relatively stable in cooking and storage.	Sunlight is the main source.

Food group 1 Food group 2 Food group 3 Food group 4 Food group 5 Food group 6

Nutrient	*Function*	*(i) Deficiency/* *(ii) Excess intake*	*Main sources*	*Proportion supplied by each food group in the 'average' UK diet*	*Effects of cooking and processing and storage*	*Other comments*
Vitamin E	Currently being researched into. Claims are made that it contributes to preserving tissues, fertility, longevity, wound healing and protecting against heart disease. Little of this has been substantiated. *RDA* No specific RDA.	Little is known.	Food group 1 – whole grain cereal foods, wheat germ, some breakfast cereals. Food group 3 – egg yolk, almonds, hazel nuts. Food group 6 – cottonseed oil, corn oil, palm oil, peanut oil, rapeseed oil, safflower seed oil, soya oil, sunflower seed oil, margarines from these oils.	Information not available.	Relatively stable in cooking and storage.	
Vitamin K	Required for the clotting of blood. *RDA* No specific RDA.	(i) Not been seen in humans. (ii) Little is known.	Food group 2 – fresh green leafy vegetables. Food group 3 – beef liver.	Information not available.	Relatively stable in cooking and storage.	
WATER SOLUBLE VITAMINS **B complex** Vitamin B1 (Thiamin)	Required for the release of energy from carbohydrates and for growth in children. *RDA* Depends on RDA for dietary energy. Varies from 0.3 mg (children under 1 year) to 1.3 mg (very active men 18–64 years). Boys 12–14 years:	(i) Severe deficiency leads to beri-beri, not often seen in the UK. First signs are appetite loss, general feeling of being unwell, weak legs, swellings in the face and legs and sometimes palpitations. Thiamin deficiency is found in the UK in alcoholics who	Food group 1 – whole grain cereal foods, some breakfast cereals, potatoes, other starchy vegetables. Food group 2 – most fruit and vegetables. Food group 3 – all the foods in this group. Food group 4 – milk, cheese, yoghurt.	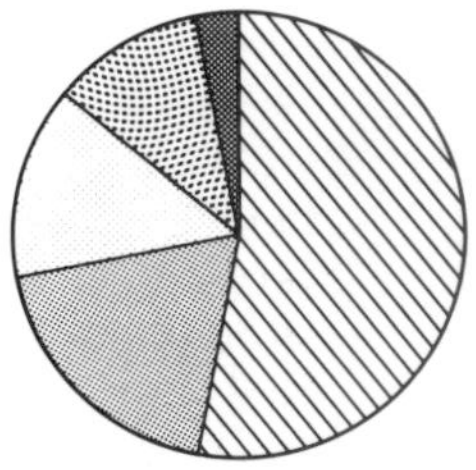 Average intake: 1.26 mg.	Soluble in water and easily destroyed by heat in neutral or alkaline solutions. Losses occur in the thawing of frozen meat, in the fluid which is lost.	

	1.1 mg. Girls 12–14 years: 0.9 mg.	have a very poor diet. (ii) Little is known.				
Vitamin B2 (Riboflavin)	Required for the release of energy from foods, especially amino acids and fats. *RDA* Depends on age. Varies from 0.4 mg (children under 1 year) to 1.6 mg (very active men 18–64 years). 12–14 years: 1.4 mg.	(i) Severe problems with deficiency are not widely known and seem only to be minor. (ii) Little is known.	Food group 1 – whole grain cereal foods, some breakfast cereals. Food group 2 – green vegetables. Food group 3 – fish, meat, eggs, pulses, nuts Food group 4 – milk, cheese, yoghurt.	Average intake: 1.77 mg.	Soluble in water and easily destroyed by heat in alkaline solutions. Destroyed by ultraviolet light (e.g. sunlight shining on transparent glass milk bottles).	
Vitamin B3 (Nicotinic acid)	Required for the release of energy from food and therefore necessary for growth. Required to keep the skin, tongue, digestive and nervous systems healthy. *RDA* Depends on age and psychological state. Varies from 5 mg (children under 1 year) to 21 mg (breastfeeding women). 12–14 years: 16 mg.	(i) Severe deficiency leads to pellagra. Sore, cracked skin, diarrhoea and nervous depression. Partial paralysis may also occur. (ii) Little is known.	Food group 1 – whole grain cereal foods, some breakfast cereals. Food group 3 – meat, liver, kidney, fish, peanuts, pulses.	Average intake: 13.7 mg.	Soluble in water, otherwise one of the most stable of the vitamins.	Nicotinic acid can be manufactured in the body from the amino acid tryptophan. 60 mg of tryptophan are needed to produce 1 mg of nicotinic acid. Nicotinic acid is found in maize but is unavailable. It can be released by soaking the maize in lime (similar to chalk).

Food group 1 Food group 2 Food group 3 Food group 4 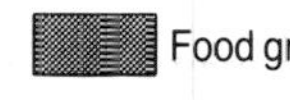 Food group 5 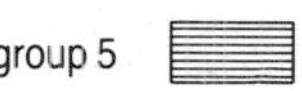 Food group 6 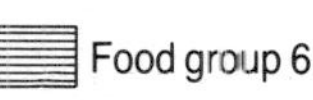 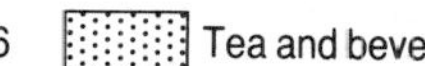 Tea and beveridges

Nutrient	*Function*	*(i) Deficiency/ (ii) Excess intake*	*Main sources*	*Proportion supplied by each food group in the 'average' UK diet*	*Effects of cooking and processing and storage*	*Other comments*
Vitamin B12 (Cyanoco-balamin)	Required for the formation of red blood cells and for amino acid metabolism. *RDA* No specific RDA.	(i) Pernicious anaemia: tiredness, run down, lethargic. (ii) Little is known.	Food group 3 – liver, meat, eggs. Food group 4 – milk, cheese.	Information not available.	Soluble in water and is destroyed by heat in alkaline solutions (e.g. heated milk).	Not present in vegetable foods, therefore vegans need to take a dietary supplement.
Biotin	Forms part of several enzyme systems including that involved in the synthesis of fatty acids. *RDA* No specific RDA.	(i) Not known except in diets consisting of very few foods. (ii) Little is known.	Found in a wide variety of foods.	Information not available.	Soluble in water.	
Pantothenic acid	Part of a co-enzyme involved in numerous reactions in the body, including the synthesis of fatty acids and cholesterol. *RDA* No specific RDA.	(i) Little evidence has been found. (ii) Little is known.	Found in a wide variety of foods.	Information not available.	Soluble in water and readily destroyed by heat in acid and alkaline solutions.	
Vitamin B6 (Pyridoxine)	Involved in the metabolism of all amino acids. Also necessary for the formation of haemoglobin. *RDA* No specific RDA although requirements may	(i) Anaemia, failure-to-thrive (in infants), depression. (ii) Little is known.	Food group 1 – whole grain cereal foods. Food group 2 – bananas. Food group 3 – meat, fish, eggs, peanuts.	Information not available.	Soluble in water.	

	be increased amongst women taking oral contraceptives.					
Folates	Necessary for the synthesis of DNA and haemoglobin. *RDA* No specific RDA.	(i) Anaemia. (ii) Little is known.	Food group 2 – green leafy vegetables, oranges, bananas, avocado pears. Food group 3 – liver, pulses, fish, beef, eggs.	Information not available.	Soluble in water and rapidly destroyed by heat in neutral or alkaline solutions.	
Vitamin C (Ascorbic acid)	Necessary for the formation of the connective tissue – collagen. Helps the absorption of iron from plant sources. Also involved in lipid, brain and muscle metabolism, resistance to infection and the detoxification of potentially harmful substances including drugs and alcohol. *RDA* Depends on age and physiological state. Varies from 20 mg (children under 1 year) to 60 mg (pregnant and breastfeeding women). 12–14 years: 25 mg.	(i) Scurvy: wounds do not heal, bruises develop easily, sores on the skin, breakdown of old wounds. (ii) Little is known.	Food group 1 – potatoes, sweet potatoes, plantain. Food group 2 – most fruit and vegetables, especially citrus fruits and berries. Food group 5 – some blackcurrant and rose hip drinks.	Average intake: 55 mg.	Very soluble in water and then easily oxidized when in alkaline solution, heated, exposed to the air or to traces of metal (such as copper in copper saucepans).	

Food group 1 Food group 2 Food group 3 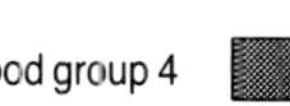 Food group 4 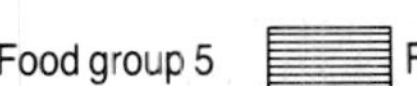 Food group 5 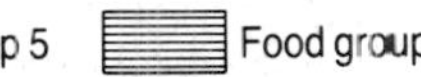 Food group 6

Nutrient	*Function*	*(i) Deficiency/ (ii) Excess intake*	*Main sources*	*Proportion supplied by each food group in the 'average' UK diet*	*Effects of cooking and processing and storage*	*Other comments*
Sodium chloride (Salt)	The exact role is not fully understood but it seems to be necessary in very small quantities. *RDA* 8 g a day, average for the whole population.	(i) Dehydration, low blood pressure, rapid pulse, dry mouth, feeling of apathy, loss of appetite and vomiting, muscular cramps. (ii) Possibly connected with an increased risk of high blood pressure. Hypernatraemia in infants.	Food group 1 – salted foods such as crisps, some breakfast cereals, bread. Food groups 2 – most canned vegetables, olives in brine. Food group 3 – meat products, canned foods, salted and smoked meats and fish. Food group 4 – cheese.	Information not available.	Added to many foods during processing.	
Potassium	May be involved with sodium in the regulation of blood pressure. Involved in muscle and brain function.	(i) Muscular weakness and mental confusion. May be connected with high blood pressure in combination with sodium. (ii) Little is known.	Food group 1 – whole grain cereal foods, starchy vegetables. Food group 2 – most fruit and vegetables. Food group 3 – fish, meat, pulses, nuts.	Information not available.	Stable.	
MINERALS Calcium	Required for the formation, growth and maintenance of healthy bones and teeth. Involved in the working of the muscles and nervous system. May be involved in control of blood pressure.	(i) Not clearly understood. May be associated with osteoporosis in later life especially among women. May be associated with increased risk of high blood pressure. (ii) Little is known.	Food group 1 – white bread (fortified). Food group 2 – broccoli tops, spring onions, parsley, spinach, watercress, rhubarb. Food group 3 – almonds, brazil nuts, egg yolk, pilchards,	Average intake: 864 mg.	Stable	Absorption may be reduced by presence of phytic acid. Vitamin D required for absorption.

	RDA Varies with age and physiological state from 500 mg (most adults) to 1200 mg. (pregnant and breastfeeding women). 12–14 years: 700 mg.		sardines, whitebait, shrimps. Food group 4 – milk, cheese, yoghurt. Food group 5 – black treacle, milk chocolate.			
Phosphorus	Involved with calcium in the production and repair of bones. *RDA* No specific RDA.	(i) Not known in the UK. (ii) Little is known.	Found in a wide variety of foods.	Information not available.	Stable.	
Iron	Essential to keep the blood healthy because it forms part of the haemoglobin in red blood cells. *RDA* Varies with the age and physiological state from 6 mg (children under 1) to 15 mg (women who are breast feeding. 12–14 years: 12 mg	(i) Anaemia. (ii) Constipation. Little else is known.	Food group 1 – some breakfast cereals, wholemeal bread and flour, white bread (fortified). Food group 2 – dark green vegetables Food group 3 – red meat, offal, almonds, pulses. Food group 5 – treacle.	Average intake: 11.1 mg.	Stable.	Absorption related to physiological need. Absorption of non-haem iron increased in presence of vitamin C. Absorption may be reduced by presence of tannin and phytic acid.

Food group 1 Food group 2 Food group 3 Food group 4 Food group 5 Food group 6

Index

Acids for preservation 140
Additives 10, 14, 48–9
Aesthetics and food 148–9
Agriculture 52
Alcohol 13
  and pregnancy 60
  and preservation 140
  and vitamin C 91
  in the diet 46–7
Allergy 49
Amino acids 72–3, 107, 115
Amylose 68
Anaemia 63
Anorexia nervosa 58–9
Antibiotics 140
Antibodies 72
Antioxidants 48

Babies and diet 56–7
Bacteria 130–1
Baking 144
Balanced diet 15–17, 20–1, 33, 51, 54–5, 65, 125
Barley 23, 85
Basal metabolic rate 66
Beans and cooking 105
Beta carotene 92
Bile salts 123
Biological value 72
Biotin 95, 101
Blanching 136
Blood pressure 10, 43
Boiling 144
Bottle feeding 56, 108–9
Bottling 138, 141
Braising 144
Brandt Commission 128–9
Bran 78
Bread 22, 79
  consumption 10
  energy density 124
  making 86
  storage 135
Breakfast cereals 23, 51
Breast feeding, 56, 60–1, 108–9

Calcium 57, 81, 104, 112
  deficiency 112
Cancer 10, 49, 78
Canning 106, 138
CAP 52
Carbohydrates 16, 68–9, 88–9, 98
Cardiovascular disease 13
Casein 115
Catalyst 18
Cellulose 78
Cereal foods 22–5
  nutritional role 76–7
Cheese 34, 110–11, 114
Chlorophyll 68
Choice 54–5
Cholesterol 70
Citrus fruits 26
Classifying foods 20–1
Coagulation 34, 86
  of milk 114–15
Collagen 90–1
Colostrum 108
Colouring 48
COMA 13, 41, 71
Combination of foods 64
Conduction 142–3
Confectionery 37
Connective tissue 90
Constipation 78
Contraceptive pill 58
Convection 142–3
Cookers 147
Cooking
  effects of 84, 96, 105, 114, 118–19, 122
  methods 142–7
Crash diets 59
Culture and choice 54–5

Dehydration 45
  of food 139, 141
Dental caries 116–7
Diabetes melitus 117
Diet
  poor quality 9
  balanced 15–7
Dietary energy 66–7, 76, 89, 99
  in milk 110
  in fats 120
Dietary fibre 13, 16, 24, 26, 28, 69, 76, 78–9, 88–9, 98
Dietary goals 12
Digestion
  protein 107
  of milk 115
  of fat 123
Digestive system 18
Disaccharides 68

E numbers 48–9
Eating patterns 50–1
Eggs 31–2
Elderly dietary needs 62–3
Empty calories 116
Emulsions 48, 122
Energy 13, 57, 116
  balance 66
  density 74, 120, 124–5
Enzymes 18–19, 88, 115
  and food spoilage 136–7
Equipment 146–7

Famine 126–7
Fats 13, 16
  animal 40
  vegetable 40
  and oils 40–1, 70–1, 120–3
Fatty acids 70, 120
Fermentation 86
Fish 31, 105–6
Flavours 48
Flour 22, 79
Fluoridation 45, 117
Folic acid (folates) 94, 97, 101
Food
  aid 126–9
  groups 20–1
  handling 132–3
  hygiene restrictions 130
  poisoning 105, 130–1
  preservation 138–41
  processors 146
  shortage 126–9
  storing 133–5
  spoilage 136–7
  technology 48
Formula milks 109
Freeze drying 139
Freezing 106, 138–41
Fructose 36, 89, 119
Fruitarians 64
Fruits and vegetables 26–9, 89, 90
Frying 122, 145
Frying pan 146
Fungi 131

Gall stones 78
Glucose 68, 87, 89
Gluten 22, 86
Glycerol 70, 120
Glycogen 69, 116
Green revolution 128
Grilling 144
Growth chart 66

Haem iron 80, 91
Haemoglobin 80
Heart disease 10, 13, 33, 41, 70, 121
Heat and preservation 138
Heat transference 142–3
Herbs and spices 149
Home preservation of food 141
Honey 36, 119
Hunger and food aid 126–9
Hydrolysis 71
Hygiene 130–3
Hyperactivity 49
Hypernatraemia 42

Infant feeding 56–7, 108–9
Invert sugar 119
Iron 32, 58, 65, 80, 104
  absorption 91
  deficiency anaemia 80
Irradiation of food 140–1

Jam making 119, 141

Karhai 146
Kidney bean 105
Kidneys 42, 44–5
Kitchen
  skills 130
  hygiene 132–3
Knives 146–7
Kwashiorkor 73

Labelling 54
Lactation 61
Lactose 36, 68, 110–11
  intolerance 111
Life style and diet 10–11
Lipases 123

Maillard reaction 86
Maize 23
Malnutrition 8, 12, 41, 74, 126–7
Malting 84–5
Maltose 68, 98
Marasmus 73
Meat 30
  alternatives 30–3
  nutritional role 99
  storage 134–5
Menstruation and diet 58
Metabolic rate 66
Micro-organisms 48, 137
Microwave 145, 147
Milk 34, 56
  consumption 35
  human 56
  products 34–5, 57, 108, 15
Mineral hydrocarbons 49
Minerals 17, 28, 75, 95, 104
Monosaccharides 68
Monosodium glutamate 49
Monounsaturated 70
Multiculture 14–15
NACNE 12, 41, 69, 71, 76, 79
Nicotinic acid (B3) 100
Nitrates 106
Non-haem iron 80, 91
Nutrients 8, 16–17
Nutrient density 60–1, 124
Nutritional recommendations 9
Nuts 31

Obesity 41, 58, 117
Offal 30
Oils 40–1, 120–3
Osteomalacia 63, 102–3
Overnutrition 8, 10, 12
Oxidation 71

Pantothenic acid 95, 101
Pasta 22
Pasteurization 138
Peer group pressure 55
Peptides 107, 115
Phosphorous 81, 104, 112
Photosynthesis 68
Phytates 81
Pickling 141
Poaching 144
Politics and food 55
Polysaccharide 68, 88
Polyunsaturated fats 70
Potassium 81, 95, 104
Potatoes 10, 23, 84
Pregnancy and diet 60–1
Preservatives 48, 136–41
Pressure cooking 144
Processed foods 10, 14, 52, 105–6, 116
Processing
  effects 84, 96, 105
  of fat 122
  of milk 114
Protein 17, 24, 32, 57, 72–3
  digestion 107
  energy malnutrition 73
  in cereals 77
  in meat 99
  in milk 110
  structure 72
Pulses 31–2, 65
  and cooking 105
Pyridoxine 95, 100

Radiation 143
Rancidity 71
RDA 12, 67, 69, 102
Refined sugar 37
Refining cereals 25, 77
Refrigerator 134–5
Religion and diet 31, 55
Retailing 53
Retinol 92
Riboflavin 101, 113
Rice 23, 84
Rickets 102
Roasting 145
Rye 23, 85

Saccharides 68
Saccharine 38
Safety 146–7
Salivary amylase 98
Salmonella 130
Salting 106
Salt in the diet 42–3, 67
Saturated fats 70, 77, 99
Saucepan 146
Scurvy 63
Semi-skimmed milk 34
Shortening 122
Simmering 144–5
Skimmed milk 34
Smoking and pregnancy 61
Smoking food 140
Snacks 38, 43
Sodium chloride 42–3
Sodium salts 139, 141
Soft drinks 37
Soya milk 34, 110
Spoilage of food 136–7
Staple foods 24, 84
Starch 16, 22, 24, 76, 88
Starchy fruits and vegetables 23
Steaming 144, 146
Sterilizing
  infant feeding bottle 109
  milk 138
Stewing 144
Storage 134–5
Strokes 10
Sucrase 98
Sucrose 36, 89, 119
Sugar 13, 16, 36–9, 68–9, 116–19
  as preservative 140
Sugary food and drinks 36–9, 116–19
Supermarkets 53
Sweeteners 38–9, 49
Sweets 37, 118
Syrup 36, 119

Taboos 54
Teenager special needs 58–9
Thiamin (B), 82, 95, 97, 101
Toddlers 56–7
Tofu 35
Tooth decay 10, 39, 116–7
Toxins 131
Trace elements 17, 75, 81, 104
Transport system 52,
Triglycerides 70
Trypsin 115

UHT 138
Undernutrition 8, 12
Unleavened bread 81

Vegans 64–5
Vegetables 26–9
Vegetarians 31, 55, 64–5
Vitamins 17, 26, 74
Vitamin A 92–3, 103, 113, 120
  B 82, 95, 100–1
  B12 64–5, 100–1
  processing 96
  C 28, 82, 90–1
  deficiency 91
  D 102–3, 113, 120
  E 82, 120
  K 93, 113
  supplementation 28, 64, 103

Water and fluids in diet 44–5
Weaning 57, 74
Wheat 85
Wholemeal flour 79
Woks 146

Yam 23
Yoghurt 34, 110–11, 114

Zinc 81, 104